THE AMERICAN DRUGGIST'S COMPLETE FAMILY GUIDE TO PRESCRIPTIONS, PILLS, AND DRUGS

THE AMERICAN DRUGGIST'S
Complete Family Guide to Prescriptions, Pills, and Drugs

----

text by

JOHN J. FRIED

and SHARON PETSKA

editors

GERARD COONEY, PHARM.D.
HOWARD LEVINE, R.PH.
HERBERT I. MINDLIN, R.PH.

editorial director

GENELL SUBAK-SHARPE, M.S.

Hearst Books
NEW YORK

LIBRARY OF CONGRESS CATALOGING-IN-PUBLICATION DATA

Fried, John J.
The American druggist's complete family guide to prescriptions, pills, and drugs / by John J. Fried and
Sharon Petska ; editors, Gerard Cooney, Howard Levine,
Herbert I. Mindlin.
p.   cm.
"Produced by G. S. Sharpe Communications, Inc."
Includes bibliographical references and index.
ISBN 0–688–12385–6
1. Drugs—Popular works.   I. Petska, Sharon.   II. Cooney, Gerard.
III.   G. S. Sharpe Communications.   IV. Title.
RM301.15.F75   1995
615'.1—dc20   94–39831
                                                               CIP

PRINTED IN THE UNITED STATES OF AMERICA

First Edition

1 2 3 4 5 6 7 8 9 10

BOOK DESIGN BY ALISON LEW

FOREWORD

IN THIS ERA of medical specialization, chances are you are seeing different doctors for different medical problems. If you're like a growing number of Americans, you also may be trying a variety of alternative therapies—herbal remedies, homeopathic preparations, and high-dose vitamins, among others. To round out the picture, you may be experimenting with diets, home remedies, or any number of other approaches aimed at improving how you feel and look.

It's also a good bet that these various practitioners have little or no inkling of the scope and nuances of your health care. This was borne out in a recent Harvard survey that found that more than one third of Americans see alternative practitioners, usually in addition to but without the knowledge of their medical doctors. Even patients who stick to one family physician often fail to share important information regarding nutritional supplements, nonprescription medications, and other aspects of self-treatment.

It's not that these patients are trying to hide something from their doctors; most simply do not realize the importance of sharing such information. Still, the consequences can be very serious indeed. The medication one doctor prescribes may interact with those prescribed by another doctor or alternative practitioner. Increasingly, drugs that once required a prescription are now available over the counter at any pharmacy or supermarket drug section. These, too, can interact with other drugs or cause serious side effects or adverse reactions. Or an herbal remedy you prescribe for yourself can interact with medications or cause problems on its own.

This is no trivial matter—misuse of medications costs thousands of lives and millions of dollars each year. But there is one health professional who can prevent these tragic and needless deaths: your pharmacist. Of all health professionals, pharmacists have the most training and knowledge about drugs, both over the counter and prescription. Yet they are among the most underutilized members of the health-care team. All too often, a patient hands a pharmacist a prescription without asking critical questions about foods to avoid, possible interactions with other medications, side effects, and what to expect and do. Perhaps your doctor answered all your questions. Even so, it's a good idea to double-check with your pharmacist—after all, doctors sometimes make mistakes or, more likely, are unaware of possible interactions with other drugs you are taking. Pharmacists are especially well equipped to spot potential problems because they keep computer medication profiles of their regular clients. You can help by making sure your pharmacist has an up-to-date list of all the drugs you are taking—including over-the-counter medications, nutritional supplements, and birth control pills—as well as any medical conditions you may have.

Increasingly, pharmacists are also a reliable source of information about such alternative therapies as homeopathic preparations, herbal products, and nutritional supplements. In fact, many of these are now being sold in pharmacies. If you are uncertain about the ingredients in a product or how it should be used, ask your pharmacist.

This *American Druggist* book is still another extension of the pharmacist's educational mission. If you need a fuller explanation of material in this book, ask your pharmacist to help you. At the same time, learn more about the educational services offered at your pharmacy. Many pharmacists offer educational booklets and computer printouts giving detailed information about how to make the best use of your drugs.

—Editors, *American Druggist*

CONTENTS

INTRODUCTION

It USED TO be that you could come away from a doctor's appointment with a fairly good understanding of the medications your favorite physician had prescribed for you. You knew that antibiotics killed bacteria, that tranquilizers calmed you down, and nitroglycerin stopped your chest pains.

But walk out of a doctor's examining room today and it is very likely that spinning within your brain are terms like *beta-blockers*, *calcium channel blockers*, *NSAID,* and *central adrenergic agonists.* And don't assume that your doctor has it any easier. Back in 1969, the physician who wanted to look up something about a specific medication—its potential side effects or its interactions with other medications you might have been taking—could turn to the *Physicians' Desk Reference* and thumb through its 900 pages to find the requisite information.

Today, the PDR, as it is known for short, is still on the doctor's bookshelf. But 25 years of steady advances in pharmaceutical science have fattened the reference book to 2,600-plus pages. The larger bulk is partially attributable to the fact that the PDR now contains references to 2,800 drugs—an increase of 10 percent over the last 25 years. And today's PDR also discusses many drugs in far greater detail than in 1969. That's because:

- Modern drugs are increasingly complicated in the way they perform in the body and combat illness.

- Increasing knowledge shows how drugs can affect the body and its many functions.

- Many patients, particularly older men and women, are now taking more than one drug at a time, increasing the chances that these medications will interact in negative ways and cause harm.

As complicated as they are, the PDR and other drug manuals provide your doctor with dependable information about the administration of medications. But what about you? Do you need an advanced degree in pharmacology if you want to take increased responsibility for your health care, if you want to know how to use medications properly, and how to avoid drug-related problems? In a word, no. But you do need to open and maintain good lines of communication with your doctor and your pharmacist. And this book is designed to help you do just that by providing handy essential information. Here is how the *The American Druggist's Complete Family Guide* is organized and how it can help you. Chapters 1 through 13 deal with a wide variety of medication-related issues including:

- **How drugs work in your body**—the way in which the body breaks down the drugs and distributes them and how drugs perform their vital functions.

- **How to take medications**—how long to take them, whether you should take them with food, what side effects to watch for and how to deal with them.

- **How to approach your medications under different circumstances**: For example, pregnancy changes many of the ground rules for taking drugs. Similarly, as we age, the body's ability to deal with drugs also changes. Chapters 6 through 8 consider these specific life stages.

- **How to stock your medicine cabinet**: Unfortunately, in many homes the medicine cabinet is a pharmaceutical version of the family attic—a place where medications that have outlived their usefulness are dumped in the hope that someday, maybe, they can again be of help. Chapter 9 will help you clean out the mess and restock the cabinet in more rational fashion.

Chapters 14 through 36 include tables for individual drugs providing detailed information about whether they come in pills, tablets, or capsules; how they should be taken; possible side effects you should look for and steps to take if they occur; precautions for older people and children; and medications with which the drug may interact.

If you are already taking a medication—prescription or over the counter—check it out in these tables: You may find information that will alter the way you are now using these products. When you have a doctor's appointment, browse through the section of drugs prescribed for your condition beforehand so you can discuss them with your doctor and pharmacist. When you get home, look up the medication. Does the information jibe with your recollection of your doctor's instructions? If not, check to make sure you have the correct information—or remember it correctly. In most instances, the following chapters and drug tables can make you feel more comfortable that you are taking your medication correctly, thus increasing the chances that it will work properly. You'll also be in a better position to spot and deal with any problems that might crop up. Furthermore, a drug table may remind you of something you should have mentioned to the doctor or it may raise a question about medication or the way you have been told to use it. Once alerted, you can call the doctor or pharmacist for more information.

A word of caution: We have made every effort to make each table as complete and precise as possible, and each has been reviewed by leading pharmaceutical experts. However, under no circumstances should you depend solely on this information to make your medical decisions—always consult your doctor or pharmacist if you have any doubts or unexpected reactions to your medication. Above all, **never stop taking a drug or change the way in which you take it without consulting your doctor or pharmacist**. That said, keep *The American Druggist's Complete Family Guide* handy—near your medications or on a kitchen shelf—as your dependable guide through the thicket of drugs you and your family are likely to use.

-1-

HOW DRUGS ARE DEFINED AND CLASSIFIED

Look in the cabinet of the average family's bathroom and you are likely to see shelf after shelf filled with a smorgasbord of medicines: Drugs to vanquish headaches, to kill infections, to soothe irritated skin, to calm nerves, and to dampen heartburn, to mention but a few common remedies. And, then, of course, there are the pills stuck away in a kitchen drawer, as well as those that are stashed in pockets and purses.

But even the best-stocked home pharmacy holds but a fraction of the thousands—about 5,000 in fact—of drugs available in the United States today. Like the medications prepared by the healers who ministered to people before the advent of modern medicine, many of today's drugs are still made from substances taken from plants or animals. Morphine and opium, for example, are extracted from the poppy plant. Many hormones, including insulin, come from domesticated animals like cows or pigs.

Today, however, many drugs can be synthesized in the laboratory and produced by the ton in pharmaceutical factories. The development of pharmaceutical science is one of the hallmarks of modern medicine. With the advances in biotechnology and the advent of new technology using cloning and recombinant genetics, we have moved across another pharmaceutical frontier. Genes control every facet of our lives by directing the production of enzymes, hormones, and other biological compounds that carry out specific duties in our bodies. With the help of recombinant genetics, researchers have been able to isolate, in animal as well as human tissues, genes responsible for manufacturing key body chemicals, including insulin and human growth hormone, making it possible to produce them artificially. Certain genes also can be taken out of their natural habitat and transplanted into selected microorganisms, most often harmless viruses or other microorganisms that can either make the hormone or substance or carry a drug to a specific target within the body. Such technology now makes it possible to turn out large quantities of growth hormone and other substances through these highly efficient biological factories. In fact, biotechnology is on the verge of allowing doctors to inject healthy genetic material directly into the body to counter certain genetic disorders such as cystic fibrosis.

The Many Facets of Drugs

Drugs are chemical substances that can cure or prevent illnesses, alleviate symptoms, act as substitutes for some natural bodily substances, or dampen the excessive production of others. And yet, when we talk about this diverse universe of chemicals, we tend to lump them all under the catchall terms *drugs* or *medicines*. At the most, we only distinguish between *prescription* drugs—those we can get only by handing the pharmacist that piece of paper a doctor has thrust into our own hands—and the *over-the-counter*, or nonprescription, products that we buy directly at a drugstore or supermarket.

But when pharmaceutical scientists look upon the universe of medical products, they see a dazzling array of products that are classified in myriad ways. Take, for example, the drug company chemist who has worked on a medication to control blood pressure. She looks up on a shelf and sees a compound known by its chemical name, **(S)-1-[N-[1-(ethoxycarbonyl)-3-phenylpropyl]-L-alanyl]-L-proline, (Z)-2-butenedioate salt (1:1)**. But if that chemist were to have visitors from the group whose job it is to approve generic names given to medications—the U.S. Adopted Name Council—they would look at the same compound on the same shelf and see **enalapril maleate**. Should the drug company representatives drop by, chances are they would refer to the medication by the proprietary or patented brand name used in the market—*Vasotec*. And your neighborhood pharmacist knows **enalapril maleate** by numerous generic equivalents as well as similar antihypertensive medications such as *Accupril, Altace,* and *Lotensin*.

Moreover, doctors and pharmacists—not to mention the FDA (Food and Drug Administration)—know that many drugs have to be defined by more than their chemical, generic, and proprietary names. The experts know that drugs also have to be defined by their potential for being abused, for being taken for the wrong psychological or physiological reasons. Drugs that have a low potential for misuse are classified as *uncontrolled substances*. But many others are classified as *controlled substances* because they are habit-forming, and as such, they can be misused and abused. Thus, prescribing by doctors and dispensing by pharmacists are closely monitored by the federal Drug Enforcement Administration (DEA) and law enforcement officials (see Chapter 10).

GOVERNMENT CONTROL

Of course, a drug's potential for abuse is not the only concern. Perhaps more important, the Food and Drug Administration has been empowered by Congress to determine whether new drugs are effective, to determine their side effects, and to weigh their risks against potential benefits. This FDA approval process is long and drawn out and may take up to ten years. In fact, the long waiting period has been severely criticized in recent years, particularly by AIDS activists who point out that the process insures that people who might benefit from a drug often die before it is allowed on the market. Moreover, other critics say that the long approval period means that drugs become available in places like Europe long before they are available to Americans and that the process is needlessly costly and adds to high drug prices in the United States.

Defenders of the FDA answer that the tortuous path to approval is meant to prevent the release of drugs like thalidomide, which when taken by pregnant women caused severe congenital defects in their babies.

Recently, though, the FDA has moved to deal with the complaints, allowing some drugs to be released for use, even if all the testing has not been finished, by patients who have no other recourse.

HOW DRUGS ARE TESTED

Researchers working on a new drug begin the testing process in a laboratory by giving it to animals. This animal testing helps researchers determine how the proposed medication might affect specific organs as well as its overall toxic effects.

Once a drug has passed the animal testing phase, a drug company can ask the FDA, through an Investigational New Drug (IND) application, for permission to test it in healthy human volunteers to see how the drug acts in the human body. If all goes well, the drug is then tested on patients—initially in small groups, and then in larger numbers—who actually have the illness the medication is intended to treat. If other drugs are already available to treat this illness, it will be compared with these drugs as well as a placebo, a sugar pill or other inert substance resembling a drug.

In ways that are not completely understood, the human mind has a pervasive influence on disease and on the way a person taking something for an illness reacts. Thus, if 100 patients are given a placebo, up to 30 of them will not only report that they feel better, but may actually show signs of improvement. Because doctors and researchers also influence the results of these tests unconsciously, drugs are usually tested in a double-blind fashion. This means that neither the patients taking the drugs nor the researchers administering them know who is taking the drug and who is getting the placebo, both of which are coded. At the end of the experimental period, the codes are revealed and the data collected from each group are reviewed. A statistical study is conducted correlating the results with the identification code numbers assigned to the patients. In order for an experimental drug to move further down the road to approval, this study must show that the real drug does better than the placebo. Everyone who has a serious illness like cancer and seeks to be admitted to a program in which an experimental drug is being tested should be aware of the double-blind testing procedure. Admission into an experimental program is not a guarantee of getting the drug under consideration.

Once a drug has shown that it is indeed effective, its manufacturer must prove that is better than existing drugs. Thus, a second round of double-blind tests begins. In these, some patients are given the new drug, other patients are administered available medications, and in some cases, a third group is given a placebo.

Once a drug passes successfully through this testing labyrinth, its manufacturer must submit a New Drug Application (NDA) to the FDA. That essentially means that FDA physicians, pharmacologists, chemists, statisticians, and other medical professionals will review all the data developed during the testing period. The FDA, moreover, will review the proposed drug label that will be placed on the bottle and package as well as that small-print pamphlet that is often found in medicine packages. If all goes well, the drug finally receives FDA approval, allowing it to be sold in pharmacies. Even after a drug has passed this stage and patients are taking the drug regularly, the FDA keeps an eye on it because even the most thorough testing program cannot foretell what will happen when many people start taking a drug for extended periods of time. Recently, for example, the FDA allowed a new drug, *Omniflox*, to be used to treat some bacterial infections. But soon after it became available nationwide, the FDA ordered it withdrawn because physicians across the nation reported that *Omniflox* was causing severe liver and kidney problems, was lowering blood sugar levels in elderly patients, and had even resulted in some deaths.

-2-

HOW DRUGS WORK IN THE BODY

YOU'VE BEEN IN the garden all day, weeding, planting, transplanting, and pruning, and now you are paying the price. Your left shoulder hurts, your back aches, and your fingers feel like stiffened claws. The roses—a holdover from a previous owner—have also provoked your allergies, causing a runny nose, itching eyes, and periodic sneezing jags.

You go to your medicine cabinet for a couple of pain-killers such as ibuprofen (*Advil, Haltran, Motrin*) and an antihistamine to take with your iced tea and a sandwich. About an hour later, after a shower and a rest, you realize that the aches have diminished, your allergies have calmed down, and you feel fine again.

Like most people, you probably take this feeling of relief for granted, never giving a second's thought to the physiological processes that made it possible for those little pills to soothe your symptoms. But here is what happened: When the medication, iced tea, and sandwich entered your stomach, digestive juices and enzymes went to work, transforming the solids into a liquid solution that then moved from the stomach into your small intestine for further digestion and distribution. Slowly and inexorably, tiny particles that were once food and medication were absorbed into the bloodstream from the stomach or small intestine. The particles that used to be ibuprofen and anti-

histamine then traveled to the liver, where they were broken down even further, and returned to the bloodstream, which carried them to their intended destinations—your aching muscles and the tissues that responded to the allergens released by the roses.

Except for topical medications that are designed to work only where they are applied, most drugs are transported throughout the body via the circulatory system. But these medicines may enter the bloodstream through many different gateways and forms in addition to the familiar pills described earlier. The lungs, the insides of the mouth and the rectum, various muscles, and many areas of the skin are all richly supplied with blood vessels. Thus, medications may be inhaled, injected into a muscle or vein, placed under the tongue, tucked between cheek and gum, inserted in the rectum, or rubbed into a patch of skin. Regardless of the form, medications are formulated so that they can readily enter the nearest blood vessel for transportation to the sites where they will exert their influence.

Some drugs—pain medications, for example—have a very broad range of action, affecting different types of tissue throughout the body. But other drugs are designed to be highly specific, to function only at the point where they are needed.

Digitalis drugs, for example, are formulated so that they influence only the complex chemical and electrical workings of the heart muscles, and have little or no effect on the muscles in your legs or other body parts.

But to really appreciate how your medications work, you need to look at your body's basic building blocks, the cells.

Cells are highly specialized according to their location and purpose. Cells in the lungs, brain, kidneys, and skin are organized to perform very specific functions. The genes of each cell dictates its specific function. But cells also are controlled by chemical and electrical messages from neighboring cells as well as from glands and organs throughout the body.

To deliver its message, a hormone or other chemical must tap into a very specific area on the cell, on a site called a receptor. The process works very much like a lock and key, with the cell's receptor acting as a lock and the hormone or chemical as the key. When the hormone or chemical finds its right key, it fits the receptor, throws the lock, and sets the cell to work. Thus, certain cells have insulin receptors that enable this hormone to perform its metabolic function; other chemicals trigger a feedback reaction that turns off hormone production or receptors.

In effect, drugs are designed to work as the equivalent of the body's natural chemical messengers. In scientific terms, a drug that locks on to a cell and stimulates it to do something is classified as an **agonist** drug. Take, as an example, vaccines. They work by inducing the cells that make up the body's immune system to increase the production of antibodies, the protein molecules that fight off specific disease-causing microorganisms. Levodopa (*Dopar, Larodopa, Sinemet*), amantadine (*Symmetrel, Symadine*), and bromocriptine (*Parlodel*)—drugs used in the treatment of Parkinson's disease—are also ago-

nist drugs. The tremors that are so characteristic of Parkinson's disease are set off because some brain cells have stopped (or slowed down) production of dopamine, a chemical that works in that portion of the nervous system where movement is regulated. The medications taken by patients who have Parkinson's disease stimulate the brain to increase the production of dopamine. Medications to treat parkinsonism also illustrate the mechanisms that are behind the side effects brought on by drugs. Dopamine, in addition to playing a key role in the neural network that controls movement, is also important to those parts of the brain that control emotions. Thus, on occasion psychiatric disorders come hand in hand with the increased dopamine production that has helped bring the tremors of parkinsonism under control.

There are drugs, however, that are designed not to stimulate cells into action, but to stop or dampen excessive cellular activity—when something in the body has gone awry and control messages are not being delivered correctly. These drugs are called **antagonists** because, in attaching themselves to a receptor, they stop a certain activity of the cell. Pain-killers inhibit the cellular response that is responsible for transmitting impulses from the injured or diseased area to that part of the brain where the impulses are interpreted as a perception of pain. In the same way, angiotensin-converting enzyme (ACE) inhibitors, which are prescribed for patients with high blood pressure or angina, act as antagonists by blocking the activity of the cells that produce the enzymes that constrict blood vessels. Anticonvulsant drugs inhibit the electric activity of brain cells that trigger epileptic seizures.

But modern drugs do far more than turn cells on or off. In numerous instances, disease, injury, genetic changes, hereditary disorders, and unexplained circumstances prevent our bodies from producing a crucial substance. If the production stoppage is temporary, **substitutive** drugs may be used until the tissue or organ that normally produces the substance recovers. For example, a woman who has been taking oral contraceptives may have lost, temporarily, the ability to produce her own estrogen. In time, she will be able to do so again but in the meantime, she may take a hormonal preparation to speed up the process.

In other instances, the body loses completely the ability to manufacture a key substance. When that happens, a drug can act as a permanent replacement. For example, your pituitary gland controls the other glands that make up the body's endocrine system by sending out hormone messengers. If the pituitary gland has to be removed or stops functioning, the person will have to take appropriate substitute pituitary hormones for life. Similarly, if your pancreas stops making insulin—resulting in diabetes—you can take replacement insulin. This does not cure your diabetes, but it can control the disease and allow you to live a normal life.

Some drugs have to have the ability to cure by destroying the microorganisms—the bacteria, viruses, fungi, and other disease-causing organisms—that share our environment and sometimes invade our bodies. Various antimicrobial or antibiotic drugs combat these organisms by interfering with their ability to form cell walls. Like a human deprived of skin, a bacterium cannot survive without its cell wall. Other drugs stop bacteria by interfering with their ability to synthesize the proteins they need to function. Still others make it impossible for the bacteria to reproduce.

Not every molecule of every drug—be it an agonist, an antagonist, a curative or a replacement medication—plays a beneficial role. Moreover, in the process of doing their work, drugs may act differently in various parts of the body and produce effects that are potentially dangerous—which we refer to as side effects or adverse reactions. For example, theophylline (*Theo-Dur, Slo-bid*) is a drug that is used by many people with asthma because it keeps the airways in the lungs open. If the dose of the drug is too high, it can also stimulate the heart and make it beat faster, which is considered a side effect of the drug. Your doctor will determine the appropriate dose of the drug for you—one that will produce the desired effect without the side effect. Some drugs, however, may produce side effects that are not dose-related and may be potentially serious. For example, penicillin (*Pen • Vee K Veetids*) can produce a series of reactions in some individuals ranging from a mild rash to anaphylactic shock even when it is used in low dosages. In such cases, alternative medicine will be prescribed.

The process of breaking down—of metabolizing or transforming, also known as biotransformation—drugs is primarily assigned to the liver, though sometimes the lungs, kidneys, blood, and intestines are also involved. The liver's goal is straightforward: to produce and put into action the enzymes that will inactivate the drug or, at the very least, break it down into components that can be easily expelled from the body. As the liver metabolizes drugs, it passes the remnants back into the circulatory system. As the blood circulates through the body, minute bits of the transformed medication may be left behind in various tissues. Thus, some of the medicine you took in the last few days may leave your body in urine, body waste, tears, and other excretions. If you are breast-feeding, some of the medicine may be dissolved in your milk. Because the metabolizing process can even transform some drugs into gas, you may expel some of the drug waste products when you exhale.

Tears, sweat, and breath, though, account for only a small part of the drugs that leave your body because as your blood passes through the kidneys, a substantial portion of the medication leftovers leaches out and, with other wastes, rides out of the body in urine.

Taking medication would be simple if every drug could be made in the same doses and dispensed to all patients in the same way. But taking medication is not that simple. Each pill, spoonful, capsule, or individual prescription has to have just the right amount of the drug. And "just the right amount" is a tricky concept, involving a host of variables. One is the drug's **therapeutic index or window**, the concentration at which the drug is likely to be the most effective. Another is the drug's **half-life**, the amount of time it takes one half of the amount of drug in the blood to leave the body.

The third variable is *you*—your overall health, age, sex, size, metabolic rate, and a host of other factors. Therapeutic index, half-life, and your physical attributes are important because they determine both the positive and negative impacts of the drugs you take. Some drugs have a narrow therapeutic index, meaning that the drugs, to be effective and safe, have to be given in very precise quantities—even a bit too much or too little can be harmful. Others have large windows, meaning that they can be given in fairly large or imprecise quantities with little risk of serious side effects.

Half-life is important because it determines the rate at which a drug can be given. Amoxicillin (*Amoxil, Trimox, Polymox*), an antibiotic in the penicillin family, has a half-life of one hour. Because it remains in the body only for a short time, it must be given several times a day to maintain its effectiveness, without the danger that it will accumulate and cause side effects. But diazepam, the active ingredient in *Valium* and other tranquilizers, has a half-life of 27 to 37 hours. Thus, it has to be given sparingly, otherwise large stores of it will

gather in the body and cause serious problems for the user.

Once drugs are inside your body, your physical makeup also influences the way they act. If you are in generally good health, your doctor will feel comfortable prescribing a full dose of a drug you need. But if you have kidney or liver disease, for example, the regimen may have to be cut back. Similarly, if you are very thin, you may need a lesser dose than a person who is overweight. If you have a slow metabolism, the rate at which medications are broken down also may be slow. As a result, a drug may linger in your body and its impact will be magnified. Conversely, if you have a fast metabolic rate, your body will transform your prescription at a rapid clip, perhaps flushing it out of your body before it can be fully effective. Again, your doctor will have to tailor drug dosages accordingly.

Of course, if you suffer side effects no matter how much your doctor fine-tunes the dosage, you and your physician will have other choices. You might:

- **Adjust the way you schedule your medication** so that you take it at a time when it is least disruptive to you. A medication that makes you a little bit drowsy and needs to be taken only once every 24 hours may well be taken at night before you go to bed. Each of us has our own internal, or biological, clock, and your individual biorhythms can alter a medication's effectiveness. This is probably most critical when you are traveling and cross several time zones. If you are taking a medication in which timing is critical—insulin, for example—ask your doctor how to adjust your dosage to stay in sync with time and biorhythm changes.

- **Switch medications** until you find the one that causes you few or no problems. Given the thousands of drugs available, this is often another choice.

- **Live with the medication's side effects**, either because there is no substitute or because the good the drug is achieving is worth whatever irksome problems it may be causing.

Remember that some side effects of a drug may be increased by other drugs being taken concurrently. If you sense a noticeable increase in a side effect from your regular medication after you begin a course of a new drug, check with your doctor or pharmacist.

-3-

- - - - - - - - - - - - - -

HOW DRUGS ARE ADMINISTERED

THE AMERICAN TOURIST on vacation in the Dordogne region of France breathed in and out as the doctor in the small village of Aynac repeatedly passed the stethoscope across his chest. The cold had suddenly invaded the tourist's airways, making each raspy breath a chore. Finally, the doctor straightened and confirmed what the tourist already knew: "It is an infection, monsieur," he said as he draped his stethoscope around his neck and reached for a prescription pad. He started to write, then stopped.

"But you are an American, no?"

"Yes." The American wheezed. "Why?"

"To know how to prescribe the antibiotic for you. The Americans, I know, do not like suppositories. I will prescribe for you some medication you can take by mouth, if you wish."

Feeling that somehow he had been insulted, the American started to speak, but the doctor interrupted.

"It is a matter of preference, monsieur," he explained.

"Americans like to take things by mouth. In France, it is the suppository that is routine."

Culture, the French country doctor was saying, is a factor in how we take our medicine. To the French, taking medicine for minor illnesses is something of a nuisance, and the best way of dealing with it is to take the drug by suppository. By contrast, Americans have an abiding faith in medication—the long shelves of over-the-counter drugs that grace every supermarket and drugstore in the United States are seldom seen in France. And, in a sense, they affirm that faith by turning it into a ritual that involves symbolic eating.

Obviously, a host of factors beyond culture influence doctors of any nationality when they prescribe a drug. Questions that must be addressed include: How can I make sure that the medication has the fastest impact possible? Will a pill or the liquid form be easier for the patient? How long does the drug have to work? How old is the patient? Is she pregnant? Is the patient taking other medications that are likely to interact with a new drug? Are there other conditions or illnesses that have to be considered?

Oral Medications

In general, the most familiar, convenient, and easiest way to take a drug is to simply swallow it in the form of a liquid, a pill, or a capsule. This oral route is also the safest because if a patient does have a severe reaction to a drug, there are ways to remedy the situation. In extreme cases, it can be flushed out with a stomach pump; in others, it may be diluted by taking extra fluids, or another drug may be given to lessen its effects or speed up its exit from the body.

Still, there are many other ways to take drugs. Some are quickly absorbed into the bloodstream through the skin or mucous membranes. Thus, a nitroglycerin pill placed under the tongue quickly dissolves and enters the bloodstream to ease or prevent angina attacks. Drugs meant to be placed under the tongue are described as sublingual. Other pills are designed to be placed between the cheek and the gum; these are known as buccal medications. *Mycelex*, an antifungal drug, is one medicine that comes in lozenges.

Injected Medications

Injections are another quick and exceedingly common form of medication. When the medicine is injected into a muscle, usually in the arm, thigh, or buttock, it is called an **intramuscular** injection. Muscles provide a route for relatively fast, steady absorption of the drug into the bloodstream. Antibiotics and vaccines are often given this way. If a faster route is needed, the drug can be injected or dripped directly into a vein; this is referred to as **intravenous,** or **IV,** administration. Potent antibiotics and anticancer drugs are often given intravenously. If a slower route is needed, the drug can be injected into the layer of fat just below the skin. This is called a **subcutaneous** injection. Insulin is an example of a drug that is usually given by subcutaneous injection.

Whatever the site and type of injection, it serves at least two purposes: to avoid the destructive effects of enzymes and acids in the digestive tract and to create medication "pools" that allow the drugs to move slowly and evenly into the

bloodstream, thus extending the time that the drug has to do its work.

Localized infections or other disorders are sometimes treated by direct application or injection of drugs. Thus, if you have a particularly stubborn bladder infection, your doctor may resort to an **intracystical** injection directly into the urinary bladder. Similarly, an **intrapleural** injection goes directly into the pleura, the membrane surrounding the lungs; and an **intraperitoneal** injection goes into the peritoneum, the membrane surrounding organs in the abdominal cavity. In addition to injections for therapeutic purposes, some also are used in making a diagnosis. **Intradermal** injections are used to place tiny amounts of a substance under the skin to test for allergic reactions. **Intra-arterial** injections transfer radioactive materials or dyes into an artery to make soft tissues visible on X rays or other scanning techniques.

Suppositories

Notwithstanding the French physician's observation that Americans are not well disposed toward suppositories, there are many instances in which U.S. doctors prescribe medication that has to be inserted into the rectum or vagina. The most obvious circumstances under which a doctor will turn to suppositories include those involving rectal or bowel disorders. For example, the most common nonsurgical treatment of hemorrhoids is a suppository or cream applied to the irritated rectal tissues, and serious bowel disorders such as colitis are often treated with steroids administered via enemas or foams. Vaginal suppositories are often used to fight yeast infections.

Suppositories can also be used to carry medication to parts of the body far removed from the bowel or vagina. Some people have trouble swallowing pills or liquids, and for them, a suppository provides a solution to this problem. Suppositories also provide a route of administration for someone who is plagued by nausea and vomiting, as might be the case for a person receiving radiation treatment. Suppositories also bypass the digestive process, which destroys certain drugs.

Inhaled Medications

Inhalation provides still another route into the body. Medications that are inhaled include:

- **Aerosols,** which are suspensions of tiny solid or liquid particles in air or gas. In some cases, corticosteroids are given in an aerosol form to treat asthma. Aerosols can also contain antihistamines or decongestants, the compounds that bring relief from allergies and sometimes colds and flu.

- **Sprays,** which are composed of fine drug particles dissolved in water. Like many aerosols, they are used to treat diseases of the nose, throat, bronchial tubes, and lungs or to help ease unpleasant effects from congestion and allergies.

Aerosols and sprays are used to administer drugs that are intended for a localized problem, such as nasal congestion, as well as drugs with more distant targets. The nose has a rich supply of blood vessels just under the surface lining, so drugs absorbed through the nasal membranes quickly reach the bloodstream and are carried throughout the body. Nitroglycerin is sometimes given in aerosol form, and an inhaled form of insulin is nearing approval. Medical gases are another category of inhaled medication. But they are used primarily to induce anesthesia, not to treat any particular illness.

There are several advantages to taking inhaled medications. In some cases, this route reduces side effects. Inhaled steroid medications used to control asthma, for example, can have fewer side effects than steroid pills because a precise amount of the medication is delivered directly to the bronchial tissues. Inhaled medications also work faster than oral drugs because they enter the bloodstream without going through the intestinal tract.

Topical Medication

Topical preparations—creams, ointments, and assorted drops—also bypass the intestinal tract and work directly on localized problems. Acne, skin infections, insect bites, rashes, some eye problems, and vaginal conditions are prime targets for these approaches. While some of these conditions are sometimes treated with shots or pills, most are better treated locally.

Transdermal Medications

These drugs are formulated to be absorbed into the bloodstream through the skin. Some are given in creams, ointments, or lotions, while others are administered by transdermal patches, special medicated tapes that slowly release a drug into the skin for absorption into the body. In some cases, the patch is placed near the site where the drug is supposed to do its work. Thus, a nitroglycerin patch is placed on the chest, somewhere around the heart. An estrogen patch (*Estraderm*), used in hormone replacement therapy for menopausal women, is taped to the abdomen. Scopolamine patches (*Transderm Scōp*), originally developed to help astronauts cope with motion sickness, are worn behind the ear. An exception is the new nicotine patch (*Habitrol, Nicoderm, Prostep*) prescribed as a stop-smoking aid, which is usually worn on the arm or chest.

Long-Acting Medications

Whereas some drugs are formulated to act instantly, others are meant to work slowly over long periods of time—hours, days, or even months and years, depending on the circumstances. All of these medications are classified as **sustained-release** or **time-release medications.** These drugs can come in capsules, skin patches, and implants to be placed under the skin. Time-release capsules contain individual pellets of a drug. As the capsule, which is made of a specially formulated coating, dissolves in the gastrointestinal tract, it slowly releases the individual pellets. Many 24-hour cold pills use this formulation. Some time-release medications are designed so that the drug, which is embedded in an insoluble synthetic core or matrix, is slowly re-

leased into the gastrointestinal tract as it passes through. Examples are *Procan SR* and *Theo-Dur* tablets. Glaucoma is sometimes treated with pilocarpine in a thin disk that is placed directly on the eye under the lower lid. In that position, the disc dissolves at body temperature and releases the drug, which improves drainage from the eye, easing the pressure inside.

Enteric coated tablets have a special protective covering that prevents them from dissolving in the stomach. Instead, they dissolve in the small intestine, where they are absorbed into the bloodstream. This form of time-release medication is used for drugs that are destroyed by stomach acids and for some kinds of aspirin and other drugs that irritate the stomach lining. One of the longest-acting medications is *Norplant,* a contraceptive that is implanted under the skin to slowly release progestin into a woman's body. The implant can be left in place for five years, or removed sooner if the woman wants to become pregnant.

Common Forms of Medications

- **Capsules**—Medication is enclosed in a cylindrical gelatin coating. Drugs are generally released from capsules faster than from tablets.

- **Drops**—Sterile solution or suspension is administered by a dropper directly into the eye, the outer canal of the ear, or the nose.

- **Inhalant and sprays**—Medication is breathed or sprayed into the nose or mouth. Some medications are formulated to escape the container in specific fixed doses, but others are allowed to escape the inhaler in random, or nonfixed, doses.

- **Injectable solutions**—Sterile solutions or suspensions supplied in ampules or bottles.

- **Liquids**—Liquid medications are available as **solutions**, a drug preparation that is already dissolved; **syrups**, which are mixed with sugar and water; **suspensions**, preparations of finely crushed drugs held in liquid; and **elixirs**, medications dissolved in alcohol and water.

- **Powders**—Ultrafine drug particles in a dry form. Depending on the specific medication, they are usually dissolved or mixed in liquids or food and taken immediately after being prepared.

- **Suppositories**—Large, bullet-shaped tablets administered either rectally or vaginally; they are designed to melt at body temperature.

- **Tablets**—Contain medication, binding substances, and disintegrating agents. Some also have added flavoring to make them taste better.

- **Topical skin preparations**—Available as **ointments**, which are spreadable greasy preparations used for local application; **creams**, which are not greasy and are used on the skin only; and **lotions**, which are solutions or suspensions used on the skin and are not as sticky as creams or ointments.

-4-

BEFORE YOU TAKE ANY MEDICATION

FOR THE MOST part, the typical visit to the doctor goes something like this: You are ushered into a small room where you sit on the examining table. Eventually your doctor enters, quickly reviews your chart, asks a few questions, and proceeds with an examination, more questions, and perhaps some tests if the nature of your problem is unclear or needs clarification. In the end, chances are you'll wind up with one or more prescription medications. Along with the prescription, the doctor is likely to outline some often rudimentary instructions and ask if you have any questions. Unless you're an exceptional patient, you can't think of anything to ask, and maybe you sense that your doctor is already edging out the door. In any case, you ask nothing—and that is a big mistake.

Anytime you take medication, you need to find out both the good it can do *and* its potential harm. The best sources for this information are your doctor and your pharmacist. Among the questions you should ask one or both are:

- **How often should I take my medicine?**

   Some drugs are taken only as they are needed. Most pain relievers, for example, are taken whenever pain—a headache, say—hits. But most other drugs are meant to be taken regularly at specified intervals. Thus, if the doctor says you should take your medicine three times a day, find out whether that means once every eight hours or three times a day during waking hours.

   If you have to take a drug four times a day, meaning once every six hours, ask if you can have any leeway in the timing of doses. If you sleep seven hours a day, will the extra hour between evening and the morning dose make a difference? If a medication has to be taken in the middle of the night, ask if there is an alternative formulation that can be taken on a more comfortable schedule.

- **How long will I need to take this medication?**

   Some medications need to be taken only a few days or a few weeks. Others, like those for tuberculosis, are taken for a year or more. Many illnesses, though, necessitate long-term, even lifelong, treatment with one or more drugs. A person with epilepsy, for example, may take anticonvulsants for years to control seizures, though some specialists now recommend that medication be tapered off once seizures are under control. People who have hypothyroidism—who do not produce enough thyroid hormones to convert nutrients to energy efficiently—need to take replacement drugs for their entire lives. Similarly, juvenile, or insulin-dependent, diabetes mellitus must be treated with replacement insulin for life. High blood pressure, or hypertension, also requires lifelong treatment in most cases. As a special rule, **you should never stop taking a drug without first consulting your doctor.** Even if your symptoms disappear, the underlying disorder may still be present, so it's vital to stick with your treatment for as long as your doctor prescribed. This is especially true of antibiotics. Even though you may feel better after a few days of taking an antibiotic for a sinus infection or strep throat, for example, some of the organisms causing the infection may still be living. Thus, if you stop taking the medication when you feel better, the remaining organisms will have a chance to start multiplying again, setting off a new round of illness. It is also unwise to take extra doses of medication without your physician's approval. "More is better" is not the case in drug therapy because too much medication can lead to the accumulation of dangerous, even toxic, levels of the drug in your body. (For more information on taking medication and following a recommended regimen, see Chapter 12.)

Many people stop taking medicine because of undesirable side effects. If side effects are troublesome, discuss them with your doctor before taking any action. A simple decrease in medication dosage or a switch to a different medication may solve the problem.

- **Should I take the medicine with meals or on an empty stomach? Are there any foods I should make a point of eating? Are there any foods I should avoid?**

Certain drugs should be taken with meals, while others are best taken on an empty stomach. In general, food delays absorption of orally administered drugs. It may be desirable, however, to eat something with a drug such as aspirin, which can irritate the stomach lining or cause nausea.

Other drugs, such as penicillin and tetracycline (*Sumycin, Achromycin, Panmycin*), should be taken on an empty stomach because certain foods inhibit or even deactivate them. Moreover, taking a drug on an empty stomach can speed up its absorption into the bloodstream and thus hasten the onset of its effects.

Your physician may advise you to eat certain foods during drug treatment. For example, some diuretics flush the mineral potassium out of the body in the course of expelling excess liquids. Because potassium is crucial to proper working of the nervous system, particularly the heart's electrical system, your doctor may recommend foods rich in potassium if you are taking a diuretic. If your doctor has prescribed griseofulvin (*Fulvicin P/G, Gris-PEG, Grisactin*), an antifungal medication, you may be advised to take it with fatty foods, which enhance its absorption.

On the other hand, some foods can diminish a drug's therapeutic effect. For example, people taking tetracycline should avoid milk and other dairy products because calcium can slow down the drug's absorption from the gastrointestinal tract into the bloodstream, thereby delaying or even eliminating the drug's effectiveness. Antacid tablets have the same effect on the absorption of tetracycline. (See Chapters 14 to 36 for specific advice on which foods and beverages to avoid with which drugs.)

• **Can I have an alcoholic drink while I am taking this drug?**

Some drugs are not impacted adversely by a moderate amount of alcohol, such as a glass of wine or a beer at a ball game. But other medications can interact dangerously with alcohol. As a general rule, abstain completely from alcohol if you are taking drugs that affect the central nervous system or make you sleepy, such as antihistamines, tranquilizers, or muscle relaxants.

• **What if I miss a dose?**

Usually, missing one dose of a drug you are taking regularly is not a problem. But in some cases, if you miss a dose, there are steps you can take to make up for the oversight. Your doctor or pharmacist will be able to recommend the right ones. If, for example, you are taking an oral contraceptive and forget to take one pill, you will probably be told that you should take it as soon as you remember and use an additional form of protection for the remainder of your menstrual cycle. If you habitually forget to take your medicines, let your doctor know—there may be some way to simplify your treatment or your pharmacist may offer practical suggestions to help you remember.

• **What side effects—allergic reactions or other adverse effects—can I expect?**

Doctors, nurses, and pharmacists routinely ask if you are allergic to any medications, and it's crucial that you report any past reactions or allergies to foods and other substances.

There are many types of allergic reactions. The most common are mild, taking the form of a rash, generalized itching, or hives. These reactions can appear within seconds (following an IV injection, for example) or may appear days after you have begun taking the medication. They usually clear up in a few days or can be treated with antihistamines, or in severe cases, steroid drugs. Even so, their occurrence should be taken as a warning against any further use of the drug since a second reaction can be worse.

A far more serious, though relatively rare, allergic reaction is **anaphylactic shock**, which can strike within minutes or, less commonly, several hours after a drug is taken. Symptoms include severe swelling of the eyes, lips, or tongue; swelling of the throat causing difficulty in breathing; widespread hives; dizziness; nausea and vomiting; and a rapid drop in blood pressure, which can lead to unconsciousness. Anaphylactic shock can be life-threatening, so medical help should be obtained immediately.

Serum sickness is another type of allergic response. It usually strikes one to three weeks *after* administration of a drug and is characterized by fever, skin rash, nausea and vomiting, and aching muscles and joints. Although the symptoms may cause discomfort, serum sickness is not as serious as anaphylactic shock and symptoms typically disappear within a week of discontinuing the drug. It can be dangerous, however, if the fever is high and certain medications are administered. If you develop such symptoms and have taken medication recently, report your symptoms to your doctor, and ask advice before taking any drug.

Of course, allergic reactions are not the only adverse effects of drugs; all medications can cause side effects, ranging from merely annoying to intolerable. Often your doctor or pharmacist can suggest ways to minimize side effects. For example, if you are taking prazosin (*Minipress, Minizide*) for high blood pressure, you can avoid the dizziness sometimes attributed to a too-rapid drop in blood pressure by taking the drug at bedtime and avoiding abrupt changes in posture, such as hopping out of bed instead of getting up in stages. If constipation is a common side effect of a drug you are taking, changes in your diet that add more fiber to your meals may help you get around the problem.

Many drugs cause drowsiness, dizziness, blurred vision, or impaired coordination. So you might be advised not to drive or operate machinery, and to schedule your medication for times when you do not need to concentrate intensely.

Some side effects lessen or disappear as your body adjusts to the drug. If possible, wait out the adjustment period to see if the situation improves. If not, ask your doctor about a lower dosage or an alternative drug.

- **What should I do if I have an adverse reaction?**

The answer should be: "Call me immediately and I'll tell you how to proceed." If you can't reach your physician or your symptoms are rapidly worsening, call for an ambulance or ask someone to take you to the nearest emergency room.

Although your doctor and pharmacist are your most reliable sources of information because they are familiar with your special circumstances, there are additional sources you can consult. One is the small pamphlet, or package insert, that should accompany your medication. If your package insert is missing, ask your pharmacist to give you a copy. Don't be intimidated by medical jargon—ask your pharmacist to explain terms you don't understand. Specific information that you'll find in the package insert includes:

- **A listing of active and inactive ingredients.** This is essential data for anyone who has allergies.

- **Special considerations and warnings.** The print may be small, but the information is crucial because it includes possible side effects; activities, drugs, or foods that should be avoided; and warnings of conditions that may be aggravated by the medication. For example, cold and allergy pills usually are contraindicated for people with heart disease, high blood pressure, diabetes, or glaucoma.

Use the same diligence when taking over-the-counter medications. Many people mistakenly assume that just because you don't need a prescription, an over-the-counter drug is harmless. Nothing could be further from the truth. Any drug is potentially harmful, if not fatal, if you are hypersensitive or if it is taken in excessive quantities, combined with other drugs, or taken in conjunction with alcohol. The same care extended to the most potent of prescription drugs should be taken with over-the-counter medications.

There are approximately 500,000 over-the-counter products available in the United States. The Food and Drug Administration has determined that prescriptions for these drugs are not necessary, and that they can be taken without a doctor's supervision. In recent years, a number of prescription drugs have been reclassified as over the counter. Some, such as topical hydrocortisone (*Cortaid*) and ibuprofen, an anti-inflammatory painkiller, have been reformulated to a lower dosage. Others, such as *Gyne-Lotrimin*, an anti-infective used to treat vaginal yeast infections, are now sold without a prescription, but a doctor's guidance is still advisable. A number of other prescription drugs are under study for reclassification, including some oral contraceptives, antibiotics, anti-ulcer compounds, and allergy medications. So, increasingly, you should take pains to educate yourself about all medications. Be especially diligent about reading all labels and instructions *before* taking any medication. This not only helps protect against side effects and adverse reactions, but also helps ensure that you are taking the correct medication for your ailment.

Remember, too, that labels on over-the-counter drugs sternly advise you to "consult a doctor if symptoms persist." This is invaluable advice.

For example, if you have headaches that just won't go away, you may have a problem that requires medical attention. Again, if you have any questions about an over-the-counter drug, don't hesitate to ask the pharmacist—that's what he or she is there for. If you have more questions after you get home, call your pharmacist, or look for the manufacturer's name and phone number on the package and get in touch with the company directly.

Be Sure to Tell Your Doctor If . . .

While it is important for you to get information from your doctor, it is also important for you to inform him or her about special circumstances in your life. For example:

- Tell the doctor if you are pregnant or if you are breast-feeding.

- Tell the doctor about other physicians and alternative practitioners you are seeing and why.

- Make it a point to tell the doctor if you are taking other medications, including vitamin and mineral supplements, nonprescription medications, and birth control pills, even if he or she does not ask.

chapter

-5-

- - - - - - - - - - - - - - - -

MONITORING DRUG THERAPY

IN MOST CASES, you can soon tell whether a drug is working: Take a pain-killer for a headache or toothache, use an inhaler to control an asthma attack, put a nitroglycerin pill under your tongue when angina flares, and the relief you experience tells you that the medication has worked. But how do you know that a medication is working if the disease is a silent one that has no symptoms, such as high blood pressure, and the effects of the medication are not readily apparent? First and foremost, you should see your doctor periodically for monitoring tests to make sure the drug is performing its function. These regular trips to the doctor or to a laboratory are also important to detect hidden adverse effects. For example, if you are taking a drug that can potentially damage your liver or kidneys, periodic blood and urine tests are essential to make sure this is not happening. If spotted early, your doctor can change your dosage or medication before permanent harm is done.

For further protection, carry a warning card or wear a bracelet describing your drug regimen. If you have to have emergency treatment, the information you carry will stop paramedics and emergency room doctors from using any drugs that are likely to conflict with the ones you are taking or that might cause a dangerous reaction when mixed with your regular prescriptions.

You can also insure that medication will work the way it should by keeping your doctor informed of any changes in your life-style. If, for example, you wish to become pregnant, inform your doctor as soon as possible. He or she can then determine whether your treatment should be stopped or changed by switching you to a different drug that is unlikely to harm a fetus. Or if there are no safe alternative treatments, your doctor might advise you to wait to conceive until your drug therapy is completed.

Special Situations

Although anyone who uses powerful medications for prolonged periods should abide by a regular schedule of checkups, there are some who must be particularly conscientious, and also learn to monitor themselves. The table at the end of this chapter lists commonly prescribed drugs and their recommended monitoring tests. In addition, diseases and regimens that fall into this category include:

- **Arthritis**. There are more than a hundred diseases that cause joint soreness, inflammation, and other symptoms of arthritis. The more serious forms, such as lupus and rheumatoid arthritis, often require high doses of nonsteroidal anti-inflammatory drugs, or even more potent medications like gold salts and steroids or other drugs that suppress the immune system. Some of these drugs hinder the production of blood cells in the bone marrow, and can cause kidney damage and other adverse effects. Regular blood tests can detect these side effects at an early stage, before they cause permanent harm.

- **Asthma**. Powerful drugs like corticosteroids and theophylline are critical in controlling asthma, but they can also cause serious side effects, especially in children. Theophylline has a very narrow dosage range—too little is ineffective and even a small overdose can cause serious arrhythmias (irregular heartbeats) and other problems. Long-term use of oral steroids hinders growth, lowers immunity, and causes weight gain, mood swings, and numerous other adverse effects. Frequent checkups to adjust dosages and monitor drug levels help keep asthma in check and minimize adverse drug effects.

- **Cancer chemotherapy**. In the public mind, the most pervasive side effects of cancer treatment are hair loss, nausea, diarrhea, and extreme fatigue. But many of the drugs used to fight malignancies can cause even more serious side effects, such as interference with the bone marrow's ability to manufacture red blood cells and damage to vital organs, including the liver, the kidneys, and the heart. Regular blood, urine, and other tests during cancer chemotherapy are essential to tailor the dosage to destroy the cancer cells without causing permanent damage to vital organs. When you begin cancer chemotherapy, your doctor will tell you how often you should come in for a checkup—make every effort to follow that schedule.

- **Diabetes**. Patients with insulin-dependent diabetes have to monitor their own blood sugar levels every day to determine that they are taking the proper dosage of insulin to keep their disease under control. They also need to see a doctor who specializes in diabetes and its complications so that diabetes-related problems such as arteriosclerosis, kidney failure, and nerve and eye damage can be spotted and treated early. Recent studies show that these measures can prevent or delay many of the diabetes complications that doctors once considered inevitable.

- **Gallstones**. Anyone undergoing drug treatment for gallstones should see his or her doctor regularly. Ultrasonography—a procedure that uses sound waves to produce images of the gallbladder and other internal structures—every six to nine months is usually recommended to study how well the drug is working.

- **Heart disease**. Heart patients often must take numerous drugs that require careful monitoring. Digoxin (*Lanoxin, Lanoxicaps*)—a purified form of digitalis, the oldest heart medication—remains an important drug for people with failing hearts. But it is also a highly toxic medication, and even a small overdose can cause vision problems, confusion, fainting, loss of appetite, and other more serious consequences. Periodic blood tests are essential to monitor blood levels of digitalis to guard against toxicity.

- **High blood pressure**. Over the last 40 years, dozens of highly effective medications to lower blood pressure (antihypertensives) have been developed. These drugs are largely responsible for the more than 50 percent decrease in the death rate from strokes and the more than 35 percent decline in heart attack deaths since the 1970s. But that is not to say that these drugs are harmless. Many of the diuretics used to lower blood pressure can reduce the body's reserves of potassium, a mineral essential to maintain the body's chemical balance. Others can raise blood sugar, interfere with production of blood cells, and cause numerous unpleasant side effects. Because there are so many classes of antihypertensive drugs, your doctor can almost always devise a safe, tolerable regimen. To do this, however, you should see your doctor at least every six months, or more often if so instructed. It's also a good idea to monitor your blood pressure at home, using an automated device sold in pharmacies and medical supply stores. If you do use a home device, take it with you each time you go in for a checkup to make sure that it is properly calibrated with your doctor's blood pressure device.

• **Hormone replacement therapy.** Replacement hormones are needed in many situations, but the most common is estrogen—with or without progesterone—for women during and after menopause to alleviate symptoms such as hot flashes and to protect against bone loss and possible heart disease. Although estrogen replacement therapy has well-established benefits, it also causes certain side effects, such as weight gain, nausea, breast soreness, mood changes, and others, as well as an increased risk of blood clots and certain cancers. Thus, any woman taking estrogen should see her doctor regularly for checkups, including a Pap smear. Younger women taking birth control pills also should have regular checkups and Pap smears. Similarly, people taking thyroid, adrenal, or pituitary hormones require careful monitoring to make sure they are getting the proper dosage.

Table 5.1

FOLLOW-UP MONITORING OF COMMONLY PRESCRIBED DRUGS

drug and common usage (Generic names or class of drugs listed first, examples in parentheses)	testing recommended or done at doctor's discretion
ACE inhibitors (benazepril, captopril, enalapril, lisinopril) for high blood pressure and heart disease	Prior to starting drug: complete blood cell counts, urinalysis with measurement of protein content and blood potassium level. While using: blood cell counts, urine protein measurements, periodic check of blood potassium.
acyclovir (Zovirax) for herpes infections	Kidney function test
albuterol (Proventil, Ventolin), adrenergic bronchodilators for asthma	Blood pressure measurements, evaluation of heart function
allopurinol (Zyloprim, Lopurin) for gout	Blood uric acid levels, complete blood cell counts, liver and kidney function tests. Eye examinations for possible cataract formation or macular damage.
amantadine (Symmetrel, Symadine) for Parkinson's disease	White blood cell counts, liver and kidney function tests, evaluation of heart function
auranofin (Ridaura), oral gold preparation for rheumatoid arthritis	Urinalyses, complete blood cell counts, liver and kidney function tests
beclomethasone (Beclovent, Beconase, Vancenase, Vanceril), steroid inhalants and sprays for asthma and hay fever	Nose, throat, mouth examinations for fungal infections
beta-blockers (atenolol, acebutolol, metoprolol, nadolol, timolol, pindolol, propranolol, and others) for heart disease and high blood pressure	Measurement of blood pressure, evaluation of heart function. With propranolol, complete blood cell counts as well.
betamethasone (Diprolene), topical steroid. In high doses can act like cortisone	Tests for blood in stool, serum electrolytes

bumetanide (*Bumex*) and furosemide (*Lasix*), loop diuretics to treat heart failure and reduce body fluid volume	Complete blood cell counts; measurements of blood levels of sodium, potassium, chloride, sugar, and uric acid; liver and kidney function tests
calcitonin (*Calcimar*), hormonal preparation for osteoporosis, Paget's disease, high blood calcium levels	Measurements of blood calcium, phosphate, and alkaline phosphatase levels; measurement of urine hydroxyproline content
calcium channel blockers (diltiazem, nifedipine, verapamil) for high blood pressure and heart disease	Evaluations of heart function, including electrocardiograms. With long term-use: liver and kidney function tests.
chlorpromazine (*Thorazine*), one of many phenothiazine preparations to treat psychotic disorders	With prolonged use: complete blood counts, blood pressure, liver function tests, eye examination, and monitoring for tardive dyskinesia and other movement abnormalities
cholestyramine (*Questran*) to lower blood cholesterol	Measurements of total cholesterol, low-density cholesterol, and high-density cholesterol; hemoglobin and red blood cell count for possible anemia
cimetidine (*Tagamet*) for peptic ulcers	Complete blood cell counts, liver and kidney function tests, prothrombin times if taking anticoagulant at same time
clomiphene (*Clomid, Serophene*) for female infertility due to ovarian failure	Prior to beginning use: complete pelvic examination and hormone studies. After use: periodic pelvic examinations, pregnancy test, kidney function tests, eye examination.
clonidine (*Catapres*) for high blood pressure	Blood pressure measurements, kidney function tests
colchicine (*ColBENEMID, Col-Probenecid, Probenecid with Colchicine*) for gout	Complete blood cell counts, uric acid blood levels to monitor status of gout, liver function tests
cortisone to treat inflammatory conditions	Blood sugar, blood in stool, blood components
dextroamphetamine (*Dexedrine*), stimulant to treat narcolepsy and childhood hyperactivity	Blood pressure, growth studies, drug dependency and abuse
diazepam (*Valium*), tranquilizer and muscle relaxant	Liver function tests

(continued)

digoxin (*Lanoxin*), digitalis preparation to treat heart failure, cardiac arrhythmias	Electrocardiograms and measurements of blood levels of digoxin, calcium, magnesium, and potassium
diphenoxylate (*Lomotil*) for diarrhea	Liver function tests
dipyridamole (*Persantine*) to reduce blood clots after heart valve replacement	Measurements of blood pressure, status of blood clotting
disopyramide (*Norpace*) for cardiac arrhythmias	Electrocardiograms, complete blood cell counts, measurements of potassium blood levels
estrogen (*Premarin*) to reduce menopausal symptoms, prevent osteoporosis	Regular examinations of the breasts and pelvic organs, including Pap smears; liver function tests
famotidine (*Pepcid*) for peptic ulcers	Complete blood cell counts
fluoxetine (*Prozac*) to treat depression	Frequent checkups to evaluate mental status; blood glucose measurements
gemfibrozil (*Lopid*) to lower high triglyceride levels	Complete blood cell counts; measurements of total cholesterol, HDL and LDL cholesterol fragments, triglycerides, and blood sugar; liver function tests
guanfacine (*Tenex*) to lower blood pressure when taken with a thiazide diuretic	Blood pressure measurements
haloperidol (*Haldol*) to treat schizophrenia and other psychotic disorders	Complete blood cell counts, liver function tests, eye examinations, electrocardiograms
hydrochlorothiazide (*HydroDIURIL, Esidrix* and others), thiazide diuretic to lower blood pressure and reduce volume of body fluids	Blood pressure measurements, complete blood cell counts, liver and kidney function tests, measurement of blood potassium
indapamide (*Lozol*), diuretic to lower blood pressure and reduce body fluid volume	Measurements of blood levels of sodium, potassium, chloride, sugar, and uric acid
ipratropium (*Atrovent*), bronchodilator for asthma	Internal eye pressure measurements for possible glaucoma

isotretinoin (*Accutane*), oral acne medication	Complete blood cell counts, including platelet count; measurements of blood cholesterol and triglyceride levels; complete eye examinations, liver and kidney function tests
ketoconazole (*Nizoral*) to treat systemic fungal infections	Liver function tests prior to long-term use and monthly once begun
levodopa (*Larodopa*) for Parkinson's disease	Complete blood cell counts; liver, kidney, and heart function tests; measurements of internal eye pressure; blood pressure measurements
liotrix (Thyrolar), thyroid hormone replacement	Thyroid and heart examinations
lithium (*Cibalith-S, Eskalith, Lithobid*) to treat manic phase of manic-depression	Regular monitoring of blood lithium levels; periodic evaluation of thyroid gland size and function; complete blood cell counts; kidney function tests
lovastatin (*Mevacor*) and simvastatin (*Zocor*) to lower blood cholesterol levels	Blood cholesterol measurements: total cholesterol, LDL and HDL fractions; liver function tests; eye examination at beginning of treatment and periodically thereafter
loxapine (*Loxitane*) to treat psychiatric disorders	With prolonged use: complete blood cell counts, liver function tests, eye examination
mebendazole (*Vermox*) to treat intestinal worms	Stool examination, blood counts
methylphenidate (*Ritalin*), stimulant used to treat childhood hyperactivity	Complete blood cell counts, blood pressure measurements, eye examinations, growth monitoring
minoxidil (*Rogaine*), topical medication to stimulate hair growth	General checkup after one month and every six months thereafter to check blood pressure and heart function
niacin (*Nicolar, Niacor*), used to lower blood cholesterol	Blood sugar, liver function tests
nicotine patches (*Habitrol, Nicoderm, Nicotrol, Prostep*) to stop smoking	Heart function tests

(continued)

nitrofurantoin (*Macrobid, Macrodantin*), antibiotic to treat urinary infections	Evaluations of pulmonary, liver, kidney, and heart function; complete blood count
nitroglycerin (*Nitro-Bid, Nitro-Dur, Nitrostat, Transderm-Nitro*) to prevent or treat angina attacks	Blood pressure measurement and heart function, periodic check of white blood cell counts
nizatidine (*Axid*), histamine H$_2$ blocker to treat peptic ulcers	Complete blood cell counts, liver and kidney function tests
nonsteroidal anti-inflammatory agents (ibuprofens [*Advil, Motrin*, etc.], *Indocin*, naproxen [*Naprosyn*], *Tolectin*, ketoprofen [*Orudis*], and others) to treat arthritis and other inflammatory disorders	Periodic blood cell counts, kidney and liver function tests
norfloxacin (*Noroxin*) to treat urinary tract infections	Liver and kidney function tests, urinalysis
penicillamine (*Cuprimine, Depen*), chelating agent to treat severe rheumatoid arthritis, Wilson's disease	Urinalysis, complete blood cell counts, liver and kidney function tests
phenelzine (*Nardil*) to treat mental disorders	Blood pressure measurements, complete blood cell counts, liver function tests
phenytoin (*Dilantin*) to treat seizure disorders	Monitoring of blood phenytoin levels; complete blood cell counts; liver function tests; measurement of blood glucose, calcium, phosphorus, folic acid, and vitamin B$_{12}$ levels
prednisone (*Deltasone, Prednisone*), systemic corticosteroid for inflammations, asthma	Frequent checkups with measurement of blood pressure, blood sugar and potassium levels; regular eye examinations; bone density studies; growth monitoring of children
probenecid (*Benemid, Probenecid, ColBENEMID*) to treat gout	Blood uric acid levels, complete blood cell counts, liver and kidney function tests
procainamide (*Procan SR, Promine, Pronestyl*), used to treat cardiac arrhythmias	Frequent checks to monitor heart rate and rhythm
ranitidine (*Zantac*) to treat peptic ulcer	Complete blood cell counts, liver and kidney function tests

sulfamethoxazole (*Gantanol*) and other sulfonamides to treat urinary and other bacterial infections	Complete blood cell counts weekly for first eight weeks, urinalysis weekly, liver and kidney function tests
sulfinpyrazone (*Anturane*) to treat gout	Blood tests to measure uric acid; kidney function studies
terfenadine (*Seldane*), antihistamine for allergies	Electrocardiograms for patients with heart disorders
theophylline (*Theo-Dur*), bronchodilator for asthma	Measurement of blood theophylline levels with high dosages or prolonged use
thiothixene (*Navane*) to treat psychotic disorders	Blood counts, liver function tests, mental function evaluation, eye examination
tocainide (*Tonocard*) to treat irregular heart rhythm	Periodic blood check, liver function tests, potassium levels, x ray, and electrocardiograms
tolazamide (*Tolinase*) and other oral hypoglycemic drugs to treat type 2, or adult-onset, diabetes	Frequent checkups to monitor blood glucose levels; heart and kidney function tests; eye examinations
tricyclic antidepressants (*Elavil, Anafranil, Sinequan, Tofranil,* and others) to treat depression	Frequent checkups to assess mental status; complete blood cell counts
ursodiol (*Actigall*) to treat gallstones	Liver function tests, periodic ultrasound examination of gallbladder
valproic acid (*Depakene*) to treat seizure disorders	Prior to starting treatment: complete blood cell counts and baseline liver function tests. Thereafter: periodic blood cell counts and liver function tests

chapter

-6-

GIVING MEDICATION TO INFANTS AND CHILDREN

As any parent knows, giving medicine to a child is fraught with anxiety and problems. First, there is the worry over the underlying need for medication. You also may be concerned whether your child is getting the proper dosage. You know that drugs sometimes affect a child differently than they do adults, which raises the specter of an adverse reaction. Finally, there's the task of simply getting a recalcitrant youngster to take the medication. In some cases, the latter looms as the most trying, so let's tackle it first.

Administering Medicine to Children

Planning, psychology, and perhaps a bit of subterfuge can go a long way toward erasing tensions associated with giving children their medicine, especially if it has an unpleasant taste. Try letting your child suck on an ice cube or an ice pop made of frozen juice immediately before giving the medicine. The cold treat not only will placate the child psychologically but, more importantly, also will numb the palate and tongue, making them less sensitive to the offending taste. If the child gags or complains about the taste, offer another ice cube or frozen juice as a postmedication chaser. Chilling the medicine itself also reduces its taste and smell. But check with your pharmacist before resorting to this tactic—some medicines should not be put in the refrigerator.

The Mary Poppins remedy of a spoonful of sugar is not generally recommended because of the potential harm to teeth. But sometimes medication can be disguised by mixing it with fruit juice, apple sauce, cereal, pudding, or baby food. Again, check with your pharmacist first, because some drugs should not be taken with foods. Don't forget a reassuring hug, which can lessen the impact of even the most bitter medicine.

If the child complains of nausea after taking medicine, offer flat, or unfizzed, ginger ale. You can get the fizz out by repeatedly pouring the drink from one glass to another.

MEDICATION FOR BABIES

Most infants cannot swallow tablets or capsules. Thus, when your doctor prescribes a medication, it is likely to be in an easy-to-give liquid form.

Even so, some medications have an unpleasant

aftertaste. If the baby fusses or refuses to open his or her mouth, gently squeezing the nostrils will force the child to open up to breathe, allowing you to insert the spoon or medicine dropper.

A teaspoon is the standard measurement for most liquid medicines. To make sure that the right amount is given, most pharmaceutical manufacturers include a measuring device—either a spoon or a special dropper—in the medicine's package. Using this measure guarantees that your baby gets the proper dosage. If there is no measuring aide, don't automatically reach for a conventional spoon without checking its accuracy. Regular teaspoons vary greatly in size. Pour the medication into a true household measuring teaspoon that holds 5 milliliters (ml) of liquid.

MEDICATION FOR OLDER CHILDREN

Children over the age of six should be able to swallow tablets, capsules, or pills. Instruct the youngster to place the tablet on the back of the tongue and then quickly take a drink of water or fruit juice. If he or she has difficulty swallowing the pill, offer it with seltzer or a carbonated drink, which works even better than plain water or juice.

If the pill still won't go down, use two spoons to crush it into a fine powder, which can be added to a spoon of applesauce or dissolved in a small amount of water. Similarly, a capsule can be opened and emptied into water or applesauce. However, don't use these tactics with time-release drugs or medication with a special enteric coating to prevent its being dissolved in the stomach. Otherwise, the medication will be absorbed too rapidly in the stomach or in the wrong part of the gastrointestinal tract. If you are not sure what kind of capsule you are dealing with, ask your physician or pharmacist.

If possible, allow an older child leeway in how to take medication. For example, youngsters old

enough to choose between alternatives can practice this skill when it comes to taking medicine. "Do you want to take your medicine with juice or water?" Or foster a sense of responsibility by setting an alarm clock so the child can remind you it's medicine time. Giving children a role in decision making invariably evokes a more cooperative response.

Of course, there will be times when even the most cooperative child will not be able to take oral medication because of nausea and vomiting. In such instances, you must resort to some other form, such as a suppository. Put a little petroleum jelly around the anal opening and gently insert the suppository into the rectum. Be sure that the pointed end of the suppository goes in first. Then hold the buttocks together for about a minute until the urge to expel has passed.

Medications that cannot be given either by the oral or the rectal route may have to be administered by injection. Following are tips on giving other forms of medication:

EYE MEDICATION. Even adults hate to have anything put in their eyes and, as a result, blink reflexively as the dropper approaches its target. To make the process easier for a child, ask him or her to lean back in a chair. Gently pull the lower lid back from the eye so that the lid forms a pouch, then direct the drops into the pouch. By making the pouch and not the eye the target, you avoid the reflexive blinking that makes it impossible to give the drops properly. For eye ointments, pull the lower lid downward, and then apply the solution or ointment to the inside of the lid. If an eye infection is being treated, it is important to avoid touching the eyelid with the container or bottle nozzle in order to prevent contaminating the medication. This will prevent transmitting the infection to the other eye.

EAR DROPS. Make sure that the medication has warmed to room temperature; cold drops can cause severe pain. It is easier if the child lies on his or her side when you put the drops in the ear, and stays in that position for two or three minutes afterward.

NOSE DROPS. Tilt your child's head backward and instruct the youngster to breathe through his or her mouth. Insert about one third of an inch of the dropper into the nostril, taking care not to touch the insides of the nose. The medication should flow to the back of the nose and not down the throat. Following instillation of the drops, keep the child's head tilted back for a few minutes to keep the medication from running out.

Adjusting Dosage for Children

Babies and children not only are smaller than adults, but their bodies also metabolize drugs differently, making it more difficult to arrive at the correct dosage. Here are some important considerations:

- Water makes up a greater percentage of body weight in children than in adults; for example, water constitutes 80 percent of a premature baby's body weight, compared to 75 percent of a full-term newborn's, 59 percent of a 1-year-old's, and 55 percent in an average adult's. Because water makes up a greater proportion of a child's weight, an infant may require more of certain drugs to reach an effective concentration. But the volume of body water is not the only consideration. Certain oral drugs—including penicillin—are absorbed more efficiently into a child's body, compared to an adult's. In addition, a baby's liver and kidneys may not be mature enough to break down and excrete a drug. Thus, drugs that are well absorbed into the body must be given in doses low enough to prevent excessive accumulation.

- Food and water move through the gastrointestinal tract more slowly in children than in adults. Children also have less gastric acid than older people, and the transport mechanisms that allow drugs to pass through the intestinal walls to reach the blood vessels are less developed in children. Thus, some medicines have to be given in higher doses in order to compensate for these differences.

- The skin of children is thinner than that of adults. Ointments, creams, and salves are absorbed into the body more readily, possibly in dangerous amounts. For example, excessive use of hydrocortisone cream, a steroid medication, can suppress growth and cause other adverse effects in young children. Therefore, these topical medications should be administered in lower doses to children than to adults.

Dosages for children of various ages are listed on the packaging of many over-the-counter drugs. If this information is not provided, ask your physician or pharmacist for guidance. In general, children over the age of 13 can tolerate about the same dosages as adults, but again, there are exceptions. For example, if your child is very much underweight, your doctor will gear the dosage to weight rather than age.

Common Childhood Afflictions

Parents invariably develop a sixth sense about the ailments that strike their children. And while experience and common sense go a long way toward coping with an illness successfully, experts advise consulting a doctor, even if the symptoms are mild. Nevertheless, here are some tips for dealing with some of the more common childhood afflictions at home.

THE COMMON COLD

Children six months old or younger should be kept away from people who have colds or the flu. A viral infection that causes a mild illness in an older child or an adult can be much more serious in an infant, causing croup, tonsillitis, and pneumonia, to name a few. If your baby does come down with a cold or flu, call your physician right away. Never give aspirin to a child of any age who has a viral infection—in this setting, it increases the risk of Reye's Syndrome, a potentially fatal brain and liver disease. And don't give acetaminophen (*Tylenol, Apacet, Liquiprin*) or any other fever or cough/cold preparation to a child three months or younger without first consulting your pediatrician.

After the age of six months, cold symptoms—runny nose, fever, loss of appetite, coughing, and sneezing, usually disappear in a few days. In most cases, there is no need for medication, particularly if the child is playing and sleeping normally. But if your child is having trouble sleeping, is coughing often and hard, or is running a fever of 102°F or higher, acetaminophen may help. Contact your doctor if symptoms persist, especially if the cough lasts more than five days, if the youngster's temperature rises to 102°F or higher, or the child complains of an earache, is sleeping more than usual, or is unusually cranky.

STREP THROAT

Colds and flu often cause a sore throat that disappears with the other symptoms. But if the sore throat comes on suddenly, is especially severe, and persists for more than two or three days, it may

well be strep throat—an illness caused by the *Streptococcus* bacterium. An untreated strep throat can cause rheumatic fever, an illness that damages the joints and heart, as well as kidney diseases like nephritis. A strep throat is easily diagnosed by a throat culture and treated with antibiotics. The usual course calls for a full ten days' medication; be sure to administer all of the pills to ensure that the infection is eradicated, even if the sore throat clears up earlier.

EAR INFECTIONS

Ear infections, which strike most often during the winter and early spring, are especially common in babies and young children. Most often childhood ear infections settle in the middle portion of the ear and are referred to as otitis media. If you suspect that your child has an infection, see your physician as soon as possible. If an examination confirms otitis media, the doctor will probably prescribe an antibiotic, which usually alleviates any ear pain in about three days. As with any antibiotic therapy, the drug should be continued for the full course of treatment—usually ten days or until the medication is used up. A follow-up visit may be needed to make sure the infection has been eradicated. Although ear infections tend to recur, take some comfort in the thought that most are eminently treatable, and most children have fewer and fewer episodes as they grow older.

FEVER

A fever is a sign that the body is mustering its defenses against an infection or some other illness. Most fevers are short-lived and harmless; it is when the temperature rises too high or the fever persists too long that you need to worry or call your doctor (see Table 6.1).

Give the child plenty of liquids to avoid dehy-

FEVER IN CHILDREN:

WHEN TO CALL THE DOCTOR

In general, you should contact your pediatrician if a fever (high or low) lasts more than two days, or in the following cases:

If child is:	and temperature is:
Younger than 3 months	100.2°F or higher
Between 3 and 6 months	101°F or higher
Older than 6 months	103°F or higher

dration; for younger children, many pediatricians recommend the use of specially formulated oral rehydration solutions such as *Pedialyte*, as plain water supplementation may not replace some of the essential electrolytes—compounds essential to controlling the body's balance of fluids—that are rapidly lost. Dress the youngster lightly to prevent overheating. Some children are especially susceptible to febrile seizures, or convulsions. If the child becomes delirious or starts to shake uncontrollably, take immediate steps to lower his or her temperature. This can be done by bathing or sponging the child with cool water.

In general, acetaminophen is the preferred medication to lower a child's fever. This drug, which also eases aches and pains, comes in a liquid formulation and dosages for children. A child's formulation of ibuprofen is also available, but it is a prescription-only medication and is not recommended for use in children less than three years of age. The advantage of ibuprofen over acetaminophen is that it is generally longer acting and it may be more effective in the management of some fevers. As noted earlier, aspirin generally is not recommended for children, especially if they have a viral illness. Whatever fever-lowering drug you use,

be sure to read the label carefully to determine the most appropriate dosage for your child. Call your doctor if you have any doubts about the dose or how often to give the medicine.

Precautions

The following precautions will help you avoid hazards related to giving children medicine:

1. **Never give a child (or anyone else, for that matter) someone else's prescription medicine.** The safety and effectiveness of many prescription drugs have not yet been established in children, and dosages must be tailored to the individual child. If your child needs a prescription, your pediatrician will issue one in the correct dosages.

2. **Ask your physician or pharmacist if there are foods or drinks that your child should avoid while taking a certain drug, whether prescribed or available over the counter.** Certain foods, including infant formulas and milk products, may interfere with the absorp-

tion of some drugs, so feeding and medication schedules may need to be adjusted accordingly.

3. **Don't insist that your doctor prescribe antibiotics if the physician believes that they are not necessary.** Overuse or misuse of antibiotics increases the risk of adverse side effects and the emergence of drug-resistant organisms. In children, unnecessary use of antibiotics can be especially troublesome. Tetracycline, for example, hinders calcium metabolism. Although this has little or no effect on an adult, it can lead to permanent staining of the teeth and a temporary inhibition of bone growth in children. Other antibiotics are potentially dangerous when given to children and should be given only when absolutely necessary and when the potential good more than offsets the possible danger.

4. **If an antibiotic is prescribed, make sure your child takes the full course.** Even if the symptoms clear up soon after the youngster starts taking the drug, follow your doctor's instructions. Otherwise, the infection may not be eradicated completely, resulting in a relapse that could be even more dangerous than the original illness because the surviving organisms could be resistant to the antibiotic.

5. **Be alert for possible drug interactions if your child is taking other medication.** Make sure your physician knows about any other medication, including vitamin supplements. Call your physician if:

• Your child repeatedly vomits the medicine.

• You think the child is having a reaction to the medicine.

• Your child develops diarrhea a day or more after starting the medicine.

   Don't panic, however. Many symptoms (skin rashes, nausea, jittery behavior) disappear if the dosage is reduced.

6. **Take steps to prevent accidental poisoning.** Thousands of children wind up in emergency rooms every year as a result of accidental poisoning from medication, including vitamin and iron pills and over-the-counter drugs. To prevent such accidental poisoning:

• Never pretend medicine is like candy. When giving medicine to a child, use its proper name, not one that makes it seem friendly or innocuous.

• Don't take your own medications in front of children. Doing so can lead children, especially the very young, to believe that medicines are desirable.

• Be sure to close the bottle properly, using the child-resistant cap. Draw skulls and bones or other scary designs on medication bottles.

• Never leave any kind of medicine where a child can get to it. The safest place is in a locked box on a high shelf in a locked closet. Never leave vitamins on the table, and check pocketbooks, briefcases, drawers, and the bathroom for any stray medicines. When visiting grandparents or a household where there are no children, ask your host to make a similar check.

• If you are called to the door or phone while you are in the process of giving a child medicine—or taking your own—take the container with you. Given a chance, a child can very quickly down the contents of a medicine bottle.

- When you are finished with any medication, empty and rinse out the container thoroughly before throwing it in the garbage. A child who finds the bottle may take any of the leftover drug.

POISONING EMERGENCIES

If, despite your best efforts, your child manages to swallow the contents of a bottle of medicine, call your local poison control center. The number is listed with other emergency numbers in the front of your telephone book. It's a good idea, however, to post the number by all telephones in your home, on your refrigerator, and where you store your medicines. Act immediately, even if your child appears normal. Not all overdoses or drug poisonings cause immediate symptoms, but a delay can be fatal. When you call the center:

- Stay calm. Be prepared to give a full description of your child's physical status: Does his or her skin feel clammy? Is there a fever? Convulsions? Change in consciousness?

- Don't induce vomiting unless you are told to do so. However, since this is often the line of first defense, you should have something on hand that will help you do that. A universally accepted emetic is ipecac, which can be obtained without a prescription. Activated charcoal is also used sometimes to counteract poison. Taken internally, the charcoal binds the drug to itself, preventing it from being absorbed into the body. You can also buy activated charcoal without a prescription, but again, don't use it unless you are advised to do so by the poison control center or your doctor.

- Don't give antidotes without being instructed to do so. This is particularly true if your child has overdosed on two or more medications. You may have antidotes for both in the house, but one may well negate the effects of the other.

-7-

TAKING MEDICATIONS DURING PREGNANCY AND BREAST-FEEDING

EVERY TIME YOU take any medication, you should pause a moment to ask yourself whether its potential benefits outweigh the risk of possible side effects or adverse reactions. At no time is this consideration more important than when a woman is pregnant or breast-feeding, because she is making the choice not just for herself, but also for her baby.

Effects of Medication on the Fetus

At one time, it was assumed that the placenta would act as a protective barrier to keep drugs and other potentially harmful substances from the fetus. Today, we know that most medicines not only pass this barrier, but also can have a profound effect on the baby because the fetal liver and kidneys cannot break down and detoxify such substances. Thus, while some compounds may have no effect on the baby at all, others can cause severe consequences, including:

- Miscarriage, prolonged labor, or premature birth
- Congenital birth defects, especially during the first trimester of pregnancy when organs are forming. (A drug or substance that causes such defects is said to be teratogenic.)

- Retarded growth, both before and after birth
- Developmental problems, ranging from learning disorders to mental retardation
- Sensory defects, including blindness and deafness
- Emotional and behavioral disorders

Table 7.1 lists drugs that can harm a developing fetus when taken by a pregnant woman, and the birth defects that may result.

Most of us assume that any drug approved by the Food and Drug Administration has gone through a rigorous testing process that includes determining whether it is safe during pregnancy. But this is not necessarily the case. The FDA requires that all new drugs be tested on pregnant animals, usually rats or rabbits, before they are approved for human use. Although rat and rabbit studies can provide valuable information on possible teratogenic effects of drugs, they cannot accurately predict the extent of such effects in humans because, physiological similarities notwithstanding, it is very difficult to extrapolate experimental findings from species to species. A drug that produces birth defects in an animal may not do so in humans, and

Table 7.1

DRUGS TO APPROACH CAREFULLY DURING PREGNANCY

drug	adverse effects on fetus and newborn
Accutane (antiacne)	Major congenital deformities, especially neurological
Alcohol	Fetal alcohol syndrome, multiple and variable birth defects, mental retardation and low birth weight; miscarriage
Anticancer drugs	Fetal death, multiple and variable serious birth defects, growth retardation
Anticoagulants (blood thinners)	Underdevelopment of cartilage and bone (especially in the nose), fetal or newborn bleeding, mental retardation and blindness, stillbirth
Anticonvulsants	Multiple and variable birth defects, mental and growth retardation, bleeding, spina bifida
Aspirin	Fetal growth retardation and birth defects with high doses; taken in the first half of pregnancy may adversely affect child's intelligence; taken near term may delay onset of labor and cause bleeding in mother and newborn; rare cases of perinatal mortality
CNS depressants (narcotics, barbiturates, tranquilizers)	Central nervous system depression during labor
Cortisone	Possibility of birth defects with large doses
Cough/cold and asthma medications	Possible enlargement of thyroid
Cytotec (antiulcer drug)	Miscarriage, bleeding
Diazepam (*Valium*)	Cleft lip

Diuretics (medications to rid the body of excess water)	Fetal growth retardation
Sedatives	High doses may cause decrease in fetal activity and withdrawal symptoms in newborn, including irritability
Sex hormones	Masculinization of a female fetus (androgens); vaginal cancers and fertility problems (DES)
Tetracycline	Impaired bone growth, discoloration of teeth and underdevelopment of tooth enamel
Thyroid drugs	Destruction of fetal thyroid gland; enlargement of thyroid
Vitamin A	Excessive doses can cause birth defects
Vitamin C	Symptoms of scurvy following birth
Zinc	Prematurity, congenital defects

vice versa. A case in point involves the tragic consequences of thalidomide, a tranquilizer and sleep aid sometimes given to pregnant women in the late 1950s and early 1960s. The drug had passed animal tests without a hint of harm to a fetus. It wasn't until hundreds of babies were born with stunted or missing limbs that the real hazards of thalidomide became apparent.

Even when potential problems are spotted during animal testing, some drugs may still be released for sale. For example, the animal studies of isotretinoin (*Accutane*), an acne drug, showed that it could cause birth defects. This was to be expected because *Accutane* is derived from a form of vitamin A, itself a powerful teratogen when taken in large doses. Despite warnings of *Accutane*'s teratogenic potential, which were included in the information supplied to physicians and patients, within a year after *Accutane* reached the market, there were reports of babies of women using the drug being born with severe birth defects, espe-

cially of the central nervous system. Since then, restrictions have been instituted to make sure that women of child-bearing age fully understand the risks of *Accutane*, and that they practice scrupulous birth control while taking it.

Many factors influence whether a drug harms a developing fetus; its chemical makeup, the dosage, extent of exposure, and stage of pregnancy, among others. Unfortunately, there is no way to determine in advance whether a drug will harm a fetus. A small amount of one drug taken at a particular stage of pregnancy can have a devastating effect, while larger amounts of the same medication taken at a different time may have no adverse effects.

In general, however, exposure during the first three months of pregnancy—the first trimester—is the most critical. This is the time of rapid cell division and the formation of organs in the fetus. By the fourth week after conception, the fetal heart begins to beat, and by the tenth week, all the major organs are formed. Even under the best of circumstances, this process is precarious. Most miscarriages occur during the first trimester. It is also the time when exposure to certain drugs, including alcohol, can cause severe congenital malfunctions. Even common drugs that ordinarily cause few problems can harm the fetus. Tetracycline (*Sumycin, Achromycin, Panmycin*), for example, can interfere with the formation of teeth, resulting in severe mottling.

Of course, hazards to the fetus do not end with the first trimester. Many drugs can exert an adverse effect throughout pregnancy. Although the various organs have been formed, they continue to develop throughout gestation, and can become stunted or damaged. In addition, some drugs have the indirect adverse effect of reducing blood flow through the placenta, thereby reducing the steady supply of oxygen and nutrients to the fetus.

Moreover, drugs don't have to be swallowed or injected to harm the fetus; some medicinal creams or ointments can also be detrimental if their active ingredients are absorbed through the skin into the bloodstream. For example, topical steroids, when used in large enough quantities, can make their way through the skin into the bloodstream and may harm the fetus.

NONPRESCRIPTION DRUGS

Most people mistakenly assume that over-the-counter drugs are safer than those requiring a prescription. This is not necessarily so—even aspirin or vitamin supplements can be harmful under certain circumstances. In addition, many drugs that once required a prescription are now available over the counter—a trend that is accelerating. Consequently, all consumers—and especially pregnant women—must be more diligent than ever in following label instructions and warnings.

Your doctor or pharmacist can advise you about the potential impact of over-the-counter drugs. If neither professional is immediately available for consultation, avoid the medication until you can get a reading on its safety. This also applies to vitamin and mineral supplements. Your doctor will probably prescribe extra iron and folic acid—two nutrients that are needed in amounts difficult to obtain from dietary sources alone. But high doses of certain other vitamins can be as damaging to a developing fetus as any drug. This is particularly true of vitamin A, a fat-soluble nutrient that is stored in the liver and fatty tissues. The Recommended Dietary Allowance (RDA) for vitamin A—800 RE—does not change during pregnancy, and dosages that exceed four or five times the RDA can cause severe birth defects and even pregnancy loss. If you are taking high doses of vitamin A, experts recommend that you stop them at least three months before attempting a pregnancy to give your body time to clear out some of the stored reserves. High doses of zinc and vitamin C are also believed to be harmful to a developing fetus.

Individual circumstances are considered when recommending nutritional supplements during pregnancy. If you are a strict vegetarian, for example, you may need extra calcium and vitamin B_{12}. For the average woman, some obstetricians approve a daily multiple vitamin preparation containing iron and folic acid that is specifically designed for pregnant women, but stress that this is unnecessary if you eat a balanced and varied diet and take the extra iron and folic acid you may not be able to get from your diet alone.

ALTERNATIVES TO MEDICATION

Discuss with your doctor any physical problems, including indigestion, aches and pains, constipation, and swelling, associated with pregnancy. Often a doctor can recommend alternatives to drugs for these and other minor complaints. For example, muscle pain may prove amenable to cold packs as an alternative to aspirin or ibuprofen. Exercise and increased fiber in your diet can help overcome constipation. Meditation and other techniques can eliminate any need for tranquilizers or sleeping pills. Taking several rest breaks with your legs and feet elevated can alleviate swelling, eliminating a need for diuretics.

WHEN MEDICATIONS ARE NEEDED

There are, of course, situations in which the benefits of a drug outweigh the potential for harm to the fetus. In such cases, let your obstetrician be your guide. Some women avoid consulting their doctor when symptoms develop for fear that a drug will be prescribed that can cause harm. This can be a grave mistake because the underlying illness may pose more of a danger than a drug used to treat it.

Obviously, the goal is to stay healthy, but if illness develops, it affects both the mother and baby. In some cases, a woman may have a chronic condition such as epilepsy, heart disease, asthma, diabetes, or hypertension. In such cases, it's a good idea to seek out an obstetrician who specializes in high-risk pregnancies. These specialists are experienced in devising regimens that will control the chronic disease while minimizing any danger to the fetus. Experts advise that women with a chronic disease consult such a physician even before pregnancy occurs. In many instances, medications or dosages may be changed, perhaps even before conception takes place. A woman who has epilepsy, for example, may be switched from her usual anticonvulsant medication to a barbiturate, which poses a lesser threat to the fetus. Or the usual medication may be continued but at a reduced dosage or on a different schedule.

Problems that develop during pregnancy also may require medication. In such cases, the safest possible medication will be prescribed. For example, an infection should be treated with a penicillin or another alternative to tetracycline.

The Special Case of Breast-feeding

Of course, the threat your medications may pose to your baby do not end with delivery; you need to be equally diligent if you are breast-feeding your infant. Pediatricians universally agree that in most instances, breast-feeding provides the best nutrition for a baby during the first few months of life, and a growing number of mothers are electing this option. In addition to providing the optimal nutrition a newborn requires to grow and develop, breast milk also contains antibodies that protect the infant against numerous infections. In addition to these nutritional and immunological benefits, breast-feeding also promotes psychological bonding between the mother and child.

Still, breast-feeding may not be advisable if you must take certain drugs that are harmful to your baby (see Table 7.2). Others, such as bromocriptine and certain hormones, can suppress breast milk production.

Some drugs, including mild pain-killers, sedatives, antibiotics, anticoagulants, and mood-altering drugs, which are frequently employed to cope with a variety of postdelivery problems, do not seem to harm babies. Even so, small amounts are found in breast milk, so they should be used in moderation. Also, you can minimize any risk by altering the timing of your breast-feeding. Since drug levels in breast milk are usually highest shortly after taking the medication, your doctor may recommend that you breast-feed first, then take your medicine. In some cases, however, a temporary halt in breast-feeding is necessary to give time for a medication to clear the body. This is true for metronidazole (*Flagyl*), an antibacterial drug, and the various radioactive dyes used in some medical tests.

In summary, to be on the safe side, always check with your doctor before taking any medication—including vitamins and other nonprescription products—during pregnancy or while breast-feeding. Always use any medication precisely as recommended. Take those drugs that your doctor recommends for a chronic or acute condition, but otherwise, resort to drug therapy only when the benefits outweigh any potential harm to your baby.

Table 7.2

DRUGS THAT CAN AFFECT BREAST-FED INFANT WHEN TAKEN BY MOTHER

drug	possible complications
Amantadine	Vomiting, urinary retention, skin rash
Anticancer drugs, Ampethopeterin	May suppress the body's immune system
Aspirin	May migrate into milk and interfere with child's blood platelets—use caution in first week after birth
Bromocriptine	Suppresses milk production
Caffeine	Drinking too much (6–8 cups/day) may make child restless or irritable and interfere with child's ability to sleep
Chloramphenicol	Possible bone marrow depression
Cimetidine	May suppress gastric acids and stimulate nervous system
Clemastine	Drowsiness, irritability, poor feeding
Ergotamine	Diarrhea, vomiting, convulsions
Erythromycin	Risk of jaundice
Gold salts	Rash, kidney, and liver inflammation
Lithium	Muscle weakness, cardiac disorders, and low body temperature
Oral contraceptives	Decreased infant weight gain, diminished quantity and quality of milk supply
Phenindione	Bleeding, allergic reactions
Propylthiouracil	Possible goiter and bone marrow suppression
Thiouracil, iodine	Hypothyroidism, goiter

-8-

SPECIAL CONSIDERATIONS FOR THE ELDERLY

IT'S NOT UNUSUAL for an elderly person to take a dozen or more different drugs every day. Some may be over-the-counter drugs to ease aching joints, constipation, indigestion, and other common problems that accelerate with aging. Others may be part of the armamentarium used to control serious medical problems, such as hypertension, heart disease, diabetes, urinary problems, or a host of other conditions that so often develop as we grow older. In fact, a recent report by the Department of Health and Human Services noted that the average American senior citizen gets some 15 prescriptions a year. Although these drugs are often lifesaving, the multiple regimens plus the natural effects of aging increase the risk of side effects and adverse reactions.

Our bodies are constantly changing throughout life. Some of these changes, especially the repair and regeneration of various cells and tissues, are essential to keep our bodies functioning properly. But as we age, our bodies undergo different types of changes—some of which are detrimental. For example, the production of key hormones and enzymes diminishes and sometimes stops altogether. Many organs, especially the liver, kidney, and others that control key functions, become less

efficient. In many cases, these changes reduce our ability to break down and metabolize various drugs.

Take the kidneys as a prime example. By the time we reach age 70, kidney function may be only half of that of a 30-year-old. Although this is still adequate for normal needs, 50 percent of peak function may not be enough to handle the burden of multiple drugs. Consequently, it may take longer than normal to clear drugs or their by-products from the bloodstream. Of course, the ability to clear drugs from the body can be compromised even further if the kidneys are diseased or there are other underlying conditions such as congestive heart failure. Examples of drugs that are cleared through the kidneys are most antibiotics and aspirin.

Another vital organ that is slowed by age is the liver, which breaks down, or metabolizes, medications so that the body can use them, and also detoxifies alcohol and other harmful chemicals so they can be expelled from the body. With age the liver not only shrinks in size, but it also functions less efficiently. The flow of blood to and from the liver may also be reduced. Of course, any underlying liver disease further decreases its ability to deal with drugs.

Still another age-related change involves the composition of body tissue itself. Older people generally have more fatty tissue—up to 20 percent more—than when they were younger, and the body also contains more water. As the amount of fat and water increases, so does the accumulation of drugs designed to dissolve in these two substances. Thus, tranquilizers, barbiturates, and many antihypertensive agents, which dissolve in fat, can reach dangerous levels in the blood. The same is true of lithium (*Cibalith-S, Lithobid, Eskalith*), which is used to treat the manic component of manic-depressive psychosis, and salicylates, the major ingredient in aspirin, both of which must dissolve in water.

All of these changes combine to reduce the efficiency of drugs and to increase the risk of side effects due to a buildup of chemicals in the body. These may include diarrhea or constipation, nausea and vomiting, loss of appetite, severe anemia, bleeding, assorted allergic reactions, and urinary problems. The accumulation of drugs can also lead to drowsiness, confusion, depression, and even dementia, the loss of mental function. All too often, the onset of these psychological and mental problems is written off as the natural consequence of aging or is mistaken for Alzheimer's disease. To make matters worse, the person suffering from these problems may be given even more medication that causes even more side effects.

According to U.S. government statistics, each year an estimated 120,000 older people are debilitated by mental impairment or neurological problems caused by drugs. Some 32,000 suffer serious falls and fractures after taking tranquilizers or sleeping pills. In all, almost 250,000 older Americans are hospitalized each year because of drug side effects, and officials of the U.S. Department of Health and Human Services think that this may be a gross underestimate. And the problem increases in proportion to the number of drugs involved.

Unfortunately, many older people suffer from multiple illnesses. A 75-year-old man with diabetes may also be under treatment for high blood pressure, heart disease, and a host of other related conditions, as well as arthritis, an enlarged prostate, and other disorders associated with aging. Similarly, his wife may be under treatment for arthritis, glaucoma, and breast cancer. Their elderly friends and relatives can reel off equally long lists of disorders requiring multiple drug regimens. Some of those drugs may cancel each other out. Others may play off each other, increasing the effect of each. And some may combine to produce highly toxic and dangerous effects.

Most doctors, of course, are aware of the special problems of medications in their elderly patients, and they take care to monitor their patients' drug reactions and to adjust their dosage to minimize the risk of adverse effects. But many older people see different physicians, often going to specialists in various disorders. These physicians may not know about drugs that have been prescribed for other illnesses. Even if a doctor asks about other medications, many patients are uncertain about the names and dosages of their medication. In addition, they may neglect to mention over-the-counter products. Problems often can be avoided by patronizing only one pharmacist who maintains a computerized record of all medications a patron is taking. But this safety check may not work for the large number of older people who are often on the move, dividing their time between summer and winter homes, visiting children in different parts of the country, or simply taking advantage of their retirement years by traveling from area to area. Even those who stay put may patronize more than one pharmacist or use discount mail order services. Whatever the reason, they inadvertently may end up taking drugs that interact with each other. Here are tips for avoiding such problems:

- **Keep each of your doctors up-to-date on treatments prescribed by other physicians.** Let's say that you have mild arthritis that you control with an occasional nonsteroidal anti-inflammatory drug prescribed by a rheumatologist. You feel that the arthritis is a minor problem compared to your high blood pressure, so you neglect to mention it to the cardiologist. But your arthritis drug, though relatively mild, can cause sodium and fluid retention, two factors that can reduce the efficacy of your antihypertensive medication. Such common problems can be avoided by making sure that each doctor knows what medications you are taking to ensure that one medication does not reduce the effectiveness of another.

- **Always keep a doctor informed of changes in body functions, no matter how minor they seem.** A change in urinary habits, for example, may signal a change in kidney function. If so, your doctor may adjust medications or dosages to reduce the kidney's workload. In another instance, some drugs prescribed for hypertension can cause unusually low blood pressure, resulting in dizziness or fainting when you abruptly stand up after sitting or lying down. A change in dosage or medication can prevent this condition, which is referred to as orthostatic hypotension. Any unusual or strong reaction to a drug warrants an immediate phone call to the doctor's office.

- **Question your doctor closely about a new prescription.** Ask what the drug is for, how it will work in your body, and what side effects it may produce. Also ask whether the medication should be taken with meals or on an

empty stomach. This is important because some drugs should enter the body slowly, and taking them with food slows their rate of absorption. Other medications should enter the bloodstream quickly, and thus should be taken on an empty stomach. The type of liquid taken with a drug may also be important—some drugs should not be taken with milk, for example, and others should not be mixed with juice.

- **Ask your pharmacist to give you a package insert or to write out complete instructions for taking a drug.** Package inserts provided by drug manufacturers often list drug interactions and special precautions for elderly patients

- **Organize the way you take your medications.** Many older people use pill dispensers that have the time and day printed on individual compartments, making it easier to remember when a drug should be taken. Notations on a kitchen calendar can also help keep track of when medicines should be taken. If you must take drugs every few hours, set an alarm clock as a reminder. At the beginning of each week, arrange the pills you need to take each day in separate labeled envelopes or compartments in a divided tray. You can then tell at a glance what medication you need to take during the course of the day.

- **Make sure you have easy access to your drugs.** For example, if arthritis makes it difficult for you to open pill bottles, ask your pharmacist to put your prescription in a container that does not have a childproof cap. Arthritis, palsy, and loss of coordination make it difficult to open these special lids, leading many patients to skip their medication rather than struggle to open a bottle or ask for help.

• **If possible, have all prescriptions filled at a pharmacy that keeps a patient's drug profile.** Doing so will increase the chances that your pharmacist will spot potentially conflicting medications, especially when prescriptions are written by different doctors.

• **Let your doctor know if you are taking any over-the-counter medications, including vitamins or other nutritional supplements.** As noted earlier, these products carry a risk of side effects and may also interfere with prescription medications.

• **Inform your doctor if you consume wine, beer, or other alcoholic beverages, even if only occasionally.** Alcohol interacts with many medications, and its use should either be avoided or timed to minimize adverse effects.

• **Ask your doctor about other forms of administration.** For example, skin patches provide a steady, low-dose administration of drugs such as nitroglycerin and estrogen, reducing the risk of side effects while producing constant benefit. Wearing a patch also liberates you from the need to remember when to take a drug.

• **Ask for time-release forms whenever possible.** These long-acting medications often can be taken only once a day, removing the need to remember to take your medicine every few hours.

• **Make sure your doctor periodically reviews your medications.** Ask your doctor's office staff to send you a postcard reminding you to bring in all your medications with you when you come in for your next appointment. This enables your doctor to review all your medications, checking for possible drug interactions and determining whether the drugs are really needed.

-9-

STOCKING YOUR HOME MEDICINE CHEST

BEFORE ADDRESSING THE details of stocking your home medicine chest, take this little test:

• Without peeking, list ten nonprescription medicines or medical supplies that you keep on hand to deal with minor illnesses or accidents.

• Run down the list and estimate how long each has been in your home.

• Which of these medications contains alcohol? Sugar?

Now go to your medicine chest, and wherever else you keep drugs, and check your answers.

If you're typical, you probably did not do well on this self-test. Most of us do not go about stocking our home medicine chest in any organized fashion. As a result, we often wind up with several bottles of one medication and, when the need arises, discover that a particular drug is either missing or unusable. Following is an organized approach to stocking and maintaining an adequate home medicine chest.

1. Start by taking an inventory of all medicines—both prescription and over the counter—that you have at home. Don't forget those tucked away in drawers, kitchen cabinets, the refrigerator, and other places.

2. Check the label and expiration date for each. With time, all medications deteriorate, particularly if they are exposed to excess humidity, high temperatures, light, and even air. Some compounds last longer than others, so the key to determining if medications are still good is the expiration date printed on their labels. If you have kept yours in their original containers and if you have stored them correctly (see No. 6), you can consider the medications to be good to that date, which allows a bit of extra time for a margin of safety. If the expiration date is missing, look for clues of possible deterioration. Does the medication have a strange odor? Has the color changed? Thickened syrups, crumbling pills, and capsules that are stuck together should be discarded. Ophthalmic ointments, creams, and drops must be sterile for use, and they should be discarded after one treatment course. A good rule is: When in doubt, throw it out. Be careful, though, about the way you dispose of old medicines. Capsules,

tablets, and liquids can all be safely flushed down the toilet. Their bottles or containers should be rinsed out thoroughly, especially if you have young children in the house. Ointments, creams, lotions, and inhalers should be bundled separately in a sealed bag and thrown out with the trash.

This cleaning-out ritual should be meticulous when it comes to prescription medications. Obviously, any that you can take on a day-to-day basis for a chronic condition such as high blood pressure should be fresh and in good supply. Otherwise, if you have followed the instructions for taking a prescription medication for a temporary condition, you should not have any leftovers. If you find some remnants, discard them. In most cases, medicine should not be kept just in case you or a member of the household seems to come down with the same ailment. A doctor should make the diagnosis and decide what medicine would be best. If you need the medication again, your doctor will give you a new prescription. Above all, throw out all medicine bottles without labels, even if you think you know what is in them. Unmarked medicine bottles are a source of danger.

3. Make a list of ailments that are common in your household. Do you suffer from periodic bouts of indigestion? Menstrual cramps? Is there a child who always seems to have cuts and scrapes? An older person who needs an occasional laxative? Then check this list against your inventory of usable medicines.

Your Home Medicine Chest

Pharmacists generally recommend the following nonprescription supplies for most households:

Basic over-the-counter medications

Acetaminophen and aspirin (for fever and pain)

Allergy medicines: a decongestant and antihistamine (for hives, hay fever, and other minor allergies)

Antacid (for simple heartburn)

Antibiotic cream and antiseptic cream

Antidiarrhea medication with pectin or bismuth

Anti-itch lotion or spray (for insect bites, poison ivy, etc.)

Cough drops and throat lozenges (for minor coughs and sore throat)

Cough syrup with expectorant (for more severe coughs)

Eye drops (for irritated, reddened eyes)

Laxative or stool softener (for occasional constipation)

Hydrocortisone cream or ointment (for hives, insect bites)

Hydrogen peroxide (for cleaning wounds)

Nose drops (for nasal congestion)

Petroleum jelly

Rubbing alcohol

Sunscreens, including lip balm

Medical supplies

Humidifier, cool mist type
Ice bag (for injured muscles, bones, and joints)
Scissors

Thermometer (oral or digital)*
Tweezers
First-aid kit

Additions for babies and young children

Acetaminophen liquid pediatric drops
Decongestant syrup
Ipecac syrup (for inducing vomiting in some types of poisoning) and activated charcoal**

Rectal thermometer*
Skin cream for diaper rash

*See box titled Kinds of Thermometers
**See box titled Poisoning Emergencies

Poisoning Emergencies

Include in your home one or both of these products:

• **Syrup of ipecac**, which induces vomiting. This is recommended for households with young children. Before administering, however, check with a poison control center or your doctor. Also, never give the solution to someone who is unconscious.

• **Activated charcoal**, which works by absorbing certain toxic substances to prevent them from entering the bloodstream. Again, check with a poison control center or doctor before using.

Kinds of Thermometers

Consumers now have a choice of at least three types of thermometers:

- **Mercury.** These thermometers may be difficult to read but are inexpensive and readily available. There are two basic types—oral and rectal.

- **Digital.** These electronic, battery-operated thermometers register temperature in easy-to-read digits. Some also emit a beep when they have registered your temperature. They are more expensive than mercury thermometers, and batteries must be replaced periodically.

- **Ear (auricular).** These newest thermometers are fast, easy-to-use, and highly accurate. The temperature sensor is inserted into the outer ear and almost instantly provides a digital reading. They are expensive but may be worth the investment in households with young children.

4. Compare your inventory and list of needed supplies against those listed in the box titled Your Home Medicine Chest.

   You are now ready to judiciously gather medicines to restock your home pharmacy. A word of caution: While it is reassuring to have a supply of things like cough syrups, sore throat lozenges, eye drops, antacids, and other over-the-counter products, use common sense when stocking up. If you've never used a laxative in your life, there's no need to buy one now "just in case." You may end up throwing out an unused bottle during your next medicine cabinet cleanup, and that's a waste of money.

   Remember, too, to check the labels when selecting products for home use. In addition to the active ingredients, note whether a product contains dyes, alcohol, sodium, or other ingredients you may not want to take. Liquid cough and cold preparations are often high in alcohol—liquid *Benadryl*, for example, is 14 percent alcohol, and *NyQuil* is 25 percent alcohol. When in doubt, consult your doctor or your pharmacist.

5. After settling on a list of medications, turn your attention to medical supplies, especially first-aid kits for both home and car. Although you can buy an assembled first-aid kit, you can save money and end up with a better collection if you assemble your own. (See boxes titled Basic First-aid Kit and First-aid Kit for Your Car for a list of basic supplies.)

Basic First-aid Kit

Make up two first-aid kits—one for your home and a second for your car. Use a small cosmetic kit that has separate compartments. Each kit should include:

Adhesive
Antibiotic ointments (e.g., bacitracin)
Bandages, including adhesive strip bandages, adhesive tape, and sterile gauze pads (several sizes), *Ace* (elastic) bandages, surgical bandages (*Steri-Strips*)
Betadine (to disinfect wounds)
Calamine lotion and antihistamine cream
Cotton balls and cotton-tip applicators
Disposable latex gloves
Elastic bandages (for sprains)
Extra pair of glasses (if needed) and sunglasses

Flashlight and fresh batteries
Ipecac syrup and activated charcoal
Isopropyl alcohol and antiseptic wipes
Magnifying glass
Multipurpose pocket knife
Oral thermometer
Pain-killers, such as aspirin or acetaminophen
Scissors
Soap (to clean hands and wounds)
Telephone numbers for doctor and poison control center
Tweezers (to pluck glass and splinters)

First-aid Kit for Your Car

In addition to a basic first-aid kit, always carry the following items in your car:

Blanket
Chemical ice packs
First-aid manual
Flashlight, batteries, and flares
Old sheet or other clean cloth that can be torn for compresses, slings, etc.

Water purification tablets or iodine
Other emergency supplies depending on the season and your destination. If you're camping or hiking in snake country, add a snakebite kit and include basic first-aid supplies in your backpack.

6. Finally, after you've assembled your home pharmacy and first-aid kit, decide where you're going to keep it.

Virtually every home comes with a medicine cabinet in the bathroom. Yet this is the one place where you should not store medications of any kind. The extremes of heat or humidity found in most bathrooms accelerate the deterioration of most if not all drugs. So save the bathroom medicine cabinet for things like toothpaste and other toiletries and find a cool, dry, dark place for your medicine.

An important criterion for choosing a good storage area is the safety of any children who live in or might visit the household. A closet shelf is usually a good choice. But even if it meets your requirements for dryness and a cool temperature, some special precautions are necessary. Medications that contain narcotics or other chemicals that may be abused should be kept in a locked box.

All drugs should be kept in their original containers, which are designed to protect the contents from light, moisture, and unnecessary exposure to air. If you need to transfer your medicine to another container, be sure to label it properly and keep the original instructions for future reference.

Except for some liquid medications like insulin and/or suppositories that melt at room temperature, the refrigerator should also be off limits to medications; it is too humid for most drugs. All medications that have to be refrigerated should be stored toward the back. If there are children in the household, put the medicine in a locked container inside the refrigerator.

Traveling with Medication

As you're assembling your home pharmacy, it might be a good idea to put together a compact version to use when traveling, especially if you spend a good deal of time away from home. Obviously, you don't want to travel with a suitcase full of drugs, but a bit of planning can forestall seeking out a pharmacy in a strange city. Obviously, you'll want to take a supply of any prescription or over-the-counter drugs that you use on a regular basis. If you're going abroad or planning an extended trip, also have your doctor write an extra prescription; then if your supply is lost or ruined, you can obtain a replacement without having to call your doctor or pharmacist. A doctor's prescription may also come in handy if customs officials question a medication or supplies, such as needles used to inject insulin or other medication.

Your progress through customs also will be greatly facilitated if all medications are in their appropriately marked containers. Otherwise, you may have difficulty explaining to a suspicious customs officer why you're carrying an assortment of pills and capsules.

When packing medications, protect glass containers with padding or Bubble-Wrap and put them in a waterproof container that will fit in your carry-on luggage. If you regularly take blood pressure or heart medication, take twice as much as you are likely to need, dividing it between two bags. If one is lost or stolen, you'll have a reserve supply. Ask your pharmacist about any special precautions to protect your medicines against extremes in heat or cold when traveling. (See box titled Your Travel Medical Kit.)

Your Travel Medical Kit

In addition to any prescription drugs that you take on a regular basis, include the following items in your travel medical kit:

Antacid

Antibiotic pills (if you are going to a remote area)

Antidiarrhea medication

Antihistamine or allergy pills

Antiseptic wipes (for minor wounds)

Bandages, including assortment of adhesive strips, gauze, and tape

Corn plasters and moleskin (for foot blisters)

Decongestant

Elastic bandage

Feminine hygiene products (for overseas travel)

Iodine or water purification tablets (if traveling to areas where water may be unsafe)

Insect repellent and hydrocortisone cream (to treat bites and stings)

Motion sickness pills

Pain-killers (aspirin or acetaminophen)

Pocket first-aid manual

Pocket knife

Scissors

Tweezers

If you are traveling with children, also include:

Ipecac syrup and activated charcoal

Rehydration solution (to avoid dehydration if diarrhea strikes)

-10-

DRUG DEPENDENCY

FOR MILLIONS OF Americans, a prescription is something of a passport to good health, or at least it helps keep a disease in check. But some prescriptions also can be passports to a personal hell. The medications they make available, while alleviating one kind of misery, create another, namely, a physiological or psychological craving. That misery is variously defined as drug abuse, drug addiction, and drug dependence, terms that most Americans normally associate with alcohol, heroin, cocaine, crack, and marijuana, among others.

Yet the abuse of prescribed medications is widespread. Though no one knows exactly how many Americans are in the ranks of abusers of legitimate drugs, experts point out that upwards of 70 million prescriptions are written every year for benzodiazepine-based tranquilizers alone. At least 2.5 million Americans take *Valium* and a dozen other similar medications for a year or more— even though most of the conditions for which they are prescribed are temporary problems and prescribing guidelines specify short-term use. The toll of such inappropriate use of prescription drugs is huge, particularly when seen in medical terms, according to a University of Toronto study and the U.S. National Institute on Drug Abuse. The Institute estimates that more than half of the patients who sought treatment for or died of drug-related problems in 1989 were actually abusing prescription drugs. University of Toronto experts estimate that "prescription drug misuse results in more North American injuries and deaths than all illegal drugs combined" and accounts for 15 percent of hospital admissions of people age 50 years or older. Just one type of prescription drug—sleep-inducing agents—is responsible for some 60 percent of drug-related emergency room visits, the Toronto researchers say. That so many emergency trips to the hospital are related to sleeping drugs is hardly surprising, given that an estimated 80 million Americans say they have trouble sleeping and that 16 million of them, at some point, use sleeping pills.

As noted in the University of Toronto report: "Anyone can develop a drug overuse problem, although there are no good 'markers' to identify those likely to do so. Some fall into the trap following legitimate use of prescription medication(s) for conditions such as migraine or arthritis. They may become dependent on the medication, seek multiple prescriptions and use too much for too long. Others likely to overuse prescribed medicines are the inveterate worriers, people with chronic anxiety or those who demand instant relief of the slightest distress."

Drugs That Cause Dependency

Predictably, the most commonly abused drugs are prescription pain-killers that contain morphine and related narcotics, tranquilizers and other psychotropic drugs, and sleeping pills (see Table 10.2).

Protecting Yourself

If it is true that virtually anyone can develop drug dependency problems, how can you avoid becoming entrapped? Experts stress that the answer lies in understanding the potential dangers and using potentially habit-forming drugs only as prescribed. People who develop drug dependency problems generally fall into one or more of three distinct categories:

- **Those who become psychologically dependent on drugs prescribed for a legitimate reason.** At some point in their lives, more than half of all Americans could benefit from medical treatment of a psychological problem, most often depression, anxiety, panic attacks, and stress. For most of these people, psychotropic medications, such as antidepressants and tranquilizers, are an appropriate treatment. After these drugs have had an opportunity to work and the patient has come to terms with the underlying problem, most patients are weaned from the medications. But others wind up with a drug dependency problem. Some feel they can cope only if they are taking their pills or are afraid that if they stop doing so, their anxiety or depression will return. One reason psychological counseling is considered an essential component of treatment is because

it offers alternatives to drug therapy.

Drugs prescribed for emotional problems are not the only drugs that lead to dependency problems; some medications used to treat certain muscle and skeletal disorders are also potentially habit-forming. A recent year-long study of medication abuse cases reported to the Rush-Presbyterian-St. Luke's Poison Control Center in Chicago found that about 11 percent were related to drugs prescribed for disorders of the skeletal muscles, especially those of the neck and back. Some of these drugs are actually tranquilizers. For example, diazepam, marketed as *Valium* and *Valrelease,* is both a muscle relaxant prescribed to treat back and neck pain and a tranquilizer used to treat anxiety. Others such as *Soma Compound with Codeine* contain a potentially habit-forming pain-killer. If you are taking a muscle relaxant for a back problem or other musculoskeletal disorder, ask your doctor and pharmacist about any potential dependency problems and how to avoid them.

- **Those who become physically dependent on medications.** Some medications work by physically changing the way in which certain cells or organs function. Some pain-killers, for example, alter the way in which nerve cells transmit pain messages or blunt the brain's perception of these messages. With time the body becomes accustomed to the medication, and reacts when it is stopped. Sometimes the reaction is mild and easily dealt with. For example, prolonged use of nose drops to control the runny nose of hay fever or a stubborn cold can result in a rebound of symptoms—perhaps even more severe than you originally experienced—when the drug is stopped.

Table 10.1

CATEGORIES OF DRUGS THAT CAN CAUSE DEPENDENCY

The drugs that could lead you to dependence are many, including some you may never suspect. The table below lists categories established by the federal Controlled Substances Act of 1970. Use it to determine which of your medications, if any, harbors a potential for making you dependent on it. Note that regulations in some states may be more stringent than federal regulations and, in such cases, take precedence.

	potential for abuse		regulations	
CATEGORY	PHYSICAL	PSYCHOLOGICAL	TYPE OF PRESCRIPTION NEEDED	NUMBER OF REFILLS/ PERIOD
C-II	High; may lead to severe dependence	High; may lead to severe dependence	Must be written in ink or typewritten and signed by physician; verbal prescriptions allowed only in genuine emergencies and must be confirmed in writing within 72 hours	None permitted
C-III	Some; may lead to low-to-moderate dependence	Some; may lead to high dependence	Verbal or written	Five renewals in six-month period
C-IV	Low; may lead to limited dependence	Low; may lead to limited dependence	Verbal or written	Five renewals in six-month period
C-V	Low; subject to some state and local regulations	Low; subject to some state and local regulations	May not be required	No limitation on refills, but quantity dispensed in 48-hour period is limited

But sometimes ending the long-term use of a drug—especially morphine or codeine—can have violent effects. Symptoms may include vomiting, agitation, trembling, anxiety, depression, diarrhea, weight loss, sleep disturbances, increased pain, and uncoordinated muscle movements. These withdrawal symptoms continue until the drug is taken again or until the body adjusts to its absence. Withdrawal can often be minimized by slowly tapering the dosage downward until the medication can be withdrawn completely.

Table 10.2

EXAMPLES OF HABIT-FORMING DRUGS

controlled substance	category	used for:	controlled substance	category	used for:
Alurate	C-III	Sedative	Nembutal	C-II	Sedative
Amytal	C-II	Sedative	phenobarbital	C-IV	Anticonvulsant
Ativan	C-IV	Antianxiety	Restoril	C-IV	Sedative
Butisol	C-III	Sedative	Ritalin	C-II	Stimulant
Centrax	C-IV.	Antianxiety	Seconal	C-IV	Sedative
codeine	C-II	Pain-killer	Serax	C-IV	Antianxiety
Cylert	C-IV	Stimulant	Soma Compound with Codeine	C-II	Muscle relaxant
Dalmane	C-IV	Sedative			
Darvon	C-IV	Pain-killer	Tranxene	C-IV	Anticonvulsant
Demerol	C-II	Pain-killer	Tuinal	C-II	Sedative
Dexedrine	C-II	Stimulant	Tylenol with Codeine	C-III	Pain-killer
Equanil	C-IV	Antianxiety	Valium	C-IV	Antianxiety, muscle relaxant
Halcion	C-IV	Sedative			
Levo-Dromoran	C-II	Pain-killer	Valrelease	C-IV	Antianxiety, muscle relaxant
Mebaral	C-IV	Anticonvulsant			
Miltown	C-IV	Antianxiety	Xanax	C-IV	Antianxiety

In some cases, abrupt withdrawal of a drug can be dangerous. This is especially true with corticosteroids such as (*Cortone; Beclovent; Medrol*); stopping the drug after long-term use can precipitate a flare-up of the original condition. More seriously, it can lead to an adrenal crisis. When you take corticosteroids for a long period, your adrenal glands come to depend on the drug and cut their production of cortisone and other essential adrenal hormones. If you suddenly stop taking the steroid medication and your body needs steroid hormones to respond to an illness or injury, the adrenal glands may be unable to supply them. This can result in shock and even death. To prevent this, your doctor will slowly wean you from the steroid medication, which nudges the adrenal glands back to normal function.

• **Those who develop tolerance for the drugs they are taking.** Drug tolerance means that the body has grown so used to the presence of the medication that ever-increasing amounts are needed for it to have an effect. This happens with some sleeping pills. In time, the doses of medication needed to induce sleep, for example, may be dangerously high. To complicate matters further, some medications can have combined effects, leading to both tolerance and psychological or physical dependence. Again, sleeping pills are a good example because some types lead to dependence as well as drug tolerance. Thus, experts agree that sleeping pills should be approached carefully and used for only a short period of time—at most, a few weeks. Otherwise, a worsening of the original sleep problem is likely to result when the drug is stopped.

The best way to avoid a problem of drug dependency is to take only those medications that are clearly indicated, and to use them as judiciously as possible. A short course of a tranquilizer, sleeping pill, pain-killer, or other potentially addictive medication can be invaluable in helping you get through a difficult period. But to avoid becoming dependent on the medication, combine the drug therapy with other treatments that can help you cope without the drug. If you are taking muscle relaxants for an acute back problem, also consider consulting a physical therapist to learn exercises designed to overcome a bad back. Alternative relaxation therapies such as meditation, yoga, and biofeedback training can help alleviate stress and anxiety. These approaches also have proven to be highly effective in pain therapy and are used in many pain clinics to help patients cut down or even end their use of addictive pain-killers. Similarly, many sleep problems are amenable to alternative solutions.

Your doctor or a sleep clinic at a local hospital can analyze your particular sleep problem and suggest alternatives to sleeping pills.

In cases in which the potential benefits of a habit-forming drug outweigh the risks of dependency or tolerance, ask your doctor how long you are likely to need the medication. While taking the drug, keep in touch with your doctor to periodically review your continued need for it. If you will be on a medication for a protracted period, discuss with your doctor the procedure you should follow for stopping it. Find out if you should decrease the dosage slowly until you have phased it out completely or switch to an alternative medication with less potential for dependency problems.

A word of caution: Be alert to potential problems, but don't let your concern keep you from taking a needed medication. For example, many doctors and patients alike undertreat severe pain such as that experienced in advanced cancer. In such cases, alleviating the pain is more important to a patient's well-being than concerns about possible addiction.

Finally, abstain from alcohol and other addictive substances when taking medications that can lead to dependency. Many of these drugs affect the central nervous system, and adding alcohol to the regimen can compound effects of the medication. This is why combining alcohol and sleeping pills or tranquilizers can result in a fatal drug overdose, even when an otherwise safe amount of the drug is involved.

Signs of Drug Dependency

Signs and symptoms of drug tolerance or dependency vary according to the medication and length of use. In general, the following signs warrant talking to your doctor about a possible problem and course of action:

- Extreme mood swings, going abruptly from feelings of euphoria to deep depression or anxiety

- Extreme changes in energy levels, with bursts of activity followed by periods of lethargy and listlessness

- Symptoms that mimic those of excessive alcohol consumption, including slurred speech, faulty judgment, lack of coordination and balance, exaggerated emotions and movements

- Sleep problems, including insomnia, bad dreams, frequent awakenings, and drowsiness

- Loss of appetite and significant loss of weight

- Excessive sweating or flushed skin

- Diarrhea

- Tremor or increasing clumsiness

- Muscle pains or cramps

-11-

AVOIDING DRUG EMERGENCIES

EVERY TIME YOU take a pill the action should set off a small but insistent warning: **Using this medication may be hazardous to health and may even kill you.**

An overstatement? Perhaps, but not by much. Experts, including researchers at the Food and Drug Administration, estimate that Americans suffer more than 36 million adverse drug reactions every year resulting in more than 600,000 hospitalizations. Older people are especially vulnerable to drug-related emergencies; according to FDA estimates, one fourth of all reported adverse drug reactions—more than 9 million a year—occur among people 60 or older. Of those hospitalized because of adverse drug reactions, 200,000 are older adults.

Of course, an adverse drug reaction can occur even when a medication is used correctly, but in most instances, misuse—either intentional or accidental—is involved. Sometimes the error rests with a simple oversight, such as inadvertently taking a double dosage or mixing the drug with another medication or substance that triggers an adverse interaction.

Individual drug sensitivities or physical characteristics may also be a factor. Take the case of a woman identified as Jane in an FDA report. Jane developed herpes zoster, more commonly re-

ferred to as shingles. She was under considerable stress at the time, and instead of seeing her regular doctor, she consulted one at a walk-in clinic. The physician explained that the disease is caused by a reactivation of the virus that causes chickenpox, and that there was no treatment other than rest and medication to alleviate pain, itching, and other symptoms. He prescribed a combination of acetaminophen and codeine. But when Jane took the drug, she became so violently ill that she had to be rushed to a hospital. Doctors quickly determined that she had suffered an adverse drug reaction, and immediate intravenous fluids and medication prevented further deterioration.

What had happened? Over the years, Jane had experienced less severe reactions to pain medications, and ultimately her doctor had figured out she could not tolerate a full adult dosage. A doctor unfamiliar with her past medical history did not know about Jane's drug sensitivity, and faced with the discomfort of shingles and the other stresses in her life at the time, Jane neglected to mention this fact.

Even reasonably healthy adults still in the prime of life who think they are following medication instructions exactly can get into serious trouble. Take, for example, the case of Maurice C. Jauchler, Jr., an apparently healthy New Orleans electronics and communications expert in his early forties. Jauchler suffered fractures of both ankles and a wrist, and even after they healed, he was dogged by pain, which he treated with *Extra Strength Tylenol.* He was careful not to exceed the recommended daily dose, until he came down with a bad case of the flu. Not wanting to take a drug that might interact with the *Tylenol* he was taking, he turned to *Maximum Strength Tylenol Sinus Medication,* again following the daily dosage limits outlines in the instructions.

What Jauchler failed to realize was that combining the two drugs actually doubled his maximum safe dosage of acetaminophen, the key ingredient in *Tylenol.* In fact, he was taking 8 grams of acetaminophen a day, exceeding the 7.5 grams a day that represents potential toxicity. Consequently, Jauchler suffered liver failure and died five days later.

Of course, this is an extreme example, but it illustrates that even the safest nonprescription drugs can be potentially lethal under certain conditions.

Take Extra Precautions When Giving Medicine to Children

Like the elderly, children are also vulnerable to adverse drug reactions. Even though most parents know that special precautions should be followed when giving children drugs, many do not extend this caution to nonprescription drugs.

A few years ago, researchers at the University of Michigan and the University of Rochester looked at 3,900 decisions some 500 parents made about giving their children over-the-counter drugs for minor illnesses. Not only were the decisions dubious in many cases, the experts concluded, but in a few instances, they were also potentially dangerous. The researchers found that parents often selected the wrong medication, gave incorrect dosages, or

gave the right dosages but for the wrong amount of time. All too often, the parents failed to read the instructions. In a comment on these findings, an FDA report asserted: "While OTC drugs generally have such a wide margin of safety that a somewhat excessive dose won't do much harm, sometimes a wrong dose—even of a children's drug—can lead to disaster."

Very young children are especially vulnerable. A cough suppressant with codeine that is safe for an older child can have severe consequences in a two-year-old or younger child. Similarly, a medication that will stop vomiting in an older child can cause a drastic drop in blood pressure in a child of three or younger.

Many drug-related emergencies among children can be traced to the mistaken belief that administering drugs will prevent the illnesses they are designed to cure. For example, many parents fret about their children's bowel function, often concluding that constipation is the problem. Resorting to regular doses of laxatives may produce more frequent bowel movements but can also create new problems that are far more serious than constipation—real or imagined. The chronic use of laxatives disrupts normal bowel function, and in children, it can cause excessive loss of fluids, upsetting the body's chemical balance.

Children are also especially vulnerable to inadvertent overdosing and drug interactions. For example, you might give a child with a cold a multisymptom cold medication to help him get to sleep. Later that night, he wakes up coughing, so you give him some cough medicine. Two hours later, the child is jittery and keeping everyone awake. The explanation is simple. Although you were careful to give him only the recommended dose of each medication, each contained ephedrine or pseudoephedrine. These ingredients are common decongestants, but they are also stimulants.

How to Avoid Drug Emergencies

Although some drug-related emergencies are unavoidable, most can be prevented by following these guidelines:

Always tell your doctor and pharmacist about:

- Any allergies you have, especially those triggered by medications, food, or food additives. Any allergic reaction to a medication, no matter how minor, could be the harbinger of a more severe reaction if you take that medication again, or one that is chemically related. Penicillin and aspirin are especially common allergens, and should be used with caution by anyone who is plagued with allergies.

- Any plans you have for becoming pregnant (or if you already are pregnant). If you are going to breast-feed your child, make that known as well.

- Any medications, including vitamins and minerals, that you take, even if only occasionally. For an extra measure of safety, put all your medications in a bag and take them with you when you have a regular medical checkup. Alternatively, ask your pharmacist to go over your medications.

- Your alcohol consumption, even if it's limited to an occasional beer or glass of wine. Because alcohol depresses the central nervous system, it adds to or exaggerates the effects of other drugs that also depress the central nervous system, including sedatives, narcotics, tranquilizers, and barbiturates. Combining a moderate or even a small amount of alcohol with a medication can intensify dizziness, impair coordination, and lead to excessive drowsiness. In some cases, combining drugs

and alcohol can even kill. Adding to the risk is the fact that some drugs take a day or more to clear out of the body. *Valium,* for example, stays in the bloodstream for up to 24 hours. Thus, if you have several drinks even if you have not taken any *Valium* that day, you still may have a drug–alcohol interaction.

- Your medical history, especially if you are seeing a physician for the first time or returning to the doctor after a long absence. Among other things, disclose if you have kidney or liver disease, high blood pressure, heart disease, asthma, or glaucoma. Also point out any relevant characteristics, such as unusual drug sensitivity, a history of seizures, or breathing problems.

You can substantially decrease your risk of a medication emergency if you ask your doctor or pharmacist a few key questions, including:

- What is this medication for and how does it work?

- How often should I take it? Specifically, find out how many times a day you should take a drug. Timing is crucial for many drugs, and failing to observe the regimen can create problems. Thus, you could be in trouble if you misinterpret an instruction to take a medication three times a day to mean taking it once every 6 hours during the 18 hours you are awake, instead of every 8 hours over a 24-hour period.

- Should I take the medication before or after meals? Whether you take some drugs with meals or on an empty stomach can affect how well they work. Some drugs should be absorbed slowly into the body, and taking them on a full stomach accomplishes this.

This tactic can also reduce the risk of side effects, such as stomach damage caused by aspirin and other nonsteroidal anti-inflammatory drugs. Other drugs should enter the bloodstream as fast as possible, and taking these drugs on an empty stomach facilitates that process.

- Are there foods I should avoid while taking the medication? Some drugs interact with certain foods. One of the most critical examples involves monoamine oxidase (MAO) inhibitors, drugs that are sometimes used to treat depression and, less commonly, high blood pressure. When these drugs are combined with foods containing tyramine, a chemical found in aged cheese, wine, and some cured meats, among others, blood pressure can rise to dangerously high levels.

- Are there some activities I should curtail while taking this drug? If you are taking a medication that makes you drowsy, or impairs coordination and alertness, you obviously should not drive a car or operate dangerous machinery.

- What side effects should I watch for? And how should I deal with them? By learning to distinguish serious side effects or adverse reactions from minor or temporary reactions, you'll feel more confident in taking the medicine, and you'll also react more reasonably and effectively to real emergencies.

Involve your pharmacist in your medical care.

- Have all prescriptions filled at one pharmacy. This will help you develop a relationship with a pharmacist at the store, making it easier for you to ask questions and seek advice. More important, each time you fill a prescription, it will become part of your medication record, enabling your pharmacist to spot potential drug interactions and other conflicts.

- If you have difficulty opening a container with a childproof cap, and there are no young children in the household, ask for a conventional lid. Some people elect to skip a dose rather than deal with the frustration of opening a bottle with a difficult cap.

Read all the instructions, especially the fine print of the manufacturer's package insert.

- Package inserts may be written in what seems to be medical jargon, but you should still take a few minutes to read carefully through this material because it contains vital information about possible side effects and adverse reactions. If you have difficulty understanding the information, ask your doctor or pharmacist to explain it.

- Always read the label on the bottle containing the medicine. Don't take it for granted that your doctor was thorough and correct in running down the instructions for taking the medicine. More important, don't take it for granted that you remember what he or she told you. Study after study has shown that a large percentage of patients—regardless of age, educational level, or medical sophistication—forget much of what a doctor tells them about their medications. That's why it's a good idea to write down instructions while you are still in the doctor's office, and review them with the doctor before you leave. This can help you spot any discrepancy between what the doctor told you and what's on the pharmacist's label.

Don't play doctor, either for yourself or for anyone else.

- Many diseases have similar symptoms. Thus, a cough can be a sign of a cold, an asthma attack, bronchitis, or a serious infection such as tuberculosis. Take medications only for the specific conditions for which they were prescribed, and if symptoms persist, see a doctor for a proper diagnosis. Similarly, never take a medication prescribed for someone else, even if you seem to have the same problem. To resist any temptation to use a drug for a new illness, dispose of any leftovers when you have completed a regimen. (There are exceptions, of course, but even then, it's a good idea to check with your doctor before self-medicating.)

- Always consult a physician before giving a child medication, particularly a child under the age of 13.

- Never assume that a medication is innocuous just because its name seems to imply that it is less dangerous than others. Nonsteroidal anti-inflammatory agents (NSAIDs) are a classic example. Given the adverse publicity surrounding the illicit use of anabolic steroids by athletes, most Americans know that these compounds are dangerous. Similarly, most of us are aware of the adverse effects of corticosteroids, which are used to treat severe asthma, inflammatory disorders, and other serious diseases. So when a person hears "non-steroidal," he or she may assume that the drug is harmless. Not so. NSAIDs play an important part in controlling arthritis and other conditions, but they can also cause numerous side effects, including nausea, cramps, indigestion, diarrhea, increased sensitivity to sunlight, nervousness, confusion, headache, drowsiness, and dizziness. Long-term use can lead to ulcers and bleeding problems, and in some people, these drugs can even interfere with the bone marrow's ability to produce blood cells. Thus, a doctor should be informed of any reactions that seem to be related to a nonsteroidal anti-inflammatory agent.

Handle medicines properly.

- Don't break tablets unless they are scored (have a dividing line in the middle) and you have been instructed to do so.

- Don't chew, crush, or dissolve enteric coated pills, those designed to dissolve in the small intestine instead of the stomach, or sustained-release preparations.

Post the telephone numbers for the nearest hospital, a poison control center, and your physician on your telephone and in key areas around the house. Make sure that any baby-sitter or caregiver for an elderly person in the household knows where these numbers are posted and how to seek help if it is needed.

-12-

ENDING DRUG TREATMENT

ORDINARILY, STOPPING A drug is as simple as taking the last pill or dose of a prescription medication for treatment of an infection or other acute illness. But there are circumstances in which going off a medication is not that simple. In fact, if you have a chronic disease such as hypertension or diabetes, you're probably going to be taking medication for the rest of your life. There are also drugs that cannot be stopped abruptly without worsening the underlying disease or bringing on withdrawal symptoms. Still, each year millions of Americans disregard their doctor's instructions and stop taking needed medication. For example, hypertension experts estimate that about half of the 60 million Americans being treated for the condition stop taking their medication within the first year of their therapy. And many of those who do continue with their therapy do not take medication often enough to control their high blood pressure.

Why do so many people put themselves at needless risk? Experts cite many reasons: Some tire of taking daily medication. Others simply forget or convince themselves that they are feeling better and no longer need to take drugs. Some stop because a drug may be causing bothersome side effects. This is especially common among men taking antihypertensive drugs that cause impotence or lethargy. Finally, the high cost of a drug puts some

patients in a position of having to choose between necessities like heat, rent, or food and medication.

The consequences of premature cessation of a drug are well known. If we stop taking an antibiotic before an infection is cured, for example, the remaining bacteria can proliferate, resulting in a recurrence of the original infection. Only this time, the bacteria may be resistant to the original antibiotic, and a different, more potent, medication that carries a risk of more serious side effects may be required.

Whatever money may be saved by stopping a drug is often lost to the increased cost of additional medical care down the road. For example, if you are among those who stop taking high blood pressure medicine, you are likely to spend as much as $125 more a year for additional medical services, including doctor's visits and medication to deal with the problems generated by high blood pressure. This may not sound like a lot, but if a premature stroke or heart attack results, the price can be astronomical compared to the annual cost of drug therapy. In fact, the total cost to the nation of prescription noncompliance is more than $100 billion a year in added doctor, hospital, and nursing home fees and in lost productivity, according to the National Pharmaceutical Council. This estimate takes into account the fact that about 125,000 Americans die prematurely every year from complications of high blood pressure.

A similar set of circumstances revolves around cholesterol-lowering medications. Some of these drugs cause constipation and other bothersome side effects. Others may be free of apparent side effects but are more expensive and necessitate periodic blood tests to make sure they are not causing liver damage. Because these drugs work silently, patients don't see any concrete evidence of improvement, even though blood tests show a lowering of cholesterol levels and, consequently, a reduced risk of heart attack. Stopping the drug may not cause immediate harm, but if cholesterol levels rise, heart attack risk also goes up.

Of course, there are many instances in which stopping a drug has more immediate consequences. In one study of patients with chronic obstructive pulmonary disease, or emphysema, almost half stopped their medications. Most did so because they felt so good that either they decided they no longer needed medication or they simply forgot to take their medicine because there were no symptoms as reminders. Of course, without medication, these breathing problems inevitably recur.

For many people with diseases such as diabetes, epilepsy, and mental illness, missing even one or two doses can cause serious, even life-threatening, problems. For someone with diabetes, coma and death can result from stopping insulin injections; for the mentally ill, it means a return of symptoms that make normal activities impossible.

Dr. Victor Kovner, an internist at St. Joseph Medical Center in Burbank, California, recently summed up a doctor's reaction to such situations: "It's frustrating when a patient doesn't follow instructions and runs into serious problems. I have seen patients become more ill as a result of not complying [with their prescription regimen], and I have certainly seen some die."

What does compliance with medication prescriptions mean? That depends.

- If you have a short-term prescription for a short-term illness, take your medication until it is completely gone, even if symptoms disappear sooner.

- If you are experiencing unpleasant side effects, talk to your doctor about them. Often, adjusting the dosage solves the problem. In other cases, an alternative medication may be prescribed. Also, some side effects are temporary or can be remedied by simple lifestyle changes. If your medication is causing constipation, for example, increasing your fiber and fluid intake and exercising more may solve the problem. If not, your doctor may recommend a stool softener.

- Talk to your doctor about how you should go about stopping a medication. As noted earlier, this simply may mean taking the final dose. With some drugs, however, you must be weaned from the medication by reducing the frequency and the amount of each dose. This tactic is used to prevent withdrawal symptoms after long-term use of habit-forming drugs. It is also used to prevent a rebound or flare-up of an underlying disease. For example, some beta-blockers, drugs commonly used to treat high blood pressure and some heart disorders, cannot be stopped abruptly because doing so can trigger angina or even a heart attack. To avoid this, doctors instruct patients to come off beta-blockers over a one- to two-week period.

Anticonvulsants also require a slow withdrawal, because stopping the drugs abruptly can lead to a recurrence of seizures. Stopping corticosteroids after long-term use also must be approached carefully. Abrupt withdrawal of the drugs can precipitate a recurrence of the underlying disease.

In summary, if your doctor or pharmacist tells you that your medication requires slow withdrawal, write down the relevant instructions and keep them with the medication. When the time comes, it's a good idea to check with your doctor or pharmacist for refresher instructions—tapering off some medications is a lot more complicated than starting them.

-13-

CONTROLLING DRUG COSTS

THE SKYROCKETING COSTS of prescription drugs is often cited as proof positive that our health care system is in need of cost containment and reform. While many new drugs may be lifesaving, their cost puts them beyond the reach of many family budgets. It's not unusual, for example, for a course of antibiotics for a relatively minor infection to cost $100 or more. New cholesterol-lowering drugs and antihypertensive medications may be more effective and cause fewer side effects than older drugs, but they are also many times more costly. There are numerous accounts of older Americans on fixed incomes who must choose between medications and food or heating fuel, with the immediate necessities of life winning out over lifesaving drugs.

Critics of the pharmaceutical industry charge that drug companies are profiteering, charging prices that far exceed those of the same medications in Europe and Latin America. The drug companies counter that over the last 50 years, drug prices have risen at a rate lower than costs of other consumer goods, and that the high prices also reflect the expense of researching and developing new drugs.

So far, the debate has done little to help consumers whose budgets are devastated by the high cost of medications, especially those that must be taken for long periods of time. This situation may be improved by health care reforms currently under consideration in Washington. In the meantime, there are measures you can take to lower your prescription costs, starting in your doctor's office.

If your doctor says you don't need medications, don't press for any. Many doctors report that they will write prescriptions for patients who insist on having a medication, even when it is not medically necessary. Ask your doctor to explain why a medication is unnecessary and how long it will take for your symptoms or disorder to subside with proper self-care. For example, low to moderate hypertension can often be controlled with weight loss, salt restriction, and increased exercise. Experts recommend a six-month trial of these lifestyle changes before instituting drug therapy.

There are also disorders that are not helped by drugs, yet many patients demand medication anyway. These include:

- **Colds and flu.** People suffering these common illnesses often ask for an antibiotic, but antibiotics have absolutely no impact on viruses. Sometimes a doctor will prescribe an antibiotic to prevent a secondary bacterial infection in patients who have asthma, chronic bronchitis, or emphysema. Otherwise, antibiotics should be reserved for bacterial illnesses.

- **Intestinal upsets.** Indigestion, heartburn, instestinal gas, and constipation are among the many gastrointestinal complaints that send patients to doctors seeking prescription medications such as *Tagamet* or *Zantac*. While these medications are highly useful in treating some disorders, they are not indicated for routine upsets. So before you seek a costly prescription drug, establish whether you really need it. Heartburn, indigestion, and similar problems are better treated with dietary and life-style changes, including reducing stress and abstaining from tobacco and alcohol. If problems persist and an ulcer or other underlying cause has been ruled out, a nonprescription antacid will usually suffice. Similarly, most constipation should be treated by diet and life-style changes rather than by taking laxatives.

- **Minor aches and pains.** Headaches, muscle tension, and lower back pain are among our most common medical complaints. Many people are convinced that only a prescription drug is strong enough to control chronic or frequently recurring pain, but many inexpensive nonprescription pain-killers are just as effective as the more expensive prescription drugs. What's more, most are a lot safer than prescription drugs when used as directed.

- **Ordinary "blues."** Antidepressant medications are indicated for clinical depression, but not for the occasional bouts of the blues that afflict all of us from time to time. Exercise or simply sharing your problems with a friend, member of the clergy, or counselor is more effective than antidepressant drugs in over-

coming feeling down in the dumps. Winter depression, or seasonal affective disorder (SAD), is now treated with light therapy instead of drugs. Unfortunately, the widespread publicity suggesting that the new antidepressant drugs such as *Prozac* enhance general well-being and performance has prompted millions of Americans to demand these medications, even though they are not necessarily clinically depressed.

If your doctor has prescribed a drug you need, but the price is exorbitant, let the doctor know. Physicians learn about new drugs from medical journals, colleagues, pharmaceutical company representatives, and other sources, but they often have no idea what a drug costs. In many instances, a far less expensive medication that is just as effective can be prescribed. In some cases, the less expensive drug is an older medication that has been eclipsed by a widely advertised new drug, even though the older drug may do the job. For example, studies show that thiazide diuretics often lower blood pressure just as effectively as the new, more costly ACE inhibitors or calcium channel blockers. But these new medications are often prescribed as the initial medication because they are perceived as causing fewer problems. Cost-conscious doctors often try a thiazide diuretic first, and if it does the job without undue side effects, fine. If not, they can then substitute one of the more expensive drugs or use a lower dosage of the diuretic along with another medication.

Consider generic drugs. Generic drugs are chemically equivalent versions of brand name drugs whose patents have run out. Since the original brand name drug was already tested for safety and effectiveness, a company that wants to bring a generic counterpart to market only has to prove to the Food and Drug Administration that its product contains the same key ingredients in identical strength and form. Because this is not as costly as the original drug testing and approval process, makers of generic drugs can offer them for much less than the original brand name drug. About 80 percent of brand name drugs have generic equivalents, with an average savings of 30 percent per prescription (although the range is 10 to 80 percent). Laws relating to dispensing generic drugs vary from state to state, but most require that pharmacists inform patients of any generic drug and dispense it unless the doctor or patient specifically requests otherwise. Medicaid and many other insurance plans specify that a generic must be dispensed if one is available.

There are instances, however, in which your physician will insist that you take a brand name drug, even though a less costly generic is available. Some anticonvulsants, for example, require you and your doctor to go through a careful trial-and-error approach to find the best drug and dosage. In such cases, your doctor will want to stick to the drug that he or she knows is likely to be the most consistent. Although generic drugs are chemically equivalent to brand name drugs, their bioequivalency—the way the drug works in your body—is not always the same.

Your physician may also want you to stay away from generics if you suffer from allergies to either medications or some of the ingredients in them, namely the binders, fillers, or flavoring agents. If you have hit on a brand name medication that does not give you trouble, it may be wiser to stick with it than to invite problems by switching to a generic with unknown inactive ingredients.

Ask your doctor if he or she has samples of a medicine being prescribed for you for the first time. Pharmaceutical representatives often give doctors free samples of drugs. Starting a new drug with such samples not only saves money, but it also gives you an opportunity to make sure the drug works for you without undue side effects or ad-verse reactions before you pay for the complete amount prescribed. If your doctor doesn't have free samples, have the pharmacist fill only part of the prescription. Then if you do have to switch drugs, you won't be stuck with a bottle full of expensive but unusable medicine.

Shop around. Prices among pharmacies vary greatly and you can save substantial amounts of money by comparing prices. Even if you have a favorite pharmacy or if you want to have all your prescriptions filled at one pharmacy, it may pay to shop around. If you are quoted a lower price than at your regular drugstore, mention that to your pharmacist. You may get a price reduction. Or it may pay to switch pharmacies. If you do fill your prescription elsewhere, make sure that your primary pharmacist enters the drug on your medication record.

- Ask your doctor if you will need the medication on a long-term basis. If so, and if you have determined that the drug works for you, buy as large a supply as possible. Buying in a larger quantity can lower your cost by 15 percent or even more. If you order a 90-day supply, ask your pharmacist about a discount.

- Check with your local community hospital pharmacy. Some hospital pharmacies fill orders for outsiders at costs lower than community pharmacies. Because hospital pharmacies buy in bulk, they are sometimes able to pass the savings on to outside customers, even though hospital patients may be charged much more for the same drugs.

- Look into mail order pharmacies. If you are taking drugs for chronic conditions such as high blood pressure, arthritis, or heart disease, you may save money by buying from a mail order pharmacy, which gets its drugs at a reduced price by negotiating with drug manufacturers. Remember, however, that buying by mail requires planning. It takes about three days to get a prescription drug by mail, so you must order a medication a week or two before your current supply runs out. For older people, the American Association of Retired Persons (AARP), (800) 456-2279, offers mail order drugs for its members. Your insurance company may provide listings of other mail order services. Before placing your order, be sure to ask the total charges, including handling and shipping. There's no point in saving $5 on the cost of a prescription if handling and shipping will cost $6. Once the order has arrived, check it immediately to make sure that you have the right medicine in the prescribed doses.

• Check your insurance coverage. Many company plans provide coverage for drugs, but employees are often unaware of these provisions or don't know how to file claims. Some plans specify preferred providers—doctors, hospitals, and pharmacies or drug chains that members can use for lower charges or increased reimbursement. For example, if you

go to the pharmacy of your choice, your medical plan may reimburse only 75 percent of your costs, but if you go to a preferred provider, your plan may increase this to 80 percent.

• Look into special programs. Some pharmaceutical manufacturers have programs under which they offer drugs to patients who otherwise cannot afford them and cannot get financial help from other sources. Bristol-Myers Squibb, for example, makes drugs available to indigent patients with cardiovascular disorders, cancer, AIDS, and infections.

• Consider volunteering for a clinical drug trial. Although many clinical trials are set up to compare a new medication against a placebo, some are also designed to establish if a new medication is better than those already on the market. If you enroll in these programs, you won't know whether you are getting the new drug or an existing one. But you will be getting free medication and perhaps regular checkups as well. Your physician may be able to guide you to such programs.

chapter

-14-

NONNARCOTIC PAIN-KILLERS AND FEVER MEDICATIONS

AT ONE TIME or another, all of us encounter some sort of discomfort—headache, back problem, muscle strain, menstrual cramps, fever, among others—that calls for pain medication. There are two major categories of analgesics, or pain-killers—narcotic and nonnarcotic. (Anesthetics, either local or general, are used to deaden pain under special circumstances, especially during surgery and dental work.) In general, doctors recommend starting with a nonnarcotic drug and, if that is insufficient, working up to a narcotic (see Chapter 15).

Although there are hundreds of choices, nonnarcotic pain-killers fall into only a few basic categories: acetaminophen (*Tylenol*, and other brands), aspirin (salicylates) and other nonsteroidal anti-inflammatory drugs (NSAIDs), and migraine preparations such as ergotamines (*Cafergot, Ergostat, Wigraine*) and methysergide (*Sansert*). Barbiturates such as butalbital are also nonnarcotic analgesics, but because they are habit-forming and potentially dangerous, their use is rather limited.

In general, pain-killers are distinguished from one another by the way in which they work in the body. Aspirin and other nonsteroidal anti-inflammatory drugs work by reducing the tissue concentrations of prostaglandins, hormonelike sub-

stances that cause inflammation and make nerves more sensitive to pain. Acetaminophen also reduces prostaglandin production, but only in the brain; thus, this drug reduces pain but does not counter inflammation. Barbiturates work by interfering with the chemical activity in the brain and communication between nerves.

Because all of these drugs act on the brain's temperature control center in the hypothalamus, all can be used to reduce a fever. In practice, however, aspirin and acetaminophen are the favored drugs to lower a fever. In recent years, some doctors have started recommending a low dose of ibuprofen (*Advil, Haltran, Motrin*), a nonsteroidal anti-inflammatory agent, as an alternative to acetaminophen or aspirin as fever-lowering medication for children because it works faster and is generally more potent than acetaminophen and safer than aspirin.

Drugs used to treat migraines are believed to work by interfering with the action of two body chemicals—serotonin and norepinephrine, compounds that play a role in the constriction and dilation of blood vessels—major factors in migraines and other vascular headaches.

Although millions of people use nonnarcotic

pain-killers—sometimes on a daily basis—none of these drugs is trouble-free. Aspirin can irritate the stomach, often severely enough to cause intestinal bleeding. Long-term heavy use can also cause ringing in the ears and hearing loss. Aspirin is given to children or teenagers only under special circumstances because it has been found to increase the risk of Reye's syndrome—a potentially fatal disease—in youngsters who have a viral infection.

While many people opt for acetaminophen or NSAIDs to avoid the potential problems of aspirin, these drugs also have side effects. NSAIDs also can cause severe gastrointestinal bleeding. Acetaminophen, while easier on the stomach, can cause severe liver and kidney problems if taken in excessive doses. Children in particular may be harmed by large doses of acetaminophen. Side effects and precautions to follow when taking common nonnarcotic pain-killers are outlined in the following tables.

drug or category:

NON-STEROIDAL ANTI-INFLAMMATORY DRUGS (NSAIDs)

condition:

PAIN, STIFFNESS, INFLAMMATION; ARTHRITIS AND GOUT, INCLUDING JUVENILE
RHEUMATOID ARTHRITIS; DIFFICULT OR PAINFUL MENSTRUATION

warning

Tell your doctor if you have or have had:
- an allergic reaction to NSAIDs, or to aspirin
- severe gastrointestinal problems like colitis or peptic ulcer
- asthma
- hypertension or congestive heart failure

drugs

GENERIC	BRAND	RX
ibuprofen	Advil, Motrin	some
piroxicam	Feldene	
naproxen	Naprosyn, Anaprox	
flurbiprofen	Ansaid	
ketoprofen	Orudis	
diflunisal	Dolobid	
others		

form/usage

CAPSULES, TABLETS, LIQUIDS, SUPPOSITORIES: Capsules and tablets should be taken with food or liquid to lessen possible stomach irritation.
Capsules and tablets may be crumbled for easier swallowing.
For liquids, follow instructions on bottle or package.
When taking an especially strong dose of NSAID (a prescription medication) by mouth, do not lie down for about half an hour.

Suppositories: Unwrap, insert pointed end into rectum first. If suppository has softened, it may be chilled in refrigerator (while still in wrap) or in cold water to harden for insertion.

when

At the same time every day.

side effects and adverse reactions	what to do
Severe allergic reaction (anaphylactic shock)	Get emergency medical help immediately.
Muscle cramps, numbness or tingling in hands or feet, ulcers in mouth, bloody stool, jaundice, mental disturbances, sore throat, urinary tract and kidney problems, abdominal pain, chills	Stop taking. Get in touch with doctor immediately.
Fatigue, mild depression, headache, dizziness, nausea, minor to moderate gastrointestinal problems, insomnia, menstrual irregularities	Continue taking, but discuss with your physician.
Sexual problems, including impotence and decreased sexual appetite	Discuss with your doctor.

special precautions	because
DRUG INTERACTIONS	
1. Angiotensin-converting enzyme inhibitors, beta-adrenergic blockers, diuretics, minoxidil, sotalol, terazosin, triamterene	1. NSAIDs may decrease their effectiveness.
2. Antiarthritis gold compounds, Tiopronin	2. May increase damage to kidneys.
3. Cephalosporin antibiotics, oral anticoagulants, other anti-inflammatory pain relievers	3. Increases risk of bleeding.
4. Antacids	4. Antacids dampen NSAIDs' pain-relief capabilities.
5. Aspirin, cortisone drugs	5. Will raise risk of stomach ulcers.
6. Thyroid hormones	6. Will increase blood pressure and heart rate.
DIET No restrictions.	
ALCOHOL and TOBACCO Avoid alcohol. No interaction with tobacco.	Alcohol could increase risk of stomach bleeding.
PREGNANCY Discuss with your doctor.	No conclusive studies about impact on fetus.

(continued)

BREAST-FEEDING

Avoid drug or avoid nursing.

Medication enters breast milk and may cause side effects in baby.

AGE FACTOR

1. Ibuprofen elixir and chewable tablets are sold in pediatric strengths for children older than three years, but these are available by prescription only. Get your physician's advice about giving children and adolescents ibuprofen.

1. Safety and effectiveness have not been established.

2. People over 60 should use cautiously.

2. Side and adverse effects may be more severe. Be on the lookout for fluid retention, dizziness, confusion, impaired memory.

MISSED DOSE

You can take a missed dose up to two hours after scheduled time. Otherwise, wait for next dose but do not double the amount taken.

OVERDOSE

Get emergency medical help immediately if patient falls into coma, has convulsions, seems to be bleeding internally, has a severe headache, or is incoherent.

STOPPING DRUG

You may have to taper off the drug slowly. Consult your doctor before stopping.

OTHERS

Do not drive or operate machinery until you have determined how medication affects you.

Some NSAIDs may cover up developing infections. Talk to your doctor if you think you have an infection because you are running a fever or if you feel weak or tired.

May increase sensitivity to sun. If you go outdoors between 10 A.M. and 3 P.M., wear protective clothing and/or sunblock.

ACETAMINOPHEN

condition:

PAIN, FEVER, AND INFLAMMATIONS

warning

Tell your doctor if you have or have had:
• an allergic reaction to this medication, or to any preservatives or foods. Combinations of acetaminophen and calcium, potassium, and sodium bicarbonate may contain about 140 mg of salt per tablet, a problem if you are on a low-salt diet.

drugs

GENERIC	BRAND	RX
acetaminophen	*Tylenol, FEVERALL, Datril*, others	No

form/usage

TABLETS, CAPSULES, EFFERVESCENT PREPARATIONS, ELIXIRS, SUPPOSITORIES, POWDERS: Tablets, elixirs, and capsules can be taken with liquid.
Powders should be mixed into liquids.
Effervescent preparations should be dissolved thoroughly in 4 ounces of cool water.

when

Not more often than every three hours as needed. Maximum dosage per day should not exceed 3 to 4 grams, the equivalent of 9 to 12 tablets.

side effects and adverse reactions

Severe gastrointestinal problems, sweating, irritability

Fatigue, rash, sore throat, blood in urine, pain in back or side

Light-headedness, trembling, decreased urine output

what to do

Get in touch with poison control center, emergency room, or doctor.

Stop taking. Get in touch with doctor immediately.

Continue taking, but discuss with your physician.

(continued)

special precautions	because
DRUG INTERACTIONS	
1. Anticoagulants	1. Increased anticoagulant effect.
2. Isoniazid	2. Possible liver damage.
DIET	
No restrictions.	
ALCOHOL AND TOBACCO	
Avoid alcohol.	Alcohol may cause drowsiness and increase risk of liver damage.
No known interaction with tobacco.	
PREGNANCY	
Discuss with your doctor.	No known impact on fetus.
BREAST-FEEDING	
No problems reported.	
AGE FACTOR	
1. Do not give to children under the age of 6 unless your doctor tells you it is okay. Children 6 to 12 years old should get one tablet three or four times a day.	1. Children may develop severe reactions; also, an adult dosage may be too large for a child.
2. People over 60 should use cautiously.	2. Adverse and side effects may be worse. Body clears the drug more slowly in older adults.
MISSED DOSE	
Take when you remember, but then wait a full three hours for the next dose.	
OVERDOSE	
Get emergency medical help immediately if patient falls into coma or has convulsions.	

STOPPING DRUG

Generally, stop taking when you feel better, though you should consult your doctor if pain does not go away within ten days, fever does not subside within three days, or a sore throat does not disappear within two days.

OTHERS

May cause anemia if taken for long periods of time. Periodic laboratory tests might be necessary to check effect on liver and kidneys.

Acute liver failure may occur with an attempted overdose with 10 to 15 grams of drug; however, liver damage can also occur with chronic ingestion of 3 to 4 grams of drug over a period of a year or more. Alcohol can exacerbate acetominophen's toxic effects on the liver.

drug or category:

ASPIRIN (SALICYLATES)

condition:

PAIN, FEVER, VARIOUS INFLAMMATORY CONDITIONS; ARTHRITIS AND RHEUMATISM; UNDER DOCTOR'S CARE, USED TO HELP PREVENT HEART ATTACKS

warning

Aspirin is a drug and must be treated with respect.

Do not take if pills smell like vinegar, a sign the drug has deteriorated.

Do not take aspirin if you have any disease that makes you bleed easily, or if you have a history of ulcers.

Tell your doctor if you have or have had:

• an allergic reaction to aspirin or a related compound before
• nasal polyps
• asthma, gout, diabetes, or lupus erythematosus

Never take more than three pills (975 mg) at one time.

Tell all doctors and dentists you consult if you take aspirin regularly.

drugs

GENERIC	BRAND	RX
aspirin	aspirin, *Anacin, Bayer, Bufferin, Empirin, Measurin, Novasen,* others; also in *Alka-Seltzer, Excedrin,* and other products	No

form/usage

TABLETS, CAPSULES, CHEWABLE TABLETS, EFFERVESCENT TAB-LETS, SUPPOSITORIES: All oral forms of aspirin should be taken with foods or with plenty of liquids. Can be taken with any nonalcoholic drink, including milk; however, taking with orange juice or other acidic beverage may increase stomach irritation.

You can crush the pills or open the capsules to make taking them easier. Extended-release capsules or tablets should be taken whole. Effervescent tablets should be dissolved in water. Suppositories, once unwrapped, should be inserted into rectum with the pointed end first.

when

Every 4, 8, or 12 hours as needed, depending on the form taken.

side effects and adverse reactions	what to do
Anaphylactic shock	Get emergency medical help immediately.
Rashes, hives, or other skin reactions; jaundice; ringing in ears	Stop taking. Get in touch with doctor immediately.
Minor gastrointestinal problems, blood in stool, thirst	Continue taking, but discuss with your physician.

special precautions	because

DRUG INTERACTIONS

special precautions	because
1. Diabetes medications, methotrexate, valproic acid, anticoagulants	1. Aspirin increases their impact, exaggerating their effect.
2. Beta-blockers, *Capoten*, probenecid and other antigout medications	2. Aspirin may decrease their effectiveness.
3. Antacids, carteolol, cortisone, sodium bicarbonate and citrate	3. They decrease aspirin's impact.
4. *Diamox*, vitamin C, Pabalate-SF	4. Will heighten aspirin's impact.
5. Tetracycline	5. Buffers in aspirin could keep antibiotic from working, take one hour before or after aspirin.

DIET
Avoid aspirin formulations high in salt if you are on a low-salt diet.

ALCOHOL and TOBACCO

special precautions	because
Avoid alcohol. No interaction reported with tobacco.	Alcohol increases chance of stomach irritation and bleeding.

PREGNANCY

special precautions	because
Avoid aspirin, especially in last three months.	Animal studies link aspirin to birth defects, but there is no evidence of such a link in humans. Limit any aspirin intake to very small doses because large-scale use of aspirin has been linked to stillbirths and death among newborns.

(continued)

BREAST-FEEDING

Avoid drug or avoid nursing.

Aspirin passes into breast milk.

AGE FACTOR

1. Do not give to children or to young people under age of 21 without instructions from a doctor.

2. People over 60 should take cautiously.

1. In youngsters, aspirin has been linked to Reye's syndrome, an often fatal disease.

2. Greater likelihood of gastrointestinal bleeding.

MISSED DOSE

For headaches and other pains, take when you remember; take next dose four hours later.
For arthritis, take a missed dose up to two hours after scheduled time. Otherwise, wait for next dose but do not double the amount taken.

OVERDOSE

Get emergency medical help immediately in case of coma, convulsions, severe gastrointestinal distress, rapid breathing, muscular twitches, or hallucinations.

STOPPING DRUG

For headaches and other minor pains, discontinue when discomfort ends.
Patients taking aspirin as part of their heart disease treatment should discuss with their doctors before stopping.

drug or category:

COMBINATION DRUGS FOR HEADACHES

condition:

MIGRAINE AND TENSION HEADACHES

warning

Do not take if you are allergic to acetaminophen, isometheptene, dichloralphenazone

Tell your doctor if you have or have had:

- an allergic reaction to this medication, preservatives, or dyes
- severe kidney or liver disease
- high blood pressure or a physical defect of the heart

drugs

GENERIC	BRAND	RX
isometheptene, dichloralphena-zone, and acetaminophen	*Midrin, Migrex,* others	Yes

form/usage

CAPSULES: Take with liquids.

when

For migraine: Two capsules at once and one capsule every hour until headache ebbs.

Do not take more than five capsules in a 12-hour period.

For tension headaches: One or two capsules every 4 hours. Do not take more than eight capsules in 24 hours.

side effects and adverse reactions

Diarrhea, vomiting, nausea, mild to moderate abdominal pain, rash, bleeding, weakness, fever, sores in mouth

Drowsiness, dizziness

what to do

Stop taking. Get in touch with doctor immediately.

Continue taking, but discuss with your physician.

(continued)

special precautions	because
DRUG INTERACTIONS	
1. Aspirin, nonsteroidal anti-inflammatory agents	1. May cause severe kidney damage, including cancer.
2. MAO inhibitors	2. May lead to sharp and sudden increases in blood pressure.
3. Phenobarbital	3. Will speed elimination of acetaminophen and decrease its effect.
4. Tetracycline	4. Will slow absorption of this antibiotic. Take two hours apart.
5. Anticoagulants	5. May increase effect of blood thinners.
6. Any drug that has an impact on behavior, causes drowsiness, or diminishes reflexes	6. Will increase impact of those medicines on alertness, reflexes, etc.
DIET	
No interactions.	
ALCOHOL and TOBACCO	
Avoid both.	Alcohol may increase damage to liver and will cause drowsiness. Tobacco decreases effect of medicine.
PREGNANCY	
Discuss with your doctor.	
BREAST-FEEDING	
Discuss with your doctor.	
AGE FACTOR	
1. Children should not take for more than five days. Adults under 60 should not take for more than ten days.	1. Long use may cause anemia.
2. People over 60 should use carefully.	2. Inefficient elimination of drug because of age may increase its impact.

MISSED DOSE
Take when you remember, take next dose four hours later. Do not double dose.

OVERDOSE
Get medical help immediately in case of coma, convulsions, or severe diarrhea.

STOPPING DRUG
Discontinue when headache abates. If headache persists for more than two days, contact your doctor.

OTHERS
Regular laboratory tests to assess drug's impact on blood and liver should be conducted.

---

drug or category:

ERGOTAMINE

condition:

MIGRAINE AND MIGRAINELIKE HEADACHES, HISTAMINE HEADACHES

---

warning

Tell your doctor if you have or have had:
- an allergic reaction to previous dose
- an infection
- cardiovascular, liver, or kidney disease

If taken in excessive amounts, drug can cause migraine headaches.

Tell your doctor if you are pregnant.

May lead to dependence.

---

drugs

GENERIC	BRAND	RX
ergotamine tartrate	*Cafergot, Migergot, Wigraine,* others	Yes

---

form/usage

AEROSOLS, TABLETS, SUPPOSITORIES

1. Aerosol is inhaled.

2. Sublingual tablets should be placed under tongue to dissolve and should not be swallowed. Tablets that contain ergotamine and other medications are to be swallowed. They can be crushed. However, combination medications in extended-release tablets should be taken whole.

when

1. One spray at beginning of headache and then 1 spray every 5 to 10 minutes. No more than 6 sprays in a 24-hour period. Do not exceed 15 sprays a week.

2. Take tablets at beginning of headache. Take 1 mg every half hour to hour as needed, but no more than 5 mg per attack. Do not take more than 5 mg per 24 hours or more than 10 mg over the course of a week.

AEROSOLS, TABLETS, SUPPOSITORIES

3. Insert pointed end into rectum. If suppository is too soft for insertion, firm up while still wrapped by running cold water over it or placing in refrigerator.

3. Use at first hint of headache.

side effects and adverse reactions

what to do

Swollen ankles or feet, rapid heartbeat, itchy skin, confusion, weakness and trembling, indigestion, anxiety, blisters, vision problems, thirst

Stop taking. Get in touch with doctor immediately.

Dizziness, gastrointestinal problems, more frequent or more painful headaches

Stop taking. Discuss with your physician.

special precautions

because

DRUG INTERACTIONS

1. Amphetamines, epinephrine, ephedrine, MAO inhibitors, pseudoephedrine

2. Cimetidine, oral contraceptives, isoniazid

3. Beta-blockers

4. Sedatives, sleeping medications, tranquilizers

5. Troleandomycin

1. Will increase blood pressure to dangerous levels.

2. Will increase impact of caffeine in medication.

3. Will constrict cardiac arteries.

4. Ergotamine will reduce their effectiveness.

5. Will magnify adverse effects of ergotamine.

DIET
No problems associated with drug. However, allergies to some foods are thought to be responsible for some migraine headaches.

ALCOHOL and TOBACCO
Avoid both.

Alcohol can make vascular headaches worse. Nicotine constricts blood vessels and could intensify impact of drug.

PREGNANCY
Avoid drug.

Drug may induce abortion.

(continued)

BREAST-FEEDING

Avoid drug or avoid nursing.

Medication passes into breast milk.

AGE FACTOR

1. Do not give to children under 12.

1. Effectiveness and safety have not been established.

2. Should be taken by people over 60 cautiously.

2. Older people are more susceptible to adverse effects.

MISSED DOSE

Take a missed dose up to two hours after scheduled time. Otherwise, wait for next dose but do not double the amount taken.

OVERDOSE

Get emergency medical help immediately in case of coma, convulsions, tingling or cold hands, muscle pain, hallucinations, rapid heartbeat.

STOPPING DRUG

Do not stop abruptly. You may have to withdraw from it slowly to prevent rebound headaches. Discuss with your physician.

OTHERS

Do not drive or operate machinery until you have determined how medication affects you.

Medication contains caffeine. Avoid or limit intake of other caffeine products if excessive caffeine is a problem for you.

METHYSERGIDE

condition:
VASCULAR HEADACHES, INCLUDING MIGRAINE AND CLUSTER HEADACHES

warning

May cause scarring in chest, abdomen, lungs, and other organs. May also cause scarring of penile tissues.
Tell your doctor if you have or have had:

- an allergic reaction to this drug
- a severe infection
- any heart or circulation problems, including high blood pressure

Tell your doctor if you are pregnant.

drugs

GENERIC	BRAND	RX
methysergide	*Sansert*	Yes

form/usage

TABLETS: Tablets may be taken with food or milk to prevent stomach irritation.

when

Dosage and frequency should be discussed with your physician.

side effects and adverse reactions

Agitation; hallucinations; itchy skin; change in heart rhythm; joint, muscle, chest, back, groin, or side pain; red face

Difficult urination, weight loss or gain, vision problems, insomnia, constipation, drowsiness, weakness in legs, mild diarrhea

what to do

Stop taking. Get in touch with doctor immediately.

Continue taking, but discuss with your physician.

special precautions

DRUG INTERACTIONS
1. Beta-blockers

because

1. May help constrict peripheral arteries.

(continued)

DRUG INTERACTIONS
2. Ergot medications

2. Combining ergot with methysergide may increase or decrease the effectiveness of either drug.

3. Narcotic-based drugs

3. Effect of narcotics will be diminished.

DIET
Avoid caffeine.
Some foods may cause allergic reactions in the form of vascular headaches.

Caffeine will diminish the effectiveness of the medication.

ALCOHOL and TOBACCO
Avoid both.

Alcohol may set off vascular headaches in some individuals.
Nicotine narrows blood vessels and will make headaches worse.

PREGNANCY
Avoid drug.

While no animal or human studies have linked the drug to pregnancy problems, the drug's maker advises that it should not be taken during pregnancy.

BREAST-FEEDING
Avoid drug or avoid nursing.

Medication moves into breast milk.

AGE FACTOR
1. Not recommended for infants or children.

1. Safety and efficacy not established. Serious side effects may outweigh benefits.

2. People over 60 should use cautiously.

2. Changes brought on in cardiovascular system and in kidney function make older people more susceptible to adverse effects.

MISSED DOSE
Wait for next scheduled dose but do not double. Resume prescribed schedule.

OVERDOSE
Get in touch with poison control center, emergency room, or doctor in case of severe gastrointestinal problems, severe thirst, or lack of coordination.

STOPPING DRUG

Discontinue drug after three weeks if it has not been effective, but discuss with doctor first.

If medication works, see your doctor after six months to discuss continued treatment. If drug is effective, prescription will probably be renewed, though you should allow four weeks to pass before starting drug again.

OTHERS

While drug prevents headaches, it is of no help once a vascular headache has set in.

Do not drive or operate machinery until you have determined how medication affects you.

Have laboratory tests done from time to time to make sure liver function and blood counts have not been affected.

-15-

ANALGESICS WITH NARCOTICS

NARCOTIC PAIN-KILLERS ARE potent prescription drugs reserved for pain that cannot be controlled adequately by nonnarcotic analgesics—for example, in cases of fractures, burns, crippling headaches, severe muscle and back injuries, heart attacks, and advanced cancer. These drugs, commonly referred to as opiates because they are chemically related to opium, include **codeine; pentazocine** (*Talwin*); **propoxyphene** (*Darvocet-N, Darvon*), a type of methadone; and **hydrocodone** (*Lorcet, Lortab*), and **oxycodone** (*Percocet, Percodan, Tylox*), stronger versions of codeine. While opiates are often given alone, they are also combined with other drugs including muscle relaxants, NSAIDs, and acetaminophen. These combinations of opiates and nonnarcotic analgesics are more effective than higher doses of one or the other.

Opiate pain-killers work through the central nervous system—the brain, the brain stem, and the spinal cord—which contains the specialized nerve cells that play a role in the way the body perceives and responds to pain. Some opiate drugs mimic the action of the naturally occurring pain-moderating chemicals in the brain. Others work by blunting the action of cells that increase the perception of pain. Most opiate drugs can be taken orally, in the form of pills or liquids, but they are also administered by injection, sometimes just under the skin or into the muscle, and sometimes directly into a vein, to provide almost immediate relief at a relatively low dose. In contrast, orally administered narcotics take 30 to 60 minutes to act.

Narcotic pain-killers, however, have to be used carefully. Although the opiate compounds work on those parts of the central nervous system that deal with pain, they also interact with brain cells that control mood, emotions, and behavior, inducing feelings of well-being and euphoria and raising a danger of psychological addiction. Moreover, they may also lead to physiological addiction, meaning that the body suffers withdrawal symptoms—fever, chills, extreme anxiety, cramps, massive diarrhea—when the drugs are no longer taken.

The potential for addiction varies from narcotic to narcotic. Hydrocodone, for example, is not considered as potentially addictive as codeine and other opiates, an assessment that is reflected in the fact that most states put fewer restrictions on its prescription than on codeine. Moreover, there is a growing sentiment within the medical community that the fear that patients on narcotic analgesics will become addicted to them has led too many doctors to underprescribe the medications, particularly for end-stage cancer patients.

The use of narcotic medications, however, carries with it other risks that must also be considered.

They also affect parts of the brain stem that control breathing, nausea and vomiting, alertness, and other vital functions. Thus, narcotic medications can cause respiratory problems, extreme drowsiness, and nausea and vomiting. Less serious, albeit annoying, problems include constipation and dry mouth. Drinking plenty of fluids, eating high-fiber foods, and taking a stool softener can alleviate these difficulties. Older people run a higher risk of these effects because their ability to metabolize these drugs may be compromised. Thus, doctors generally prescribe narcotic analgesics in the lowest effective dose and for as short a period as possible.

drug or category:

CODEINE

condition:

MODERATE TO SEVERE PAIN

warning

Do not take if you are having an asthma attack or have suffered a severe head injury.

Tell your doctor if you have or have had:

- an allergic reaction to any codeine drug, or to any food dyes or preservatives
- liver, kidney, or gallbladder problems
- a convulsive disorder
- emphysema or bronchitis

Codeine products have some potential for becoming habit-forming.

drugs

GENERIC	BRAND	RX
codeine	*Tylenol with Codeine, others*	Yes
oxycodone	*Percocet, Percodan, Tylox, others*	
hydrocodone	*Lorcet, Lortab, others*	
Also: butalbital with codeine	*Fiorinal with Codeine*	

form/usage

INJECTIONS, TABLETS, DROPS, LIQUIDS, SUPPOSITORIES, SOLUTIONS, TRANSDERMAL PATCHES:

Take with food or liquid to reduce potential stomach irritation.

Tablets can be crushed, capsules can be opened.

Drops and liquids should be diluted in a beverage.

For transdermal patches and suppositories, follow instructions on package.

when

As needed, but not to exceed once every four hours.

side effects and adverse reactions

Irregular heartbeat, breathing difficulties

what to do

Get emergency medical help immediately.

side effects and adverse reactions

Prolonged constipation, severe abdominal pain, gastrointestinal upsets

Depression, dizziness, fatigue, headache, dry mouth, ringing in ears, inability to work well mentally, constipation, minor abdominal pain

what to do

Stop taking. Get in touch with doctor immediately.

Continue taking, but discuss with your physician.

special precautions

DRUG INTERACTIONS
1. Antidepressants, anticholinergics, carbamazepine, carteolol, cimetidine, ethinamate, guanfacine, methyprylon, molindone, nabilone, other narcotics, phenothiazines, sedatives, sleep medications, tranquilizers

2. Clozapine, MAO inhibitors, selegiline

DIET
No restrictions.

ALCOHOL AND TOBACCO
Avoid alcohol if possible, or use extreme caution. No interaction with nicotine.

PREGNANCY
Avoid medication.

BREAST-FEEDING
Avoid drug or avoid nursing.

because

1. Codeine medications increase their effect.

2. May cause severely toxic effects, including seizures, coma, and death.

Codeine can heighten impact of alcohol, and alcohol increases the ability of codeine drugs to depress brain activity.

Some indications that some codeine medications can cause birth defects if taken during the first six months of pregnancy. Codeine taken toward the end of pregnancy may cause withdrawal symptoms in the newborn.

Drug passes into breast milk.

(continued)

AGE FACTOR

1. Do not give to children under two years of age.

2. People over 60 should start drug in small doses, then increase slowly.

1. Drug can cause dangerous respiratory depression.

2. To be safe, older people need to determine what levels they can tolerate without getting drowsy or dizzy or experiencing other problems.

MISSED DOSE

Take when you remember, but wait four hours before taking again.

OVERDOSE

Get emergency medical help immediately if patient falls into coma or has convulsions, suffers breathing difficulties, has constricted pupils or unexplained sweating, or cannot be roused from sleep.

STOPPING DRUG

May be discontinued if pain goes away.

Do not use for more than one week. If you don't get pain relief, contact your physician.

If after stopping you have insomnia, are irritable, have dilated eye pupils, or feel weak, contact your doctor.

OTHERS

Some products are mixed with other pain-killers, including acetaminophen or aspirin. Consult your doctor if you are allergic to these medications or are taking them in other prescriptions.

PROPOXYPHENE

condition:

MILD TO MODERATE PAIN

warning

Should not be taken by suicidal or addiction-prone persons.

Tell your doctor if you have or have had:

• an allergic reaction to this medication or acetaminophen, or to preservatives or dyes

• asthma or kidney or liver disease

Tell your doctor if you are going to have any kind of surgery within two months.

Could lead to psychological and physical dependence.

Could cause anemia in children if used more than five days and in adults if taken for longer than ten days.

For warnings concerning acetaminophen, including side effects, see Chapter 14.

drugs

GENERIC	BRAND	RX
propoxyphene	*Darvocet-N* (with acetamino-phen), *Darvon*	Yes
meperidine	*Demerol*	
hydromorphone	*Dilaudid*	
morphine	*Astramorph, Roxanol*	

form/usage

TABLETS, CAPSULES, DROPS, LIQUIDS:

Tablets and capsules should be taken with liquid.

Tablets may be crushed and capsules opened and taken with liquid or food.

when

As needed, but no more often than every four hours.

side effects and adverse reactions

Prolonged constipation, jaundice, sleep disturbances, itchy skin, blood in urine, vision troubles, breathing difficulties

Depression, dry mouth, fatigue, agitation, constipation

what to do

Stop taking. Get in touch with doctor immediately.

Continue taking, but discuss with your physician.

(continued)

special precautions

because

DRUG INTERACTIONS

1. Anticonvulsants, antidepressants, antihistamines, muscle relaxants, sleeping drugs, tranquilizers, warfarin drugs

2. Anticonvulsants

3. Tetracyclines

4. Nitrates

5. Selegiline

1. Propoxyphene increases the sedating effect of these drugs.

2. Combination of these two drugs can cause neurologic problems, including coma.

3. Propoxyphene may slow absorption of this antibiotic. Take drugs 2 hours apart.

4. May cause excessive drop in blood pressure.

5. Combination of these two drugs may be toxic and cause coma or seizures.

DIET

No restrictions.

ALCOHOL and TOBACCO

Avoid alcohol.
No interactions with tobacco.

Medication increases alcohol intoxication.

PREGNANCY

Avoid drug.

Can lead to dependence on the drug by baby.

BREAST-FEEDING

Discuss with your doctor.

Drugs passes into breast milk, but no adverse effects in nursing babies have been linked to it.

AGE FACTOR

1. Do not give to children under 12 for longer than five days.

2. Adults older than 60 should use cautiously.

1. Could cause anemia.

2. Body handles drug less efficiently and excessive amounts could cause dizziness or constipation.

MISSED DOSE

Take when you remember. Do not double dose. Do not take the next dose for four hours.

OVERDOSE
Get emergency medical help immediately in case of convulsions, confusion, severe dizziness or drowsiness, or breathing difficulties.

STOPPING DRUG
If you don't get relief, stop taking after two days; otherwise, stop taking when you feel relief.

If, after stopping, you develop dilated pupils or insomnia, or are irritable or weak, notify your doctor.

OTHERS
Do not drive or operate machinery until you have determined how medication affects you.

-16-

ANTIARTHRITIC DRUGS

If you suffer from aching joints, you are not alone; 37 to 40 million Americans suffer from some form of arthritis—a general term covering more than a hundred different rheumatic disorders. The sufferers include:

- An estimated 16 million people with osteoarthritis, or degenerative joint disease, which is characterized by aching joints

- About 2.5 million who have rheumatoid arthritis, a systemic disease that affects joints and sometimes internal organs

- Some 250,000 children with juvenile rheumatoid arthritis

- Almost 2 million men who have painful attacks of gout, a metabolic disorder that results in a buildup of uric acid, crystals of which settle in joints and other body tissues

- More than 300,000 who have ankylosing spondylitis, more commonly known as spinal arthritis, which afflicts mostly men

- Some 131,000, mostly women, who have systemic lupus erythematosus, an autoimmune disease that affects connective tissue in the joints, skin, and other organs

The National Institute of Arthritis and Musculoskeletal and Skin Diseases reports that for most people, the symptoms of arthritis usually come and go. But on any given day, almost 5 million people have painful and debilitating arthritis attacks, and almost 3 million people are either partially or completely disabled by some form of arthritis. Fortunately, most arthritis sufferers can find at least some relief from a wide array of antiarthritic medications, including:

- **Nonsteroidal anti-inflammatory drugs (NSAIDs)** (see Chapter 14).

- **Gold salts, such as gold sodium thiomalate** (*Myochrysine*) **and aurothioglucose** (*Solganal*). These compounds can be taken orally in capsules or injected, though how they alleviate arthritis is unknown. In those patients whom gold helps, the first signs of relief may not be apparent for at least three months. Moreover, many patients have reported that eventually the treatments lose their effectiveness.

- **Penicillamine** (*Cuprimine, Depen*), a byproduct of penicillin, a drug used primarily as a chelating agent to remove excess copper from the body. How it works against rheumatic arthritis is unknown, but some researchers theorize that it interferes with the autoimmune reaction that causes joint inflammation.

- Gout medications like **allopurinol** (*Zyloprim*), which reduces uric acid production, and **probenecid** (*Benemid*), a uricosuric, or drug that increases excretion of uric acid in the urine, prevent attacks. **Sulfinpyrazone** (*Anturane*) also increases uric acid excretion and, when used long-term, may prevent attacks of gout. **Colchicine** is prescribed to halt attacks that do occur.

- **Corticosteroids,** such as cortisone (*Cortone*) and prednisone (*Deltasone*), which reduce the production of prostaglandins and other body chemicals responsible for causing inflammation.

No one argues that arthritis patients should suffer needlessly, but some experts contend that Americans spend some $1 billion a year on arthritis medications they don't really need. For example, some take expensive prescription nonsteroidal anti-inflammatory agents when less costly nonprescription drugs, including aspirin, might be just as effective. Nondrug treatments, including weight loss and exercise conditioning, could also reduce the need for drugs and their high risk of side effects, which range from intestinal upsets to potentially severe liver and kidney disorders and anemia. Steroids in particular have numerous adverse side effects, including weight gain, bleeding problems, bone loss, thinning of the skin, cataract formation, reduced immunity, and mood swings.

ALLOPURINOL

GOUT (LONG-TERM MANAGEMENT AND PREVENTION)

warning

Tell your doctor if you have or have had:
- an allergic reaction to progestin medication, preservatives, or dyes
- hemochromatosis
- liver or kidney disease
- epilepsy
- blood disorders or bone marrow disease

During early part of treatment gout attacks may increase, but they will eventually decrease.
Do not take while in the midst of a gout attack.

drugs

GENERIC	BRAND	RX
allopurinol	*Zyloprim*, others	Yes

form/usage

TABLETS: May be taken with food or liquid.
Tablets may be crushed.

Drink up to 3 quarts of liquid each day.

when

Same time every day.

side effects and adverse reactions

Sore throat, fever, unexplained bruising or bleeding, jaundice, skin sympttoms

Minor gastrointestinal problems, tingling or numbness in limbs, drowsiness

what to do

Stop taking. Get in touch with doctor immediately.

Continue taking, but discuss with your physician.

special precautions	**because**
DRUG INTERACTIONS	
1. Vitamin C	1. High doses of vitamin C could cause kidney stones and other problems while this medication is taken.
2. Thiazide diuretics	2. Could cause kidney damage.
3. Chlorthalidone, ethacrynic acid, furosemide, indapamide, metolazone	3. Will lessen effect of allopurinol.
4. Ampicillin	4. May cause skin problems.
5. Anticoagulants, azathioprine, chlorpropamide, mercaptopurine, theophylline	5. Their effect may be increased.
6. Antidiabetics	6. Will increase elimination of uric acid.
7. Iron supplements	7. Iron may accumulate in body.
DIET	
You may need a special, low-purine diet.	Foods high in this compound contribute to formation of uric acid.
ALCOHOL and TOBACCO	
No interactions reported.	
PREGNANCY	
Avoid drug, especially during first three months. During last six months, use only if absolutely necessary.	Human and animal studies are inadequate to ensure safety during pregnancy.
BREAST-FEEDING	
Avoid drug or avoid nursing.	Drug passes into breast milk and may affect baby.
AGE FACTOR	
1. Children should be monitored closely while on drug.	1. Could cause blood disorders. Increases toxicity of chemotherapy drugs used against cancer.
2. People over 60 should use conservatively at beginning of therapy.	2. Kidneys are less efficient and clear less of drug than in younger adults.

(continued)

MISSED DOSE

If you are taking one dose a day, you can take missed dose up to six hours after scheduled time. Otherwise, wait for next dose. Do not double the amount.

If you are taking multiple doses each day, you may take up to three hours later. If longer, wait until next dose. Do not double amount taken.

OVERDOSE

Get in touch with poison control center, emergency room, or doctor if you believe you have taken too much of this medication.

STOPPING DRUG

Do not stop taking, even if you feel better. Discuss with your doctor how to come off drug.

OTHERS

Do not drive or operate machinery until you have determined how medication affects you.

You should have periodic laboratory tests to monitor blood cell activity, liver and kidney functions, uric acid levels.

Even though there is no clear-cut link between allopurinol and eye problems, periodic eye exams are recommended.

ADRENAL CORTICOSTEROIDS

condition:

JOINT INFLAMMATION AND PAIN

warning

Tell your doctor if you have or have had:

- an allergic reaction to progestin medication, or to any preservatives or dyes
- tuberculosis, herpes, or fungus infection
- bone, heart, liver, or kidney disease, or ulcers
- blood clotting problems, high blood pressure
- glaucoma, thyroid problems, myasthenia gravis

Effects of drugs will linger for up to two years. All doctors and surgeons you consult should be told you are or have been taking cortisone or prednisone. You may want to carry a card or wear a medical alert bracelet to inform emergency medical care personnel that you are or have been on these drugs.

drugs

GENERIC	BRAND	RX
cortisone	*Cortone*	Yes
prednisone	*Deltasone,* others	

form/usage

TABLETS, CAPSULES, LIQUID: Take with food or liquid to avoid stomach irritation.

Tablets may be crumbled and capsules opened.

when

Once a day or once every other day.

side effects and adverse reactions

Irregular heartbeat, rashes, blood clots, blood in stool, vision changes, fever, cramps

Changes in mood, inability to sleep, acne, mild gastrointestinal problems, slow healing of wounds

what to do

Stop taking. Get in touch with doctor immediately.

Continue taking, but discuss with your physician.

(continued)

special precautions	because
DRUG INTERACTIONS	
1. Aspirin, oral contraceptives, estrogens, indomethacin	1. Increase effect of cortisone and prednisone.
2. Anticonvulsants, antihistamines, barbiturates, chloral hydrate, cholestyramine, colestipol, ephedrine, glutethimide, mitotane, phenobarbital, rifampin	2. Decrease effect or absorption of cortisone and prednisone.
3. Anticholinergics, sympathomimetics	3. May cause glaucoma.
4. Anticoagulants, cholinergics, insulin, isoniazid, potassium supplements	4. Their effects will be decreased.
5. Vaccines, cyclosporine	5. Increase risk of viral or bacterial infections.
6. Diclofenac, ketoprofen, phenylbutazone, NSAIDs, oxyphenbutazone	6. Increase risk of stomach ulcers and bleeding.
7. Amphotericin B, chlorthalidone, digitalis, diuretics, ethacrynic acid, furosemide, indapamide, potassium supplements	7. Decrease effectiveness of potassium; potassium depletion.
DIET	
No restrictions.	
ALCOHOL and TOBACCO	
Avoid both.	Alcohol increases risk of stomach ulcers. Tobacco could increase effect of cortisone and prednisone and cause toxicity.
PREGNANCY	
Avoid medication.	Potential harm to fetus.
BREAST-FEEDING	
Avoid drug or avoid nursing.	Drug passes into breast milk and may affect baby.
AGE FACTOR	
1. Use cortisone and prednisone in children only under medical supervision.	1. Can interfere with growth if used too long.

AGE FACTOR

2. Older adults should use both drugs cautiously.

2. Side and adverse effects could be more intense than in younger adults and could make diabetes and ulcers worse. Could also contribute to bone loss and cataract formation.

MISSED DOSE

If you are taking several doses a day, you can take a missed dose up to two hours after scheduled time. Otherwise, wait for next dose but do not double the amount taken.

If you are taking only one dose a day, wait until your next scheduled dose. **Double the amount taken.**

OVERDOSE

Get emergency medical help immediately if patient goes into heart failure, has convulsions, retains fluids, or has headaches.

STOPPING DRUG

You must finish current prescription even if disorder or illness symptoms disappear. Discuss with your doctor.

OTHERS

Cortisone and prednisone can lower immunity and resistance to infections.

Both drugs may cause recurrence of tuberculosis.

Periodic laboratory tests might be necessary to check effect on blood pressure and potassium levels. Complete eye exams are also recommended, as are x rays in the case of patients who have had tuberculosis.

GOLD COMPOUNDS

condition:

PAIN, TENDERNESS, AND SWELLING IN ACTIVE RHEUMATOID ARTHRITIS

warning

Tell your doctor if you have or have had:
- an allergic reaction to other gold medications, or to preservatives or dyes
- ulcerative colitis or a blood or bone marrow disorder
- liver or kidney disease
- lupus erythematosus, skin disease, Sjögren's syndrome

Tell your doctor if you are pregnant or planning to have a child.

Can reduce red and white blood cells; can cause liver damage.

drugs

GENERIC	BRAND	RX
auranofin	*Ridaura*	Yes
aurothioglucose	*Solganal*	
gold sodium thiomalate	*Myochrysine*	

form/usage

CAPSULES, INJECTIONS: Take with food or full glass of water or milk to reduce chances of stomach irritation.

Do not open capsule.

when

One 6-mg dose every 24 hours or two 3-mg doses every 12 hours. If no relief after six months, dosage can be increased to three 3-mg doses (a total of 9 mg) every 24 hours.

side effects and adverse reactions

Severe allergic reaction (anaphylactic shock)

Abdominal pain, tingling in arms and legs, fatigue, bad taste in mouth, flushing, bloody urine, severe gastrointestinal problems

Muscle or joint pain, stomach cramps, constipation, hair loss, pink eye

what to do

Get emergency medical help immediately.

Stop taking. Get in touch with doctor immediately.

Continue taking, but discuss with your physician.

special precautions	**because**
DRUG INTERACTIONS	
I. *Dilantin* (phenytoin)	I. Some gold compounds may increase *Dilantin's* blood levels and effects.
2. Isoniazid, tiopronin, penicillamine, nonsteroidal anti-inflammatory drugs, cyclosporine	2. Increase risk of damage to liver and kidneys.
DIET No restrictions.	
ALCOHOL and TOBACCO Use alcohol with caution and watch for any gastro-intestinal problems. No interaction with tobacco reported.	Alcohol could irritate stomach lining.
PREGNANCY Avoid drug.	While no adverse effects on fetus have been seen, the drug maker recommends that it not be taken during pregnancy.
BREAST-FEEDING Avoid drug or avoid nursing.	Drug makes its way into breast milk.
AGE FACTOR I. Do not give to children under 12.	I. Efficacy and safety have not been established.
2. Adults over 60 should use cautiously.	2. Body tolerates gold compounds less and less with advancing age. Start with small doses and note reactions as you increase the amount taken.
MISSED DOSE Take when you remember, then go back to regular schedule. If you remember after six hours have lapsed, wait for next regularly scheduled dose. Do not double dose.	

(continued)

OVERDOSE
Get emergency medical help immediately in case of delirium, numbness and tingling in hands and feet, confusion.

STOPPING DRUG
Do not stop permanently without discussing with your doctor. In any case, you must finish your current prescription.

OTHERS
Drug may not show impact for three to six months.

Periodic laboratory tests might be necessary to check effect on blood count and liver and kidney function.

drug or category:

PENICILLAMINE

condition:
ARTHRITIS

warning

Tell your doctor if you have or have had:
- an allergic reaction to preservatives or dyes
- rheumatoid arthritis
- kidney disease
- blood disorders as a result of previous treatment with penicillamine

drugs

GENERIC	BRAND	RX
penicillamine	*Cuprimine, Depen*	Yes

form/usage

TABLETS, CAPSULES: Take on an empty stomach.

when

One hour before meals or two hours after. Should also be taken at least one hour before any snack, drink, or medicine.
Do not take within two hours of taking vitamins with iron or iron pills.

side effects and adverse reactions

Vision disturbances, sores in mouth and throat, skin eruptions, breathing difficulties, fever, swollen feet or legs, pain in joints, nausea, loss of taste

Diarrhea, mild stomachache, loss of appetite

what to do

Stop taking. Get in touch with doctor immediately.

Continue taking, but discuss with your physician.

(continued)

---

special precautions	because
DRUG INTERACTIONS	
1. Anticancer medications	1. Increased risk of side effects.
2. Aspirin and aspirinlike drugs	2. Interfere with penicillamine.
3. Anticoagulants, indomethacin, ketoprofen, antibiotics, antivirals	3. Penicillamine will increase their levels in the blood and perhaps their effects.
4. Probenecid	4. Probenecid may will decrease effectiveness of penicillamine.
DIET Avoid coffee or other drinks with caffeine.	Will decrease effectiveness of drug.
ALCOHOL and TOBACCO Avoid alcohol. No problems reported with tobacco.	Alcohol interferes with drug.
PREGNANCY No negative interactions reported.	
BREAST-FEEDING No problems reported.	
AGE FACTOR 1. Drug acts same in children as in adults. 2. Probably has same effects in people over 60 as in younger adults.	

MISSED DOSE
You can take a missed dose up to 12 hours after scheduled time. Otherwise, wait for next dose but do not double the amount taken.

OVERDOSE
Get emergency medical help immediately in case of convulsions, coma, extreme nervousness, breathing problems.

STOPPING DRUG

Do not stop taking even if you feel better until you have talked with your doctor. You may have to come off drug slowly.

OTHERS

Do not drive or operate machinery until you have determined how medication affects you.

Periodic laboratory tests might be necessary to check effect on liver and kidneys, to check blood uric acid level, and to track blood count.

drug or category:

URICOSURICS

condition:

CHRONIC (CONTINUING) GOUT TREATMENT AND PREVENTION

warning

Tell your doctor if you have or have had:
- an allergic reaction to this medication, or to preservatives or food additives
- kidney disease, including stones
- ulcers
- diseases of blood marrow or blood

drugs

GENERIC	BRAND	RX
probenecid	*Benemid,* others	Yes

form/usage

TABLETS: May be taken with food or liquid. Tablets may be crumbled.

when

Once a day, at the same time every day.

side effects and adverse reactions

Aching joints; swelling of feet, legs, or face; sore throat; blood in urine or other bleeding problems; pain in lower back

Red face, dizziness, itching, urination problems, headache, minor gastro-intestinal problems

what to do

Stop taking. Get in touch with doctor immediately.

Continue taking, but discuss with your physician.

special precautions

DRUG INTERACTIONS
Clozapine, flecainide, gold medications, immunosup-pressants, oxyphenbutazone, phenylbutazone, quinine, tiopronin, tocainide

because

Will reduce production of red blood cells and could affect red blood cells themselves.

DIET
No interactions.

--   --

ALCOHOL and TOBACCO
Avoid alcohol   Alcohol increases impact of drug.
No problems reported with tobacco.

--   --

PREGNANCY
Avoid medication.   May cause birth defects.

--   --

BREAST-FEEDING
No problems reported.

--   --

AGE FACTOR
1. No studies done with children, but effects same
as in adults.

2. Older adults should use cautiously.   2. Medications can cause a vast array of problems
                                                       in older adults, ranging from mouth and throat
                                                       problems to unusual bleeding.

--   --

MISSED DOSE
If you are taking one dose every 12 hours, take a missed dose as soon as you remember. If you don't remember until the next day, wait until your next regular dose. Do not double the amount taken.

If you are taking several doses a day, you can take a missed dose up to 2 hours after scheduled time. Otherwise, wait for next dose but do not double the amount taken.

OVERDOSE
Get emergency medical help immediately in case of coma, convulsions, or blood in sputum after coughing.

STOPPING DRUG
As you see fit.

OTHERS
You should have periodic tests to determine if your kidney and liver are affected by the drug. Blood counts and urinalysis are also recommended.

SULFINPYRAZONE

condition:

GOUT (MAY ALSO ACT AS A PREVENTIVE)

warning

Tell your doctor if you have or have had:

- an allergic reaction to this medication, oxyphenbutazone, or phenylbutazone, or to preservatives or food additives
- kidney disease, including stones
- ulcers
- blood diseases

drugs

GENERIC	BRAND	RX
sulfinpyrazone	*Anturane*, others	Yes

form/usage

TABLETS, CAPSULES: May be taken with food or liquid.

Tablets may be crumbled. Capsules may be opened.

when

Discuss schedule with your doctor, then take at the same times every day.

side effects and adverse reactions

Blood in stool or urine, urination difficulties, painful joints, increase in gout symptoms

Mild gastrointestinal upset, pain in lower back, rash

what to do

Stop taking. Get in touch with doctor immediately.

Continue taking, but discuss with your physician.

special precautions

DRUG INTERACTIONS

1. Allopurinol, anticoagulants, antidiabetics, cephalexin, cephradine, penicillin, sulfa drugs

2. Aspirin and aspirinlike drugs

because

1. Effect of these drugs is increased.

2. May cause increased bleeding.

DRUG INTERACTIONS

3. Aspirin, *Pepto-Bismol*, cholestyramine, diuretics

3. Decrease effect of sulfinpyrazone.

4. Oral contraceptives

4. Bleeding between periods.

5. Thioguanine

5. May require that sulfinpyrazone dose be increased.

DIET

Avoid coffee and other drinks with caffeine.

Effect of medication is decreased.

ALCOHOL and TOBACCO

Avoid alcohol.
No problems reported with tobacco.

Effect of medication is decreased when taken with alcohol.

PREGNANCY

No negative interactions reported.

BREAST-FEEDING

No problems reported.

AGE FACTOR

1. Drug has not been studied in children.

2. People over 60 should use cautiously.

2. Adverse and side effects may be worse in older people.

MISSED DOSE

You can take a missed dose up to two hours after scheduled time. Otherwise, wait for next dose but do not double the amount taken.

OVERDOSE

Get medical help immediately if patient has convulsions, is in a coma, or has breathing difficulties.

STOPPING DRUG

Do not stop taking even if you feel better until you have talked with your doctor. You may have to come off drug slowly.

OTHERS

Have regular laboratory tests to monitor blood and urine.

PROBENECID AND COLCHICINE

GOUT

warning

Tell your doctor if you have or have had:
- an allergic reaction to this medication, or to preservatives or food additives
- blood, heart, gastrointestinal, kidney, or liver disease
- problems with alcohol

drugs

GENERIC	BRAND	RX
probenecid and colchicine	*ColBENEMID*, others	Yes

form/usage

TABLETS: May be taken with food or liquid.

Tablets may be crumbled.

when

Discuss with your doctor. Take at same times every day.

side effects and adverse reactions

Increased urination or urination problems, severe gastrointestinal problems, back pains, unexplained weight changes, bleeding problems, mood or behavior changes

Dizziness, hair loss, gum problems

what to do

Stop taking. Get in touch with doctor immediately.

Continue taking, but discuss with your physician.

special precautions

DRUG INTERACTIONS
Amphotericin B, anticancer drugs, anticoagulants, anticonvulsants, oral antidiabetics, anti-infectives, any anti-inflammatory or antipain medication, antipsychotics, azathioprine, captopril, carbamazepine, cy-

because

All these drugs interact with probenecid and colchicine medications and can cause side effects. In some cases, moreover, the listed drugs can interfere with antigout medications; in other cases, the effective-

DRUG INTERACTIONS

clophosphamide, enalapril, flecainide, flucytosine, gold salts, imipenem-cilastatin, indomethacin, interferon, ketoprofen, lisinopril, maprotiline, mercaptopurine, methotrexate, nitrofurantoin, penicillamine, phenylbutazone, pimozide, plicamycin, procainamide, promethazine, radiation therapy, sulfasalazine, thyroid medications, tocainide, tricyclic antidepressants, trimeprazine, zidovudine

ness of the listed drugs is diminished by the antigout prescription.

DIET

1. Avoid coffee and other drinks with caffeine.

2. Avoid herbal teas.

1. Will interfere with medication.

2. Will heighten effect of medication excessively.

ALCOHOL AND TOBACCO

Avoid alcohol.
No problems reported with tobacco.

Alcohol will interfere with medications.

PREGNANCY

Avoid medication.

Mary cause harm to fetus.

BREAST-FEEDING

No problems reported.

AGE FACTOR

1. No studies done with children.

2. People over 60 should use cautiously.

2. Adverse and side effects of colchicine may be worse in older people.

MISSED DOSE

You can take a missed dose up to 12 hours after scheduled time. Otherwise, wait for next dose but do not double the amount taken.

OVERDOSE

Get emergency medical help immediately if patient falls into coma, suffers breathing difficulties, is extremely nervous, or has severe gastrointestinal reactions.

(continued)

STOPPING DRUG
You may not have to finish prescription if symptoms disappear, but check with your doctor.

OTHERS
Stop taking if drug causes severe stomach upset.

Do not drive or operate machinery until you have determined how medication affects you.

Drug may cause decrease in sperm count. Discuss with your physician if you are in the process of planning a family.

Discuss with your doctor regular laboratory tests to check blood count, because medication may cause anemia. Tests may also be needed to check liver and kidney functions and blood uric acid levels.

-17-

DRUGS TO TREAT CONVULSIONS AND PARKINSON'S DISEASE

As YOUR EYES pass over this page, complex inter-actions in various parts of your brain translate the images into words, the words into phrases and sentences, and all of them into the abstract processes we know as ideas and thought. As you turn a page, your brain goes into action to control the muscle movements necessary to accomplish your goal. These and millions of other activities and bodily processes depend upon the smooth movements of electrical signals and chemicals known as neuro-transmitters along the pathway of nerves that make up the brain. When all works well, you don't give the functions a second thought. But when this mam-moth communications process goes awry, trouble follows. For example, when the electrical signals burst forth in random or excessive spurts, you may suffer a seizure or a convulsion. Other malfunctions cause disorganized thoughts and uncontrolled movement. Some of these problems are hereditary; others result from head injuries, infections, cerebral palsy, mental retardation, and tumors.

Some convulsions are generalized seizures, af-fecting the whole body, while others are limited to a limb or eye or some other part of the body. Some convulsions cause a loss of consciousness;

others leave the person wide awake or produce confused behavior or an eerie stillness.

In another kind of movement disorder—Par-kinson's disease—the abnormality is in the work-ings of the chemical messenger dopamine. In the brain, dopamine moderates the activity of the nerve cells that control muscle movement. But for unknown reasons, in Parkinson's disease the cells that manufacture dopamine either slow down or stop its production. As a result, muscle activity goes out of control, resulting in the tremors and stiffness that are characteristic of the disease. As more and more dopamine-producing cells are crippled or die, the tremors and stiffness spread, forcing the person with the disease to stoop and shuffle. Some half a million people, mostly over age 55, develop Par-kinson's disease each year, and one third suffer loss of mental abilities as well as various physical disa-bilities.

The drugs used to treat convulsions and Parkinson's disease do not produce cures, but they can help bring them under control by re-storing some balance to the brain's electrical and chemical systems. Common anticonvulsant drugs include:

- **Barbiturates, phenytoin** (*Dilantin*) **and ethosuximide** (*Zarontin*), a succinimide. Researchers believe these drugs reduce seizures by interfering with or stopping the movement of electrical messages along the brain's nerves or by making nerve cells less receptive to messages. (For tabular information on barbiturates (*Donnatal*), see Chapter 31.)

- **Valproic acid (***Depakene***)** and tranquilizers like the benzodiazepines, which probably work by spurring additional production of gamma-aminobutyric acid, a neurotransmitter that the body uses to reduce electrical messages. The tranquilizers are usually reserved for seizure patients who do not respond to other medications. (For tabular information on benzodiazepines, see Chapter 22.)

To determine the most effective drug for each patient, and the dosage at which it works best and causes the fewest side effects, doctors ask the patient to try several different medications. Once the trial-and-error process has yielded the best drug, the patient must have periodic tests to make sure that the drug is present in the blood at the right levels. Fifty to 85 percent of people who have convulsions find that just one drug will control their seizures, making it possible for them to pursue normal lives. But if one drug does not work, doctors often recommend that a second one be added. Combination drug therapies help about half of those patients who do not respond to one drug alone. Anticonvulsants are available as tablets, capsules, injections, and suppositories, and are usually taken once a day. Side effects and adverse reactions may include severe liver and kidney damage, blood disorders, and lesser problems like temporary confusion.

In treating Parkinson's disease, the goal is to increase brain levels of dopamine. However, dopamine cannot be administered directly because it is unable to cross the blood-brain barrier, a system that affords the brain extra protection against outside substances. But a substance that the brain uses to make dopamine—dopa—can cross the blood-brain barrier, and **dopa-based medications** (levodopa—*Dopar, Larodopa, Sinemet)* improve mobility and reduce rigidity in patients with Parkinson's disease. Unfortunately, these drugs can cause severe psychiatric reactions and cardiac arrhythmias, and a large percentage of patients eventually develop uncontrolled movements. Some of the newer Parkinson's drugs have fewer side effects, and doctors can often reduce symptoms and side effects by combining or changing drugs.

drug or category:

LEVODOPA

condition:
PARKINSON'S DISEASE

warning

Tell your doctor if you have or have had:
- an allergic reaction to this medication, or to any preservatives or foods
- liver or kidney problems or ulcers
- skin cancer

Tell your doctor if you are likely to have surgery with general anesthesia in the near future.

Do not take this drug if you have uncontrolled narrow-angle glaucoma, or if you have taken an MAO inhibitor within two weeks.

drugs

GENERIC	BRAND	RX
levodopa	*Sinemet, Dopar, Larodopa*	Yes

form/usage

CAPSULES, TABLETS: Should be taken with high-carbohydrate foods, but not with protein, if possible.

Tablets may be crumbled. Extended-release tablets may be cut in half but should not be crushed.

when

Same times every day.

side effects and adverse reactions

Increases in blood pressure, headaches, inability to sleep, skin problems, heart rhythm irregularities, spasms of eyelids, fainting, involuntary body movements

Anemia, pain in abdomen, constipation, fatigue, vision problems, change in urine color, minor gastrointestinal problems, emotional changes

what to do

Stop taking. Get in touch with doctor immediately.

Continue taking, but discuss with your physician.

(continued)

special precautions	because

DRUG INTERACTIONS

1. Anticonvulsants, high blood pressure medications, haloperidol, methyldopa, molindone, papaverine, phenothiazines, phenytoin, rauwolfia, vitamin B_6

2. Other antiparkinsonism drugs, guanfacine

3. Albuterol

4. Tricyclic antidepressants

1. Will decrease levodopa effects.

2. Increase effect of levodopa.

3. May cause heart rhythm irregularities.

4. May cause drops in blood pressure, leading to feelings of fainting or weakness, when getting out of bed or a chair.

DIET

No restrictions, though high-protein foods should be avoided when drug is taken.

Protein may interfere with absorption of levodopa.

ALCOHOL and TOBACCO

No problems reported.

PREGNANCY

Avoid drug during first three months. Take only if absolutely necessary during last six months.

Drug has caused fetal abnormalities in animal experiments.

BREAST-FEEDING

Avoid drug or avoid nursing. Discuss with your doctor.

Medication will migrate into breast milk and could affect child.

AGE FACTOR

1. Avoid giving drug to children under 12.

2. No problems reported.

1. Safety of levodopa for those under age 12 has not been established.

MISSED DOSE

You can take a missed dose up to two hours after scheduled time. Otherwise, wait for next dose but do not double the amount taken.

OVERDOSE

Get emergency medical help immediately in case of coma, or if patient is confused or has hallucinations, an irregular heartbeat, severe gastrointestinal problems, or involuntary muscle movements.

STOPPING DRUG

Do not stop taking until you have finished prescribed amount and you have discussed this with your physician.

OTHERS

Do not drive or operate machinery until you have determined how medication affects you.

May cause decrease in sexual desire in men and women; may cause painful and long-lasting erections and may interfere with ejaculation.

Periodic laboratory tests might be necessary to check blood count, measure eye pressures, and determine blood pressure reactions to sitting, lying down, and standing.

Your physician may need to make periodic adjustments in your medication dosage over long-term usage.

drug or category:

PHENYTOIN

condition:
SEIZURES

warning

Tell your doctor if you have or have had:
- an allergic reaction to this medication, or to any preservatives or foods
- heart or liver problems, low blood pressure, diabetes

drugs

GENERIC	BRAND	RX
phenytoin	*Dilantin*, others	Yes

form/usage

TABLETS, CAPSULES, INJECTIONS, ORAL SUSPENSION:
May be taken with food or liquids.

Tablets may be crumbled. Take capsules whole.
Be sure to shake suspension thoroughly before taking.

when

One to several times a day. Follow your doctor's instructions.

side effects and adverse reactions

Bleeding problems, jaundice, abdominal pain, vision problems, hallucinations, rash

Inability to sleep, swollen breasts, headache, diarrhea, gum problems, constipation, vomiting, sedation and tiredness, impaired coordination

what to do

Stop taking. Get in touch with doctor immediately.

Continue taking, but discuss with your physician.

special precautions

DRUG INTERACTIONS
Cortisone drugs, anticoagulants, oral contraceptives, barbiturates, many others. Discuss with your doctor.

because

Toxic effects and potentially dangerous drug interactions.

DIET

No restrictions. Discuss need for vitamin and mineral supplements with your doctor.

ALCOHOL and TOBACCO

Avoid alcohol.

No problems reported with tobacco.

Alcohol enhances sedating effects of phenytoin.

PREGNANCY

Avoid drug.

Drug has caused fetal abnormalities in animal experiments. There have been reports of increased risk of fetal deformities in humans.

BREAST-FEEDING

Avoid drug or avoid nursing.

Medication will migrate into breast milk and could affect child. Discuss with your doctor. If you do take phenytoin, keep a close eye on baby for any possible side effects.

AGE FACTOR

1. Children should be observed carefully.

2. People over 60 should take cautiously.

1. Children may be prone to drug toxicity, which includes walking, speech, and behavior problems.

2. Drug may cause side effects more readily than in younger adults and may have to be taken in smaller amounts.

MISSED DOSE

If you are taking medication once a day, take missed dose as soon as you remember that same day. If you don't remember until next day, take the next scheduled dose, but do not double the amount taken.

If you take drug several times a day, take missed dose as soon as you remember, up to four hours before your next dose. If it is less than four hours before next scheduled dose, wait until next dose, but do not double amount taken.

OVERDOSE

Get emergency medical help immediately in case of coma or if patient suffers breathing difficulties or has trouble walking or talking.

(continued)

STOPPING DRUG

Do not stop taking even if you feel better until you have talked with your doctor. You may have to come off drug slowly over several months.

OTHERS

Do not drive or operate machinery until you have determined how medication affects you.

In about 10 percent of patients, medication will cause decreased sexual desire or impotence.

May increase sensitivity to sun. If you go outdoors between 10 A.M. and 3 P.M., wear protective clothing and/or sunblock.

Periodic laboratory tests might be necessary to check blood phenytoin levels, blood count, serum albumin, liver function, and levels of vitamins and minerals. X rays to check on bone density may also be required.

---

drug or category:

SUCCINIMIDE

condition:

CONVULSIONS; ALSO USED FOR SEIZURES MARKED BY MOMENTARY BREAK IN THOUGHT AND ACTIVITY

---

warning

Tell your doctor if you have or have had:
- an allergic reaction to this medication, or to any preservatives or foods
- heart, blood, or kidney disease
- serious emotional or psychiatric illnesses

---

drugs

GENERIC	BRAND	RX
ethosuximide	*Zarontin*	Yes

---

form/usage

CAPSULES AND SYRUP: Can be taken with food.

when

According to schedule prescribed by your doctor.

---

side effects and adverse reactions

Bleeding problems, emotional disturbances, sore throat

Swollen lymph nodes, gastrointestinal problems, pain in stomach, headache, moodiness, fatigue

what to do

Stop taking. Get in touch with doctor immediately.

Continue taking, but discuss with your physician.

---

special precautions

DRUG INTERACTIONS
1. Tricyclic antidepressants, antipsychotic drugs
2. Haloperidol

because

1. Could cause seizures.
2. Could decrease effect of haloperidol.

(continued)

DIET
No restrictions.

ALCOHOL and TOBACCO
Avoid alcohol.
No problems expected with tobacco.

Alcohol may enhance sedating effect of succinimide; may also cause seizures.

PREGNANCY
Avoid drug during first three months. Take during last six months only if absolutely necessary.

Drug has caused fetal abnormalities in animal experiments. There have been reports of increased risk of fetal deformations in humans.

BREAST-FEEDING
Avoid drug or avoid nursing.

Medication will migrate into breast milk and could affect child. Discuss with your doctor. If you do take phenytoin, keep a close eye on baby for any possible side effects.

AGE FACTOR
1. Drug will not cause side effects in children different from those that may arise in adults.

2. In people over 60, this drug is not likely to cause side effects that differ from those seen in younger adults.

MISSED DOSE
You can take a missed dose up to three hours after scheduled time. Otherwise, wait for next dose but do not double the amount taken.

OVERDOSE
Get emergency medical help immediately if patient goes into a coma.

STOPPING DRUG
Do not stop taking until you have talked with your doctor. If you come off drug, you may have to do so slowly.

OTHERS

Do not drive or operate machinery until you have determined how medication affects you.

Be sure to check with your doctor regularly to determine if the amount and frequency of dose needs to be changed.

Periodic laboratory tests might be necessary to check effect on liver and kidney functions.

drug or category:

VALPROIC ACID

condition:
CONVULSIONS

warning

Tell your doctor if you have or have had:
- an allergic reaction to this medication, or to any preservatives or foods
- liver, kidney, or bleeding problems
- myasthenia gravis

Tell your doctor if you are planning to have surgery or become pregnant.

drugs

GENERIC	BRAND	RX
valproic acid	*Depakene*, others	Yes

form/usage

TABLETS, CAPSULES (REGULAR AND SPRINKLE), SYRUP:
Tablets and regular capsules should be taken whole. Contents of sprinkle capsules can be put on food. Syrup can be taken with milk or water but should not be mixed with carbonated drinks.

when

One hour before meals. However, to prevent stomach irritation, may be taken with food.

side effects and adverse reactions

Vision problems; swollen feet, ankles, or abdomen; skin or bleeding problems

Fatigue; emotional, gastrointestinal, or menstrual problems

what to do

Stop taking. Get in touch with doctor immediately.

Continue taking, but discuss with your physician.

special precautions

DRUG INTERACTIONS
1. Anticoagulants, aspirin, dipyridamole, sulfinpyrazone

because

1. May cause bleeding.

DRUG INTERACTIONS
2. Depressants such as MAO inhibitors antihistamines, muscle relaxants

3. Clonazepam

4. Clozapine, flecainide, tiopronin, tocainide

5. Isoniazid

6. Primidone, *Tegretol*, phenobarbital

2. Increases sedative effect.

3. Seizures may be lengthened.

4. Production of red blood cells may be diminished.

5. May cause liver damage.

6. Possible toxicity; may exacerbate some side effects on central nervous system.

DIET
No restrictions.

ALCOHOL and TOBACCO
Avoid both.

Alcohol causes sedation.
Tobacco can decrease effect of valproic acid.

PREGNANCY
Avoid drug.

Drug has caused fetal abnormalities in animal experiments. There have been reports of increased risk of fetal deformations in humans.

BREAST-FEEDING
Avoid drug or avoid nursing.

Medication will migrate into breast milk and could affect child. Discuss with your doctor. If you do take valproic acid, keep a close eye on baby for possible side effects.

AGE FACTOR
1. Drug should be given to children very cautiously.

2. People over 60 years of age should use with care.

1. Valproic acid may cause Reye's syndrome. Children with mental retardation or other brain-related problems may be at high risk for liver damage.

2. Could cause confusion, sedation, and balance problems.

(continued)

MISSED DOSE

You can take a missed dose up to three hours after scheduled time. Otherwise, wait for next dose but do not double the amount taken.

OVERDOSE

Get emergency medical help immediately if patient goes into coma.

STOPPING DRUG

Do not stop taking until you have talked with your doctor. You may have to come off drug slowly.

OTHERS

Do not drive or operate machinery until you have determined how medication affects you.

Periodic laboratory tests are required to keep track of your blood count and liver and kidney functions. Tests may also be done before you begin taking medication.

chapter

-18-

ANTIDEPRESSANTS

FROM TIME TO time, all of us feel sad or down in the dumps, but in a few days, whatever led us to feel depressed works itself out, and things look brighter. This transient sadness should not be confused with clinical depression—a disabling disease that afflicts millions of people.

Mental health experts estimate that at any one time, at least 10 million Americans are suffering from depression serious enough to require medical treatment. The disease is more common in women than in men; experts estimate that 25 percent of women will suffer a serious depression in their lifetimes, compared to 10 percent of men. Men, however, are more likely to commit suicide, a major risk of depression.

While the causes of clinical depression are unclear, researchers believe that brain chemicals called neurotransmitters play a key role in emotional and psychological upheavals. There are scores, if not hundreds, of different kinds of neurotransmitters, but they have two main missions— to turn nerve cells on or off, thereby regulating how the brain directs many of the body's physical activities, and also how it perceives the world. It is now believed that imbalances in at least three neurotransmitters—serotonin, dopamine, and norepinephrine—can be linked to the onset of clinical depression.

Heredity is also thought to play a role in depression. Researchers who have studied identical twins have found that if one twin suffers from depression, there is a 70 percent chance that the other will be similarly affected, even if he or she was raised in a different household.

Depression occurs at any age, but is most common between the ages of 25 and 44. Still, we now know that babies can be afflicted by depression, as can the elderly. Gerontologists estimate that at least 5 percent of people 65 years or older who live independently may be suffering a serious depression, and among those in nursing homes, up to 25 percent may be afflicted. Despite the prevalence of depression, it often goes undiagnosed. For example, 85 percent of senior citizens see doctors at least once a year, but physicians fail to spot and treat depression in a large majority of their older patients.

The symptoms of clinical depression—pervasive feelings of sadness and low self-esteem, inability to cope with daily life, sleep problems, changes in eating habits, loss of interest in sex and other pleasurable activities, among others—often disappear by themselves after 6 to 12 months. In some cases, the depression alternates with unexplained euphoria, a condition referred to as manic-depression or bipolar affective disorder. For some

135

people, the depression does not recur, while others suffer frequent relapses.

Until the 1960s, depression was either ignored or treated by psychotherapy, and many severely depressed people were institutionalized. All this changed dramatically with the development of highly effective antidepressant medications such as:

- **Tricyclics** such as amitriptyline (*Elavil*)

- **Fluoxetine** (*Prozac*) and **sertraline** (*Zoloft*)

- **Monoamine oxidase (MAO) inhibitors** such as isocarboxazid (*Marplan*)

- **Lithium** (to treat the manic phase; see Chapter 22)

Although the precise role of the neurotransmitters in depression is not fully understood, the drugs prescribed to treat it work by influencing levels of neurotransmitters in the brain or their action on brain cells. Fluoxetine (*Prozac*) and sertraline (*Zoloft*)—the newest and most widely prescribed antidepressants—work by increasing serotonin levels in the brain. Tricyclics, among other things, increase the action of norepinephrine and dopamine by interfering with chemical reactions that would otherwise decrease their effectiveness. MAO inhibitors block monoamine oxidase, an enzyme that blocks norepinephrine, serotonin, and dopamine. Lithium salts, a mineral, tone down the euphoric phase of manic-depression.

The drugs, which most often are taken orally once a day, elevate and stabilize moods, but at different rates. For example, many tricyclic antidepressants take several weeks to begin working. Others provide relief in as little as two weeks. Often, a single drug, given in a standard dose, will achieve good results. But determining which drug works best, as well as optimal dosage, may require some trial and error.

Side effects of antidepressants are always a concern. Lithium administration must be closely monitored because even a slight overdose can cause problems including drowsiness, muscle twitching, and even a potentially fatal toxic reaction. MAO inhibitors can trigger abrupt mood swings and, if given to someone with schizophrenic tendencies, can lead to psychosis. When taken with aged cheese, pickled herring, red wine, and other foods high in tyramine, a sudden and dangerous rise in blood pressure may occur. Tricyclics can cause hallucinations, convulsions, and tremors. *Prozac*, today's most favored antidepressant because of its low potential for side effects, also has its downside—it can exacerbate Parkinson's disease, and it also suppresses the appetite.

In the early 1990s, *Prozac* briefly received unfavorable publicity after several reports of suicide among patients taking it. However, researchers note that virtually all antidepressant medications prompt patients to consider suicide as they begin to recover and are capable of making decisions—both good and bad. Researchers point out that there is a simple solution: Monitor the patient more closely until recovery is completed. If advisable, another drug may be substituted.

drug or category:

FLUOXETINE

condition:
DEPRESSION; MAY ALSO BE USED FOR OBSESSIVE-COMPULSIVE DISORDERS

warning

Tell your doctor if you have or have had:
- an allergic reaction to this medication, or to preservatives or food additives
- liver or kidney problems
- Seizures or Parkinson's disease

Tell your doctor if you are pregnant or are planning to become pregnant.

Do not take concurrently with MAO inhibitors.

drugs

GENERIC	BRAND	RX
fluoxetine	*Prozac*	Yes

form/usage

CAPSULES
With or without food.

Capsules may be opened and contents mixed with juice.

when

In the morning.

side effects and adverse reactions

Chills, pain in joints, excitability, hallucinations, swollen lymph glands, vision difficulties, chest pains, stomach pain, rapid heartbeat

Gastrointestinal difficulties, decreased appetite, fatigue, inability to sleep, unusual sweating

what to do

Stop taking. Get in touch with doctor immediately.

Continue taking, but discuss with your physician.

special precautions

DRUG INTERACTIONS
1. Anticoagulants, digitalis, MAO inhibitors, tryptophan

because

1. May cause agitation, confusion, convulsions, high blood pressure.

(continued)

DRUG INTERACTIONS

2. Central nervous system depressants

2. May increase depressant effect of CNS drugs and *Prozac*.

DIET

No restrictions.

ALCOHOL and TOBACCO

Avoid alcohol.
No problems with tobacco reported.

Alcohol can increase depression, cause toxicity.

PREGNANCY

No negative interactions reported, but drug should be used only if absolutely necessary.

No evidence of fetal harm was found in animals, but in humans, no adequate well-controlled studies have been done.

BREAST-FEEDING

Avoid medication or avoid nursing.

It is not known if drug migrates into breast milk.

AGE FACTOR

1. Not recommended for children.

1. Safety and effectiveness not established.

2. Adults over 60 should use cautiously.

2. Older people may have greater reactions to medication than younger adults.

MISSED DOSE

You can take a missed dose up to two hours after scheduled time. Otherwise, wait for next dose but do not double the amount taken.

OVERDOSE

Get emergency medical help immediately if patient has seizures, has violent vomiting spells or is agitated or has a severe skin reaction or breathing difficulties.

STOPPING DRUG

No problems expected if you stop before prescription runs out; however, discuss with your doctor.

OTHERS

Do not drive or operate machinery until you have determined how medication affects you. May interfere with erections in males and orgasm in men and women.

MONOAMINE OXIDASE INHIBITORS

condition:
DEPRESSION

warning

Do not combine MAO inhibitors: it may lead to convulsions and death.
Tell your doctor if you have or have had:
- an allergic reaction to this medication, or to any preservatives or foods
- a drinking problem
- heart disease, angina
- asthma or other respiratory diseases
- diabetes or high blood pressure
- kidney, thyroid, liver, or Parkinson's disease
- headaches

Medication may cause you to feel more energetic and full of health than before. If you have heart disease, do not increase your exercise regimen unless you have checked with your doctor.
Diabetics should closely monitor blood sugar levels.

drugs

GENERIC	BRAND	RX
isocarboxazid	*Marplan*	Yes
phenelzine	*Nardil*	
tranylcypromine	*Parnate*	

form/usage

TABLETS
May be taken with food or liquid.

Tablets may be crumbled.

when

Discuss with your doctor, then take at same time every day.

side effects and adverse reactions

Fainting, dilated pupils, chest pains, skin problems, slurred speech, change in urine color, headaches, gastrointestinal problems, hallucinations, nightmares, stiff neck, sensitivity to light

what to do

Stop taking. Get in touch with doctor immediately.

(continued)

side effects and adverse reactions

Lower sex drive, inability to sleep, constipation, increased desire for sweets, fatigue

what to do

Continue taking, but discuss with your physician.

special precautions

because

DRUG INTERACTIONS

1. Anticholinergics, bupropion, central nervous system depressants, ethinamate, fluoxetine, indapamide, insulin and oral antidiabetics, methyprylon, nabilone

1. Effect and side effects of these drugs will be increased.

2. Amphetamines, tricyclic antidepressants, beta-blockers, buspirone, dextromethorphan, furazolidone, guanadrel, guanethidine, levodopa, maprotiline, methyldopa, methylphenidate, narcotic pain-killers, phenylpropanolamine, pseudoephedrine, sympathomimetics, tryptophan

2. Will cause increases in blood pressure, perhaps to dangerous and life-threatening levels.

3. Anticonvulsants

3. May change the way they work.

4. High blood pressure medications, diuretics

4. May cause blood pressure to fall too low.

5. Clozapine

5. Excessive impact on central nervous system.

6. Cyclobenzaprine

6. Avoid completely because it can lead to seizures and high fever.

DIET
Your doctor or pharmacist should supply list of foods not be eaten with these medications. Generally, it is wise to avoid aged or fermented foods, smoked foods, excessively ripe fruit, caffeine-laden drinks or snacks (including chocolate).

Some foods, combined with MAO inhibitors, can cause a sudden and dangerous rise in blood pressure.

ALCOHOL and TOBACCO
Avoid alcohol, especially red wines. No reactions to tobacco reported.

With MAOs, alcohol can cause a dangerous rise in blood pressure.

PREGNANCY

Avoid drug.

Drug has caused fetal abnormalities in animal experiments. There have been reports of increased risk of fetal deformations in humans.

BREAST-FEEDING

Avoid drug or discuss with your doctor.

Medication will migrate into breast milk. No reports of effect on nursing babies.

AGE FACTOR

1. Discuss with your doctor.

1. No informational studies have been done with children.

2. Patients over 60 should use cautiously.

2. Medication may cause dizziness. Older patients react more strongly to drug.

MISSED DOSE

You can take a missed dose up to two hours after scheduled time. Otherwise, wait for next dose but do not double the amount taken.

OVERDOSE

Get emergency medical help immediately if patient falls into coma; suffers breathing difficulties, heart rhythm disturbances, or sweats; or has extreme changes in mood or behavior.

STOPPING DRUG

Do not stop taking even if you feel better until you have talked with your doctor. You may have to come off drug slowly.

OTHERS

Do not drive or operate machinery until you have determined how medication affects you.

Use caution getting up. Medication may cause dizziness or fainting when you get up from a chair or bed.

Users of this medication are often advised to carry a card informing emergency personnel of the fact. Periodic laboratory tests might be necessary to check effect on liver and kidney functions and blood pressure.

May increase sensitivity to sun. If you go outdoors between 10 A.M. and 3 P.M., wear protective clothing and/or sunblock.

drug or category:

SERTRALINE

condition:

DEPRESSION; MAY ALSO BE PRESCRIBED FOR OBSESSIVE-COMPULSIVE DISORDERS

warning

Do not take if you have taken an MAO inhibitor within two weeks.

Tell your doctor if you have or have had:

- an allergic reaction to this medication, or to any preservatives or foods
- a bad reaction to antidepressant drugs
- kidney or liver problems
- Parkinson's or convulsive disease

Tell your doctor if you are or are planning to become pregnant.

drugs

GENERIC	BRAND	RX
sertraline	Zoloft	Yes

form/usage

TABLETS

Should be taken with food.

Tablets may be crumbled.

when

Schedule is determined by your doctor.

side effects and adverse reactions

Skin problems, headache, vision problems, confusion, tremors, hallucinations, numbness or tingling in arms or legs

Dry mouth, bad taste in mouth, minor gastrointestinal problems, inability to sleep, inability to concentrate

what to do

Stop taking. Get in touch with doctor immediately.

Continue taking, but discuss with your physician.

special precautions

DRUG INTERACTIONS

I. Diazepam, tolbutamide, anticoagulants, antidiabetics

because

I. Sertraline may increase their effects.

DRUG INTERACTIONS
2. MAO inhibitors

2. Could cause dangerous reactions, including sei-zures and sudden increase in blood pressure.

DIET
No restrictions.

ALCOHOL and TOBACCO
Avoid alcohol.
No interaction with tobacco reported.

While no interactions have been noted, manufac-turer recommends that patients on *Zoloft* should not drink.

PREGNANCY
Avoid drug.

Drug has caused fetal abnormalities in animal exper-iments. Insufficient information about effect in hu-mans.

BREAST-FEEDING
Avoid drug or avoid nursing.

Insufficient information about presence in breast milk or effect on baby.

AGE FACTOR
1. Do not give to children.
2. Older adults may have to pay special attention to adjustments in dosage to prevent liver or kidney problems. However, all patients will need gradual increases in dosage to determine optimal levels.

1. Safety and effectiveness had not been estab-lished in children under 12.

MISSED DOSE
Take drug when you remember, unless it is almost time for your next dose. Do not double next dose.

OVERDOSE
Get emergency medical help immediately if patient has seizures.

STOPPING DRUG
Discuss with your doctor; however, it is not likely that there will be problems if the drug is stopped before prescription is finished or if you don't continue after prescription runs out.

(continued)

OTHERS

Do not drive or operate machinery until you have determined how medication affects you.

May cause sexual problems, including delayed ejaculation and inhibited female orgasm.

May increase sensitivity to sun. If you go outdoors between 10 A.M and 3 P.M., wear protective clothing and/or sunblock.

drug or category:

TRICYCLIC ANTIDEPRESSANTS

condition:
DEPRESSION, BEDWETTING, OBSESSIVE-COMPULSIVE DISORDERS

warning

Tell your doctor if you have or have had:
- an allergic reaction to this medication, or to any preservatives or foods
- a history of alcohol or drug abuse
- asthma
- blood illnesses, urination problems (including benign prostatic hypertrophy)
- heart, kidney, gastrointestinal, or liver disease
- glaucoma or high blood pressure
- mental illness

If you are scheduled for surgery or dental work, inform the doctor that you are taking a tricyclic antidepressant.

drugs

GENERIC	BRAND	RX
amitriptyline	*Elavil*, others	Yes
imipramine	*Tofranil*, others	
nortriptyline	*Pamelor*, others	

form/usage

SYRUPS, TABLETS, CAPSULES:
Capsules, syrups, and tablets may be taken with liquids.

when

Drugs are usually taken at bedtime. If you have been told to take your medication during the day, avoid taking it around mealtime or with snacks because many foods, from bread to peanut butter, interfere with proper absorption of tricyclics.

side effects and adverse reactions

Shaking, involuntary muscle movements, skin problems, swollen breasts, vision difficulties (including eye pain), pain, chills, pain in joints

what to do

Stop taking. Get in touch with doctor immediately.

(continued)

side effects and adverse reactions	**what to do**
Loss of sexual desire, strange dreams, stuffy nose, headache, gastrointestinal problems, sweating, sleeplessness, desire for sweets	Continue taking, but discuss with your physician.
Dry mouth	Try sugarless candy or gum. If condition persists, discuss with your doctor or dentist.

special precautions

because

DRUG INTERACTIONS

1. Anticoagulants, anticholinergics, antihistamines, barbiturates, tranquilizers, bupropion, central nervous system depressants, ethinamate, fluoxetine, methyprylon, metyrosine, molindone, nabilone, narcotics, sedatives, sympathomimetics

1. Effect and side effects of these drugs will be increased.

2. Cimetidine, dextrothyroxine, methylphenidate, phenothiazines

2. Increase tricyclic effect.

3. Clonidine, guanabenz, guanethidine, methyldopa, phenytoin

3. Effects of these drugs will be decreased.

4. Clozapine

4. Central nervous system toxicity.

5. Disulfiram, ethchlorvynol

5. May cause delirium.

6. Furazolidone, levodopa

6. Increase blood pressure.

7. Procainamide, thyroid hormones

7. Could cause irregular heart rhythm.

DIET
Avoid taking with meals or snacks.

Many foods interfere with tricyclic absorption.

ALCOHOL and TOBACCO
Avoid both.

Alcohol and tricyclics combined increase intoxication.
Nicotine may decrease effectiveness of medication.

PREGNANCY
Avoid drug.

There have been reports of increased risk of fetal deformations in humans.

BREAST-FEEDING

Avoid drug or avoid nursing.

Medication will migrate into breast milk and could affect child. Discuss with your doctor. If you do take these medications, keep a close eye on baby for any possible side effects.

AGE FACTOR

1. Give to children cautiously.

1. Children may react to medication more strongly than adults. Watch for disturbed sleep, fatigue, nervousness. Side effects usually disappear in time. Discuss with your doctor.

2. Patients over 60 should take cautiously.

2. Older people, too, are likely to react more strongly to medication than younger adults. May cause fatigue, vision problems, constipation.

MISSED DOSE

If you are on a once-a-day schedule and you miss a dose, check with your doctor.

If you are taking several doses a day, take the one you missed as soon as you remember, unless it is nearly time for your next scheduled dose. If so, wait until that dose, but do not double amount taken.

OVERDOSE

Get emergency medical help immediately if patient falls into coma, has convulsions, suffers breathing difficulties, has an irregular heart rhythm, or runs a fever.

STOPPING DRUG

Do not stop taking even if you feel better until you have talked with your doctor. You may have to come off drug slowly. Effects of medication linger up to a week after last dose.

OTHERS

Do not drive or operate machinery until you have determined how medication affects you.

May increase sensitivity to sun. If you go outdoors between 10 A.M. and 3 P.M., try to avoid bright sunlight and wear protective clothing and/or sunblock.

Medication may cause dizziness, light-headedness, and even fainting when you get up from a chair or bed; avoid getting up in one quick motion.

-19-

ANTI-INFECTIVE DRUGS

SOME INFECTIVE MICROORGANISMS—what we commonly call germs—are barely one hundred thousandth of an inch in diameter. The giants among them may be large enough to occupy half of a human blood cell. But all of them—fungi, bacteria, viruses, and parasites—can do damage that is vastly disproportionate to their size. Some cause upper respiratory infections that range from mild chest colds to severe pneumonia. Others cause relatively minor illnesses like herpes cold sores and athlete's foot, but some are responsible for deadly diseases like polio and AIDS. Depending upon the organism, they invade the body through the bloodstream, mucous membranes, skin, eyes, gastrointestinal tract, or any portal that offers protection and sustenance.

Until this century, infectious diseases were our leading cause of death, a distinction they still hold in many underdeveloped countries. But the development of an armamentarium of highly effective antimicrobial drugs, especially antibiotics, has given us an important edge in fighting these diseases.

Types of Anti-infective Drugs

The first antibacterial agents were **sulfa drugs,** introduced in 1935. These drugs—now referred to as sulfonamides (*Gantanol, Renoguid*)—were developed from a red industrial dye (prontosil) and became standard medications during World War II. Unfortunately, many organisms quickly developed resistance to sulfonamides, which limits their use. Now they are used mostly to treat urinary tract infections, although some are highly effective against skin, eye, and outer ear infections.

Antibiotics were originally derived from molds and other botanical substances, although most are now synthesized from chemicals. The first antibiotic was **penicillin,** introduced in 1941 although it had been discovered accidentally some years earlier by Sir Alexander Fleming, a British scientist. Various forms of penicillin remain our most widely used antibiotics, but in recent decades, they have been joined by these general classes of drugs.

The Problem of Growing Resistance

Doctors and researchers are increasingly alarmed by problems of growing resistance to some of our most common antibiotics. Resistance develops when microorganisms survive exposure to an antibiotic and then reproduce millions of offspring resistant to that drug. Improper use of antibiotics— taking the drugs when they are not indicated or failing to complete a course of treatment— accounts for mounting resistance. Researchers also cite overuse of antibiotics by dairy farmers and meat growers as another source of resistance. Farm animals fed antibiotics leave behind drug-resistant organisms in milk and meat. When we consume these products, the organisms enter the intestinal tract and pass their resistance on to the organisms that reside there.

Hospital patients are especially vulnerable to antibiotic-resistant infections, resulting in about 20,000 deaths a year and contributing to another 60,000 fatalities, according to the U.S. Centers for Disease Control and Prevention.

Infections that are becoming more difficult to treat because of drug resistance include:

- Staphylococcus, a potential cause of blood poisoning; resistant to all but one antibiotic, vancomycin

- Tuberculosis, with 20 percent of strains now resistant to isoniazid, the first-choice drug

- Gonorrhea, with most strains now resistant to penicillin

- Enterococcus, an intestinal infection

- Pneumococcus, which is now resistant to five types of antibiotics, including penicillin

---

- **Cephalosporins** such as cefaclor (*Ceclor*) and cefadroxil (*Duricef*), which are similar to the penicillins and effective against numerous infections. They are often used when there is penicillin resistance (see box titled The Problem of Growing Resistance) or a stronger antibiotic is needed.
- **Erythromycin** (*ERYC, E.E.S., Erythrocin*, and others), which is used for some of the same problems as the penicillins and cephalosporins, but which seems to be especially effective against the bacteria that cause strep throat, pneumonia, venereal disease, and amebic dysentery.

- **Tetracylines** (*Sumycin, Achromycin, Panmycin*), which work against the greatest number of infectious agents; their use is often limited by drug resistance.
- **Aminoglycosides,** such as neomycin and streptomycin, are also broad-spectrum antibiotics, but because they carry a significant risk of side effects, their use is rather limited. Also, some, such as streptomycin, are given only by injection.
- **Lincosamides,** such as clindamycin and lincomycin, can cause severe intestinal problems and are reserved for serious infections that do not respond to other antibiotics.

• **Ciprofloxocin** (*Cipro*) is often used for urinary, lower respiratory, and bone infections.

Anti-AIDS Drugs

The effort to find drugs effective against AIDS has been a frustrating—and largely unfruitful—one. However, there are medications now being used that seem to ameliorate for a time at least some of the illness's effects. The more popular drugs being used at the moment are **zidovudine** *(Retrovir)*, more popularly known as **AZT**; and **fluconazole** (*Diflucan*), which is used to treat some of the fungal conditions that come as a result of the body's lowered ability to fight off infections. **Ganciclovir** (*Cytovene*) has been helpful in the treatment of viral eye infections in patients with AIDS.

Antifungal and Antiviral Drugs

The burgeoning science of anti-infectives has also developed the medications needed to fight the fungi that cause annoying problems like athlete's foot, and the parasites that can cripple and kill with illnesses like malaria. In contrast, most viral infections are not vulnerable to anti-infective drugs, although **acyclovir** (*Zovirax*) and **amantadine** (*Symmetrel*) are effective against some strains.

Mechanisms of Action

Antibiotics attack microbes in different ways. Penicillin and cephalosporins inhibit bacteria from building protective walls around themselves. Erythromycin and tetracycline interfere with reproduc-

tion. Antifungal drugs interfere with the enzymes the organisms need to survive. Some drugs used to treat parasitic infestations make their way into the bodies of the organisms, and others make it impossible for parasites to use the sugars they need for food; still others insinuate themselves into the parasite's genetic materials and impair their ability to reproduce.

Antivirals like acyclovir work by interfering with the virus's ability to reproduce. How medications like amantadine work against viruses is unknown, although some researchers theorize that they strengthen human resistance against certain viruses.

Potential Side Effects

In addition to the problem of drug resistance, antibiotic use increases our vulnerability to an overgrowth of yeasts and other organisms that inhabit our bodies. This occurs when the drugs kill the beneficial bacteria that maintain a healthy balance of internal microorganisms. Thus, antibiotic therapy often sets the stage for yeast infections in the mouth, intestinal tract, rectum, and vagina.

Other side effects of antibiotics range from severe allergic reactions to diarrhea, nausea and vomiting, rashes, and other relatively minor problems.

Antifungals sometimes cause mild allergic reactions and vomiting, but otherwise are relatively safe drugs. Medications used to kill parasites sometimes cause dizziness, blurred vision, abdominal pain, and diarrhea, but again, are quite safe.

Antiviral agents may cause nausea, acne and hair loss, light-headedness, allergic reactions, and some mild pain or burning at the site where they are administered.

drug or category:

CEPHALOSPORINS

condition:
INFECTIONS

warning

Tell your doctor if you have or have had:
- an allergic reaction to this medication, or to any preservatives or foods
- an allergic reaction to penicillin
- bleeding disorders
- kidney, liver, or gastrointestinal problems

Medication may cause diarrhea. Consult your doctor and do not take antidiarrheals unless specifically told to do so.

Medication may interfere with blood test for sugar. Diabetics should not change diet or antidiabetic medications on the basis of results or tests done while taking this drug. Consult your doctor.

drugs

GENERIC	BRAND	RX
cefaclor	Ceclor	Yes
cefadroxil	Duricef	
cefuroxime	Ceftin	
cephalexin	Keflex	

form/usage

TABLETS, CAPSULES, ORAL SUSPENSIONS, INJECTIONS:
May be taken with or without food.

when

Generally, either one hour before eating or two hours after meals.

side effects and adverse reactions

Severe allergic reaction (anaphylactic shock)

Itching in rectum, white spots on mouth (or vagina), mild diarrhea

what to do

Get emergency medical help immediately.

Continue taking, but discuss with your physician.

(continued)

special precautions

because

DRUG INTERACTIONS

1. Anticoagulants, probenecid

2. Erythromycin, chloramphenicol, clindamycin, tetracyclines

3. Nonsteroidal anti-inflammatory agents

1. Cephalosporins increase their effects.

2. Decrease effectiveness of cephalosporins.

3. Increase risk of ulcers.

DIET

Generally, no restrictions, but food may decrease absorption if medication is taken within two hours of eating.

ALCOHOL AND TOBACCO

Avoid alcohol and any medications containing alcohol (cough medicines, for example) while taking cephalosporins and for several days after you have stopped prescription.

No interaction reported with tobacco.

Alcohol may cause severe gastrointestinal problems, heart rhythm abnormalities, headaches, or fainting.

PREGNANCY

Discuss with your doctor.

Drug has caused problems in animal experiments, including fetal defects and pregnancy difficulties. There have been no reports of increased risk of fetal deformations in humans.

BREAST-FEEDING

Discuss with your doctor.

Medication will migrate into breast milk and could affect child.

AGE FACTOR

In children over age of one and in older adults, cephalosporins reportedly do not act differently than they do in others.

MISSED DOSE

It is important that you do not miss a dose. However, if you are on a one-dose-a-day schedule, take the missed dose as soon as you remember, take the next one 10 to 12 hours later, then return to regular schedule. Do not double any dose.

If you are taking two doses a day, take missed dose as soon as you remember and the next dose five to six hours later, then return to regular schedule. Do not double dose.

OVERDOSE

Get in touch with a poison control center, emergency room, or doctor if there are severe neurological and gastrointestinal problems, including blood in stool.

STOPPING DRUG

Do not stop taking even if you feel better until you have finished prescription.

drug or category:

ERYTHROMYCIN

condition:
INFECTIONS

warning

Tell your doctor if you have or have had an allergic reaction to this medication, or to preservatives or food additives.

May cause diarrhea. Consult your doctor and do not take antidiarrheals unless specifically advised to do so.

drugs

GENERIC	BRAND	RX
erythromycin	ERYC, Ery-Tab, E-Mycin, others	Yes
erythromycin ethylsuccinate	E.E.S., EryPed, others	
erythromycin stearate	Erythrocin, My-E, others	

form/usage

CAPSULES, TABLETS (INCLUDING CHEWABLE FORMS), ORAL SUSPENSIONS: May be taken with food to prevent stomach irritation.

Chewable tablets must be chewed (or crushed) thoroughly before swallowing. Regular tablets may be crushed as well. Extended-release formulations must be taken whole.

For all other formulations, follow instructions of doctor or those on package.

Liquid forms should be stored in refrigerator.

when

If doses are to be taken four times a day, that means every six hours. Consult with your doctor if this disturbs your sleep pattern.

side effects and adverse reactions

Loss of hearing, jaundice, diarrhea, cramps, vomiting, skin problems

Feelings of fatigue, dry or itchy skin, nausea

what to do

Stop taking. Get in touch with doctor immediately.

Continue taking, but discuss with your physician.

special precautions	**because**
DRUG INTERACTIONS Theophylline, cyclosporine	May increase effectiveness of these drugs.
DIET 1. Avoid wine. 2. Don't have any acid fruit or juice within one hour of taking medication. 3. Avoid drinks with caffeine.	1. Will decrease effect of medication. 2. Will decrease effectiveness of drug. 3. Erythromycin will increase toxicity of caffeine.
ALCOHOL AND TOBACCO Avoid alcohol. No negative interaction with tobacco reported.	Alcohol combined with erythromycin can increase risk of liver damage.
PREGNANCY Discuss with your doctor.	Has been reported to cause liver damage in some pregnant women; however, no harm reported to fetus.
BREAST-FEEDING No problems reported, although drug does pass into breast milk.	
AGE FACTOR Reactions of children and older adults to medication are not significantly different from reactions reported among others.	

MISSED DOSE

Take a missed dose as soon as you remember, but do not double amount.

If you are on a twice-a-day schedule, after you have taken the missed dose, wait five to six hours before taking next dose. Then return to regular schedule.

If you are on a schedule of three or four doses a day, after you have taken the missed dose, wait five to six hours before taking next dose. Then return to regular schedule.

(continued)

OVERDOSE
Get in touch with poison control center, emergency room, or doctor if you have severe gastrointestinal problems.

STOPPING DRUG
Do not stop taking even if you feel better until you have finished the prescription.

OTHERS
In rare cases, medication has been reported to cause hearing loss.

Erythromycin may increase the risk of liver damage. You may require tests to determine effect on liver.

PENICILLINS

condition:
INFECTIONS

warning

Tell your doctor if you have or have had:
- an allergic reaction to this medication, or to preservatives or food additives
- kidney disease

Penicillin can cause diarrhea. Tell your doctor if this happens and do not take antidiarrheal medicine unless told to do so.

Medication may interfere with blood test for sugar. Diabetics should not change diet or antidiabetic medications on the basis of results of tests done while taking this drug. Consult your doctor.

If you are allergic to penicillin, carry a medical information card stating so.

drugs

GENERIC	BRAND	RX
amoxicillin	*Amoxil, Augmentin, Polymox*, others	Yes
penicillin V	*Pen•Vee K, Veetids*, others	

form/usage

CAPSULES, TABLETS (INCLUDING CHEWABLE), ORAL SUSPENSIONS, INJECTIONS: May be taken on empty stomach with 8 ounces of water.

Some types of penicillin should not be taken within an hour of acid fruits, juices, or drinks.

Regular tablets may be crushed. Chewable tablets should be chewed thoroughly before swallowing. Capsules should not be opened. Liquids should be taken with a cold nonacidic drink.

Keep oral suspensions in refrigerator.

when

Preferably an hour or two before eating.

(continued)

side effects and adverse reactions

Severe allergic reaction (anaphylactic shock)

Bleeding, sore throat, cramps, convulsions, blood in urine, swelling of face and ankles

Mild gastrointestinal problems, change in coloration of tongue

what to do

Get emergency medical help immediately.

Stop taking. Get in touch with doctor immediately.

Continue taking, but discuss with your physician.

special precautions

DRUG INTERACTIONS
1. Beta-blockers

2. Chloramphenicol, erythromycins, loperamide, paromomycin, sodium medications, tetracyclines, troleandomycin

3. Oral contraceptives

4. Probenecid

DIET
No restrictions.

ALCOHOL AND TOBACCO
No problems reported.

PREGNANCY
No reported problems in humans. No problems in animals in doses up to 25 times the usual amount given to humans.

BREAST-FEEDING
Avoid drug or avoid nursing.

because

1. May cause anaphylactic shock (extreme allergic reaction).

2. Effectiveness of penicillin, of other drugs, or of both may be decreased.

3. Decreased contraceptive effectiveness

4. May increase effectiveness of probenecid and penicillins.

Penicillins can pass into breast milk and cause allergic reactions, diarrhea, and other problems in infant.

AGE FACTOR

1. Children should be watched for diarrhea.

2. Older adults may experience itching skin.

If either of these conditions occurs, stop taking and get in touch with doctor or pharmacist.

MISSED DOSE

Take it as soon as you remember, but do not double amount. If you are on a twice-a-day schedule, after you have taken the missed dose, wait five to six hours before taking next dose. Then return to regular schedule.

If you are on a schedule of three or four doses a day, after you have taken the missed dose, wait five to six hours before taking next dose. Then return to regular schedule.

OVERDOSE

Get in touch with poison control center, emergency room, or doctor if there are severe gastrointestinal or neurological problems.

STOPPING DRUG

Do not stop taking even if you feel better until you have finished the prescription.

OTHERS

In rare instances penicillins may cause dizziness.

You may need laboratory tests to check on blood count and kidney function.

drug or category:

TETRACYCLINES

condition:
INFECTIONS

warning

Tell your doctor if you have or have had:
- an allergic reaction to this medication, or to any preservatives or foods
- kidney or liver disease
- water diabetes

If you are scheduled to have surgery with general anesthesia, inform the surgeon (or dentist) that you are taking tetracyclines.

drugs

GENERIC	BRAND	RX
tetracycline	*Sumycin*, others	Yes
minocycline	*Minocin*	

form/usage

TABLETS, CAPSULES, LIQUIDS: Should be taken on an empty stomach. May be taken with some food to avoid stomach irritation, but avoid milk or other dairy products. Tablets can be crushed and capsules opened.

when

One hour before meals or two hours afterward.

side effects and adverse reactions

Severe allergic reaction (anaphylactic shock)

Rash, severe headaches or feeling of pressure in head, vision problems, rectal and genital itching, severe gastrointestinal problems, mouth rash, discoloration of infant's or child's teeth

Vaginal discharge, thirst, increased need to urinate, darkened tongue, gastrointestinal problems, dizziness, fungal infections

what to do

Get emergency medical help immediately.

Stop taking. Get in touch with doctor immediately.

Continue taking, but discuss with your physician.

special precautions	because
DRUG INTERACTIONS	
1. Antacids, calcium supplements, choline and magnesium salicylates, magnesium salicylates, laxatives with magnesium, sodium bicarbonate, iron supplements	1. If you are taking tetracyclines by mouth, do not use these products within one to two hours of taking medication because they may interfere with effect. Iron supplements should not be taken within two to three hours of tetracycline.
2. Oral contraceptives with estrogen	2. May not work effectively with medication.
3. Anticoagulants, digitalis, lithium	3. Effects of drugs may be increased.
4. Cefixime, desmopressin, penicillin	4. Effectiveness of drugs is diminished.
5. Cholestyramine, colestipol	5. Decrease tetracycline effect.
6. Tiopronin	6. May increase toxicity, damaging liver.
7. Etretinate	7. Tetracyclines may cause increased reactions to etretinate.
DIET	
Avoid milk and other dairy products within one to two hours of taking drug.	Dairy products interfere with absorption of medication.
ALCOHOL AND TOBACCO	
Avoid alcohol. No problems reported with tobacco.	Alcohol may increase risk of liver damage.
PREGNANCY	
Avoid drug during last five months.	Animal studies show that drug may cause abnormalities such as tooth discoloration, retarded skeletal development, and even fetal death.
BREAST-FEEDING	
Avoid drug or avoid nursing.	Medication will migrate into breast milk and affect child.
AGE FACTOR	
1. Do not give to children under eight years old.	1. Drug will discolor teeth, slow bone growth.

(continued)

AGE FACTOR

2. Adults over 60 should use cautiously.

2. Older adults may have to take the drug in smaller doses. May cause rectal itching.

MISSED DOSE

It is important not to miss a dose. However, if you are on a one-dose-a-day schedule, take the missed dose as soon as you remember, and take the next one 10 to 12 hours later; then return to regular schedule. Do not double any doses.

If you are on a two-a-day schedule, take the missed dose as soon as you remember, and the next dose five to six hours later; then return to regular schedule. Do not double dose.

If you are taking the drug three or more times a day, take the missed dosage as soon as you remember, and take the next dose two to four hours later. Do not double dose.

OVERDOSE

Get in touch with poison control center, emergency room, or doctor in case of severe gastrointestinal reactions.

STOPPING DRUG

Do not stop taking even if you feel better until you have finished medication.

OTHERS

May increase sensitivity to sun. If you go outdoors between 10 A.M. and 3 P.M., wear protective clothing and sunblock.

Periodic laboratory tests might be necessary to check blood count and liver and kidney function.

Tetracyclines degrade over time into harmful substances. It is important to discard any old capsules or tablets that may be in your medicine chest.

CIPROFLOXACIN

condition:

INFECTIONS, ESPECIALLY OF URINARY AND LOWER RESPIRATORY TRACTS AND BONES

warning

Tell your doctor if you have or have had:

- allergic reactions to this medication or to similar drugs
- liver or kidney function problems
- a stroke or any nervous system problems

Tell your doctor if you are taking probenecid or theophylline.

drugs

GENERIC	BRAND	RX
ciprofloxacin	Cipro	Yes

form/usage

TABLETS: Take with a full glass of water. Should be taken on an empty stomach but may be taken with food.

Tablets may be crushed.

when

Two hours after meals, or according to your doctor's instructions.

side effects and adverse reactions

Severe allergic reaction, including fainting

Gastrointestinal problems, including diarrhea and vomiting; restlessness, confusion, hallucinations; blood in urine or pain while urinating; vision problems

Mild rash, inability to sleep, headache

what to do

Get emergency medical help immediately.

Stop taking. Get in touch with doctor immediately.

Continue taking, but discuss with your physician.

(continued)

special precautions	because
DRUG INTERACTIONS	
1. Antacids, probenecid	1. May cause kidney problems. Antacids containing aluminum or magnesium may interfere with drug's effectiveness. Probenecid may increase effect of drug.
2. Theophylline, cyclosporine	2. Effect of theophylline and cyclosporine may be increased and lead to toxicity. May also cause central nervous system problems.
DIET	
No problems reported.	
ALCOHOL AND TOBACCO	
Avoid both.	Could cause central nervous system toxicity.
PREGNANCY	
Avoid drug.	Inadequate information about effect, but animal studies show abnormal bone development in fetus.
BREAST-FEEDING	
Avoid drug or avoid nursing.	Drug migrates to breast milk.
AGE FACTOR	
1. Not recommended for children.	1. May impair bone development.
2. Older adults should use with caution.	2. In older adults, side effects and adverse reactions may be increased.

MISSED DOSE

Take as soon as you remember, up to two hours after scheduled dose. Otherwise, wait for next dose, but do not double the amount taken.

OVERDOSE

Get emergency medical help immediately in case of convulsions.

STOPPING DRUG

Don't stop taking without consulting your doctor. You may have to come off drug slowly.

OTHERS

Do not drive or operate machinery until you have determined how medication affects you.

May cause eye sensitivity to sun. Wear sunglasses outdoors.

Inform doctors that you are taking this drug because it could interfere with accuracy of some laboratory tests.

---

drug or category:

ZIDOVUDINE (AZT)

condition:
HIV INFECTION

Warning

Does not cure AIDS and does not decrease risk of transmitting HIV virus to others.
Tell your physician if you have or have had:
• an allergic reaction to this medication, or to preservatives or dyes
• anemia
May suppress bone marrow activity.

---

drugs

GENERIC	BRAND	RX
zidovudine	*Retrovir*	Yes

---

form/usage

CAPSULES, SYRUP, INJECTIONS: Should be taken on an empty stomach, but may be taken with food to reduce stomach irritation. However, avoid taking with high-fat foods.

Capsules may be opened and medication mixed with food.

If you take the syrup, use a precise measuring spoon to determine dose.

when

Dosage must be tailored by your physician because of the potential risk of side effects.

---

side effects and adverse reactions

Swollen tongue or lips, twitching, tremors, confusion, speech difficulties

Severe gastrointestinal problems, unusual bleeding

Minor gastrointestinal problems, headache, insomnia, nervousness, skin problems, muscle aches, fever, sweats, shortness of breath, tiredness

what to do

Get emergency medical help immediately.

Stop taking. Get in touch with doctor immediately.

Continue taking, but discuss with your physician.

special precautions	because
DRUG INTERACTIONS	
1. Acetaminophen, aspirin, benzodiazepines, cimetidine, indomethacin, morphine, probenecid, sulfonamides	1. May increase zidovudine toxicity.
2. Acyclovir	2. Lethargy.
3. Drugs that suppress bone marrow activity, clozapine, levamisole, tiopronin	3. May cause bone marrow poisoning.
4. Ganciclovir, thioguanine	4. Toxicity of both drugs is increased.
5. Ribavirin	5. Decreases effectiveness of zidovudine.
DIET No interactions.	
ALCOHOL AND TOBACCO No problems reported.	
PREGNANCY Consult your physician. Your physician may recommend AZT during pregnancy if you are HIV-positive to reduce the possibility that the virus will be transmitted to the fetus.	Animal studies have not linked AZT to birth defects; however, no human studies have been done.
BREAST-FEEDING Avoid drug or avoid nursing.	Not known if drug migrates to breast milk.
AGE FACTOR 1. Babies may need lower dose.	1. Insufficient data exists to recommend a dosage for infants and the effects are unkown.
2. Older adults may require lower doses.	2. Decreased kidney function slows elimination from body.
MISSED DOSE Take when you remember, unless close to time of next dose; then wait for next scheduled dose. Do not double dose.	

(continued)

OVERDOSE

Get emergency medical help immediately in case of seizures, inability to walk correctly, uncontrollable vomiting.

STOPPING DRUG

Do not stop taking without consulting your doctor.

OTHERS

Do not drive or operate machinery until you have determined how medication affects you.

You may need periodic blood tests to check for anemia.

drug or category:

FLUCONAZOLE

condition:
FUNGAL INFECTIONS, INCLUDING AIDS-RELATED FUNGAL CONDITIONS (TREATMENT AND PREVENTION); ALSO USED FOR MENINGITIS

warning

Tell your doctor if you have or have had:
- an allergic reaction to this drug or similar medications
- kidney or liver problems

Advise your dentist that you are taking this drug.

drugs

GENERIC	BRAND	RX
fluconazole	*Diflucan*	Yes

form/usage

TABLETS: Take on an empty stomach, but may be taken with food to avoid stomach irritation. May be taken with milk.

Tablets may be crushed to ease ingestion.

when

Once daily.

side effects and adverse reactions

Allergic reactions, including severe skin rashes or blistering

Gastrointestinal problems, including vomiting, diarrhea, and nausea; headaches; mild skin reactions

what to do

Stop taking. Get in touch with doctor immediately.

Continue taking, but discuss with your physician.

(continued)

special precautions

because

DRUG INTERACTIONS

1. Antidiabetes drugs

1. Fluconazole may increase their action and lead to hypoglycemia.

2. Cyclosporine, phenytoin, warfarin

2. Drug may increase their effects.

3. Rifampin

3. May decrease effectiveness of fluconazole.

DIET

No interactions with any foods or beverages.

ALCOHOL AND TOBACCO

No problems reported.

PREGNANCY

Consult with your doctor.

No information on effects of drug on pregnant women. However, drug has caused fetal abnormalities in rat studies.

BREAST-FEEDING

Avoid drug or avoid nursing.

Unknown whether drug migrates to breast milk.

AGE FACTOR

1. For children under 13 consult with your doctor.

1. Safety and effectiveness have not been established in children.

2. Older adults may require lower doses.

2. Decreased kidney function may slow elimination from body.

MISSED DOSE

Take a missed dose as soon as you remember, up to two hours after scheduled time. Otherwise, wait to take your next dose, but do not double amount taken.

OVERDOSE

Get in touch with a poison control center, emergency room, or doctor if you exhibit paranoid behavior and develop hallucinations, or if you think you have accidentally taken exceeded dosage.

STOPPING DRUG

Don't stop taking without discussing with your physician.

OTHERS

Your doctor may recommend periodic liver or kidney function tests.

drug or category:

GANCICLOVIR

condition:

VIRAL EYE INFECTIONS IN PATIENTS WITH COMPROMISED IMMUNE SYSTEMS, INCLUDING THOSE WITH AIDS

warning

Tell your physician if you have or have had:
- an allergic reaction to this medication or acyclovir, or to preservatives or dyes
- kidney disease

drugs

GENERIC	BRAND	RX
ganciclovir	*Cytovene*	Yes

form/usage

when

INJECTIONS: Under your doctor's supervision.

side effects and adverse reactions

what to do

Blood in urine or stool or other unexplained bleeding, pain in bones, chills, fever

Stop taking. Get in touch with doctor immediately.

Minor gastrointestinal problems, rash, confusion, fatigue, weakness

Continue taking, but discuss with your physician.

special precautions

because

DRUG INTERACTIONS
1. Dapsone, pentamidine, flucytosine, vincristine, vinblastine, *Adriamycin*, amphotericin B, trimethoprim/sulfa combination drugs

1. May cause toxicity.

2. Imipenem, cilastatin

2. May cause seizures.

DRUG INTERACTIONS
3. Probenecid, other drugs that have impact on kidneys

3. Ganciclovir could accumulate in the kidneys.

DIET
No major interactions.

ALCOHOL AND TOBACCO
No major interactions.

PREGNANCY
Avoid drug.

May lead to fetal abnormalities.

BREAST-FEEDING
Avoid nursing and do not resume breast-feeding until 72 hours after drug has been discontinued.

Drug will migrate into breast milk and harm infant.

AGE FACTOR
1. Give to children only if benefits outweigh risks.

1. Long-term use is associated with increased risk of cancer.

2. People over 60 should use cautiously.

2. Decreased kidney function in older people may increase side effects by slowing elimination from body.

MISSED DOSE
Consult your physician.

OVERDOSE
Get emergency medical help immediately in case of disturbed heart rhythm, psychotic reactions, or coma.

STOPPING DRUG
Do not stop taking without consulting your physician.

OTHERS
You may need periodic laboratory tests to check for possible anemia and other blood problems, as well as periodic eye exams to test your vision.

Because drug is associated with birth defects, men and women should use barrier contraceptives during therapy.

drug or category:

ACYCLOVIR

condition:

VIRAL INFECTIONS

warning

Tell your doctor if you have or have had:
- an allergic reaction to this medication, or to any preservatives or foods
- kidney or nerve disease

drugs

GENERIC	BRAND	RX
acyclovir	*Zovirax*	Yes

form/usage

CAPSULES, TABLETS, SUSPENSION, OINTMENTS: Tablets and capsules may be taken with food or liquid. Suspension may be taken with liquid.

Tablets may be crushed and capsules may be opened.

Use ointment as directed.

when

As directed by your doctor or label. For herpes, should be taken as soon as possible after disease erupts.

side effects and adverse reactions

Stomach pains, severe gastrointestinal problems, bloody urine, breathing problems, confusion, dizziness, inability to sleep

Skin problems, headache, diarrhea, pain in joints

what to do

Stop taking. Get in touch with doctor immediately.

Continue taking, but discuss with your physician.

special precautions	**because**
DRUG INTERACTIONS	
1. Interferon, methotrexate	1. Oral acyclovir will cause neurological problems in combination with these drugs.
2. Antibiotics, probenecid, tiopronin, and other drugs that can have an impact on kidneys	2. Oral acyclovir will increase risk of kidney damage.
DIET	
No problems reported.	
ALCOHOL AND TOBACCO	
No problems reported.	
PREGNANCY	
Avoid drug.	Studies of effects on pregnant women are inconclusive.
BREAST-FEEDING	
Avoid oral forms of drug or avoid nursing (ointments pose no problems).	Medication will migrate into breast milk and could affect child. Discuss with your doctor.
AGE FACTOR	
Side effects in children and people over 60 have not been shown to be significantly different from those experienced by young adults.	

MISSED DOSE

Take a missed dose up to two hours after scheduled time. Otherwise, wait for next dose but do not double the amount taken.

You may apply ointments as soon as you remember.

OVERDOSE

Get emergency medical help immediately if patient has hallucinations, seizures, kidney failure.

STOPPING DRUG

Do not stop taking even if you feel better until you have finished prescription.

(continued)

OTHERS

If used for herpes, keep affected area clean and dry. Use gloves when applying. Keep out of eyes.

Check with your doctor if symptoms do not improve within a week.

Periodic laboratory tests might be necessary to check effect on kidneys.

---

drug or category:

AMANTADINE

c o n d i t i o n :

TO PREVENT OR TREAT TYPE A INFLUENZA (WILL NOT WORK AGAINST OTHER FLUS, COLDS, OR OTHER VIRAL INFECTIONS); ALSO USED ALONE OR IN COMBINATION WITH OTHER DRUGS TO TREAT PARKINSON'S DISEASE

warning

Tell your doctor if you have or have had:
- an allergic reaction to this medication, or to any preservatives or foods
- kidney or liver disease
- ulcers
- mental illness or emotional problems

Amantadine may worsen eczema, frequency of seizures.

drugs

GENERIC	BRAND	RX
amantadine	*Symmetrel, Symadine*	Yes

form/usage

CAPSULES, SYRUP: May be taken with food or liquids to lessen stomach upset.

Syrup should be mixed into a beverage.

when

Take at beginning of flu season or as soon as you have been exposed to Type A flu.

side effects and adverse reactions

Rash, fever, rolling of eyes, heart rhythm disturbances, slurred speech, urination difficulties, hallucinations

Constipation, headaches, light dizziness, loss of appetite

Dry mouth

what to do

Stop taking. Get in touch with doctor immediately.

Continue taking, but discuss with your physician.

Try sugarless candy or gum. If condition persists, discuss with your doctor or dentist.

(continued)

special precautions	**because**

DRUG INTERACTIONS

1. Amphetamines, anticholinergics, diet pills, levodopa, sympathomimetics

2. Parkinson's drugs, antihistamines, phenothiazines, tricyclic antidepressants

1. Will increase effect of amantadine and may also cause agitation.

2. Will result in nightmares, hallucinations, confusion, and other mental disturbances.

DIET

No restrictions.

ALCOHOL AND TOBACCO

Avoid alcohol. No problems reported with tobacco.

Alcohol combined with amantadine will increase intoxication.

PREGNANCY

Avoid drug.

Drug has caused fetal abnormalities in animal experiments.

BREAST-FEEDING

Avoid drug or avoid nursing.

Medication will migrate into breast milk. Effects on baby are not known.

AGE FACTOR

1. Children over one year of age react to drug in same manner as adults.

2. People over 60 should use cautiously.

2. Adverse and side effects may be worse in older people. Risk of vision problems, problems with urination, constipation, and confusion is increased.

MISSED DOSE

Take a missed dose as soon as you remember, up to four hours after scheduled time. Otherwise, wait for next dose but do not double the amount taken.

OVERDOSE

Get medical help immediately if patient has convulsions, heart rhythm irregularities, psychotic episode, drop in blood pressure.

STOPPING DRUG

If you are taking the drug for Parkinson's disease, do not stop taking even if you feel better until you have talked with your doctor.

If you are taking drug for flu, wait until 48 hours after last traces of illness have disappeared before stopping.

OTHERS

Do not drive or operate machinery until you have determined how medication affects you.

Parkinson's patients who get relief from amantadine should be careful to get back to regular physical activity slowly in order to give sense of balance and coordination a chance to adjust. If medicine seems to become less effective as time goes by, check with your doctor to have dose changed.

Getting up from a sitting or lying position may make you dizzy. Rise slowly from bed or chair. Check with your doctor if condition does not improve after a few days.

Periodic laboratory tests might be necessary to check white blood cell count and liver and kidney function. You may also need tests to evaluate heart function.

-20-

ANTIHYPERTENSIVE DRUGS

BLOOD PRESSURE IS the amount of force that is exerted against an artery wall as blood flows through it. When you have your blood pressure measured, your doctor records two numbers, such as 120/80. In this case, 120 represents the systolic pressure, the maximum amount of force that is exerted when the heart contracts and pumps blood into the circulation, and 80 is the diastolic pressure, or the amount of force exerted when the heart rests momentarily between beats.

At least 50 million Americans—or one fourth of all adults—have high blood pressure, according to 1994 statistics from the American Heart Association. By age 65, about half of all Americans have high blood pressure—defined by a reading above 140/90—with women slightly outnumbering men. African Americans are also more likely to have high blood pressure than Caucasians.

High blood pressure, or hypertension, is often referred to as a silent killer because it does not produce symptoms in its early stages. In fact, it is estimated that 35 percent of the people who have hypertension are unaware that they have elevated blood pressure. More than half of those with high blood pressure are untreated, 28 percent are inadequately treated, and only 21 percent have their high blood pressure under control.

The toll of untreated high blood pressure is well known; hypertension is the leading cause of stroke and also a major risk factor for a heart attack. High blood pressure can also cause kidney failure, an effect that is especially devastating to African-Americans between the ages of 24 and 44, who are 18 times more likely to suffer kidney failure induced by high blood pressure than whites.

Still, great strides have been made to control this disease since 1951, when the first antihypertensive drug was introduced. Since then, dozens of highly effective antihypertensive medications have become available, and today physicians can devise a regimen for almost all hypertensive patients that lowers their blood pressure with minimal side effects. Of course, not all people with mild to moderate high blood pressure actually need drugs; in some cases weight loss, increased exercise, and salt restriction can return blood pressure to normal. Eventually, however, even these people may require drugs.

Classes of Antihypertensive Drugs

- **Diuretics.** These are among the oldest antihypertensive drugs and are still widely used, although today they are usually prescribed in low doses with other antihypertensive drugs.

There are two major types of diuretics to treat high blood pressure—the **thiazides,** such as *HydroDIURIL, Hygroton,* and *Esidrix,* and the **loop diuretics**, such as *Lasix* and *Bumex.* Both lower blood pressure by removing excess fluids and sodium from the body, thereby reducing the total volume of blood. The thiazides, which are the more widely used, act on the network of tubules that transport urine in the kidneys. The more potent loop diuretics work in the loop of Henle—the area where waste products are filtered from the blood. A new class of diuretics are the indolines, which not only increase excretion of salt and water, but also relax the walls of small arteries. These drugs include indapamide (*Lozol*).

- **Beta-adrenergic blocking drugs,** or simply, **beta-blockers.** These are the second most prescribed antihypertensive drugs. They work through the autonomic nervous system and lower blood pressure by slowing the heart rate and the force of the heart beat. Beta-blockers are also prescribed to treat angina because they reduce the amount of oxygen needed by the heart muscle, thereby alleviating chest pains that develop when the coronary arteries cannot supply adequate blood to the heart muscle (see Chapter 25). Propranolol (*Inderal*) is the oldest beta-blocker, but at least a dozen more, including atenolol (*Tenormin*) and metoprolol succinate (*Toprol-XL*), are now available.

- **Calcium channel blockers.** These drugs lower blood pressure by blocking the entry of small amounts of calcium into the blood vessel wall. Muscles need calcium in order to constrict; when calcium is blocked, vessels widen, or dilate, lowering blood pressure. The blockers include diltiazem (*Cardizem*),

nifedipine (*Procardia*), verapamil (*Calan*), and others.

- **Angiotensin-converting enzyme (ACE) inhibitors.** These medications block the production of angiotensin II, a body chemical that constricts blood vessels and raises blood pressure. ACE inhibitors include captopril (*Capoten*), enalapril (*Vasotec*), and others.

- **Vasodilators.** These drugs act directly on the blood vessels to dilate them, or open them wider, allowing more blood to flow through the arteries with less pressure. Hyralazine (*Apresoline*) is the oldest member of this class. Vasodilators are usually given with a beta-blocker, or a diuretic, and some, such as nitroprusside (*Nipride*), are given by injection to lower pressure rapidly during a hypertensive crisis.

- **Alpha-blocking drugs.** These block nerve receptors on the blood vessel walls that constrict the arteries. Prazosin (*Minipress*) is the most used drug in this class. Terazosin (*Hytrin*) is also an oft-used alpha-blocker.

- **Peripheral adrenergic antagonists.** These drugs lower blood pressure by blocking the release of norepinephrine—a body chemical that raises blood pressure in response to stress—from the sympathetic nerve endings. Drugs in this category include reserpine, a drug made from the rauwolfia plant, which herbalists in India have used for centuries as a sedative.

- **Centrally acting drugs,** or **central alpha-blockers.** These medications lower blood pressure by blocking some of the nerve impulses from the brain to the sympathetic nervous system, thereby dilating the small peripheral arteries. These drugs include methyldopa (*Aldomet*), clonidine (*Catapres*), and guanabenz (*Wytensin*). They are usually used with a diuretic or other antihypertensive.

- **Potassium supplements.** Patients taking diuretics often need to take extra potassium—a mineral essential for proper heart and muscle function—because diuretics can wash it out of the body along with salts and fluids. Increasing your intake of high-potassium foods like bananas, tomatoes, and grains is insufficient to supplement your potassium levels, so your doctor may recommend potassium supplements.

Although these drugs do not cure hypertension, once the right medication or combination is found, they lower blood pressure enough to cut the risk of stroke, heart attacks, and other complications. Fine-tuning is needed, however, to minimize side effects, which include light-headedness, sleep problems, depression, lethargy, increased sun sensitivity, and sexual dysfunction. Even if side effects develop, do not stop taking the medications. Instead, talk to your doctor—a different dosage or alternative drug usually solves the problem.

Remember, too, that in 95 percent of cases, hypertension is a lifelong disease without an identifiable cause. This means that the drugs usually must be taken for life. Exceptions are some cases of secondary hypertension that are caused by a treatable disorder or circumstance such as a narrowed renal artery in a kidney or the use of birth control pills.

ANGIOTENSIN-CONVERTING ENZYME (ACE) INHIBITORS

condition:
HIGH BLOOD PRESSURE (HYPERTENSION), CONGESTIVE HEART FAILURE

warning

Tell your doctor if you have or have had:
- an allergic reaction to this medication, or to any preservatives or foods
- diabetes, systemic lupus erythematosus
- kidney or liver disease
- cardiovascular problems, including heart attack or stroke

Do not take diet pills, asthma medications, antihistamines, or sinus medications since they can increase blood pressure.

Be sure to tell doctors or dentists that you are taking this medication if you are scheduled for surgery.

drugs

GENERIC	BRAND	RX
captopril	Capoten	Yes
enalapril	Vasotec	
lisinopril	Prinivil	

form/usage

TABLETS, INJECTIONS: Take on an empty stomach.

when

One hour before eating, unless otherwise directed by your doctor.

side effects and adverse reactions

Severe allergic reaction (anaphylactic shock); swollen face, feet, or hands

Rash, inability to taste food; changes in heartbeat, dizziness, chest pain, confused mental processes, sore throat, cloudy urine, fever, or chills

what to do

Get emergency medical help immediately.

Stop taking. Get in touch with doctor immediately.

(continued)

side effects and adverse reactions

Mild headache, mild gastrointestinal problems, pain in abdomen

what to do

Continue taking, but discuss with your physician.

special precautions

because

DRUG INTERACTIONS
1. Other antihypertensives, beta-blockers, carteolol, diclofenac, guanfacine, nimodipine, nitrates, pentoxifylline, sotalol

2. Amiloride, potassium iodide, spironolactone, triamterene

3. Chloramphenicol

4. Pentamidine, tiopronin

5. Terazosin

1. Increased antihypertensive effect or sudden and severe drop in blood pressure.

2. May lead to excessive potassium levels.

3. May increase potassium levels in blood.

4. Bone marrow damage; kidney damage.

5. Effect of terazosin may be decreased.

DIET
Avoid salt.

Salt can contribute to fluid retention and increase blood pressure.

ALCOHOL AND TOBACCO
Avoid alcohol.
No problems reported with tobacco.

Alcohol could contribute to excessive drop in blood pressure.

PREGNANCY
Avoid drug.

Drug has caused fetal abnormalities and other problems in animal experiments. There have been reports of increased risk of fetal problems in humans, as well as low blood pressure, kidney failure, and other problems in newborns.

BREAST-FEEDING
Discuss with your doctor.

Medication will migrate into breast milk and could affect child.

AGE FACTOR

1. Should be given to children under close medical supervision.

2. People over 60 should use cautiously.

1. Safety and effectiveness not established in children. Drug is given at a weight-adjusted adult dosage.

2. Adverse and side effects may be worse in older people.

MISSED DOSE

You can take a missed dose up to two hours after scheduled time. Otherwise, wait for the next dose but do not double the amount taken.

OVERDOSE

Get emergency medical help immediately if patient falls into coma; has convulsions, very low blood pressure, or chills; or faints.

STOPPING DRUG

Do not stop taking until you have talked with your doctor. You may have to come off drug slowly.

OTHERS

Do not drive or operate machinery until you have determined how medication affects you.

Getting up from a sitting or lying position may make you dizzy. Rise slowly from bed or chair. Check with your doctor if condition does not improve after a few days.

Drug may make you more sensitive to heat. Be careful in hot environments and ask doctor for guidance on taking hot showers or baths.

May increase sensitivity to sun. If you go outdoors between 10 A.M. and 3 P.M., wear protective clothing and/or sunblock.

Periodic laboratory tests might be necessary to check blood counts, urine protein levels, and blood potassium.

Constipation may occur within the first month of starting the drug. Try a high-fiber diet to relieve the constipation, or seek advice from your doctor or pharmacist.

drug or category:

ALPHA-BLOCKERS (TERAZOSIN)

condition:

HIGH BLOOD PRESSURE (HYPERTENSION)

warning

Tell your doctor if you have or have had:
- an allergic reaction to this medication, or to preservatives or food additives
- excessive blood pressure drops in response to other medications
- a stroke or other circulation problem in the brain
- liver or kidney disease

Tell your doctor if you have surgery scheduled soon.

You should not take this medicine if you are depressed or if you have heart disease but are not taking a beta-blocker.

Drug may cause impotence.

drugs

GENERIC	BRAND	RX
terazosin	*Hytrin*	Yes

form/usage

TABLET: Take with liquid or food.
Tablet may be crushed.

when

Once a day, preferably at bed-time.

side effects and adverse reactions

Chest pain, dizziness, or fainting when you get up from a chair or bed; gastrointestinal problems

Pain in back or joints, vision problems, weight gain as a result of retaining fluids, mild headache, fatigue

what to do

Stop taking. Get in touch with doctor immediately.

Continue taking, but discuss with your physician.

special precautions	**because**
DRUG INTERACTIONS	
1. Diclofenac, estrogens, loop diuretics, NSAIDs, other antihypertensives, sympathomimetics	1. Decrease effectiveness of medication.
2. Lisinopril	2. Increases effect of medication.
3. Nicardipine, nimodipine	3. Can cause severe fall in blood pressure.
DIET	
1. Avoid too much salt.	1. Increases water retention.
2. Avoid caffeine.	2. Decreases effect of medication.
ALCOHOL AND TOBACCO	
Use alcohol very cautiously. Avoid tobacco.	Alcohol could increase impact of medication. Nicotine could intensify heart disease.
PREGNANCY	
Discuss with your physician.	While no sufficient, well-controlled studies have been done in humans, drug has caused fetal problems and fetal death in animals.
BREAST-FEEDING	
Discuss with your doctor.	Drug passes into breast milk. Baby should be monitored closely for effects if you do use medication.
AGE FACTOR	
1. Use in children only under close medical supervision.	1. Safety for children under 12 has not been determined.
2. Adults over 60 should use cautiously.	2. Side effects and adverse reactions may be more pronounced.
MISSED DOSE	
Take when you remember. Do not double dose.	
OVERDOSE	
Get emergency medical help immediately if patient falls into coma, suffers breathing difficulties, has slow heartbeat, or faints.	

(continued)

STOPPING DRUG

Do not stop taking even if you feel better because high blood pressure often involves no symptoms. Discuss with your doctor.

OTHERS

Do not drive or operate machinery until you have determined how medication affects you.

Getting up from a sitting or lying position may make you dizzy. Rise slowly from bed or chair. Check with your doctor if condition does not improve after a few days.

You should have periodic checkups to make sure medication is working.

drug or category:

BETA-BLOCKERS

condition:

HIGH BLOOD PRESSURE (HYPERTENSION), ANGINA, CARDIAC ARRHYTHMIAS, MIGRAINE PREVENTION

warning

Tell your doctor if you have or have had:
- an allergic reaction to this medication, or to preservatives or foods
- allergies, including hay fever and asthma
- respiratory problems, including bronchitis and emphysema
- heart, liver, or thyroid disease
- depression

Medication may cause blood sugar to fall. Diabetics should consult their physician.

drugs

GENERIC	BRAND	RX
atenolol	Tenormin	Yes
metoprolol succinate	Toprol-XL	
metoprolol tartrate	Lopressor	
nadolol	Corgard	
propranolol	Inderal	

form/usage

TABLETS, EXTENDED-RELEASE CAPSULES, LIQUIDS: Should be taken with liquids, but can be taken with food.

Tablet may be crushed. Capsule may be opened.

when

At mealtimes.

side effects and adverse reactions

Severe shortness of breath, rapid heartbeat, continuous palpitations and intermittent loss of consciousness

what to do

Get emergency medical help immediately.

(continued)

side effects and adverse reactions

Sore throat, rash, inability to sleep, nightmares, pain in chest or joints, very slow pulse

Impotence, dry eyes, constipation, fatigue, tingling or feeling of cold in hands or feet, depression, confusion, stomach pain, frequent dreams or nightmares

what to do

Stop taking. Get in touch with doctor immediately.

Continue taking, but discuss with your physician.

special precautions

DRUG INTERACTIONS
1. ACE inhibitors, other antihypertensives, betaxolol eye drops, calcium blockers, clonidine, diazoxide, guanabenz, levobunolol eye drops, nitrates, propafenone, timolol eye drops

2. Antidiabetics, barbiturates, insulin, molindone, narcotics, reserpine, verapamil

3. Antihistamines, sympathomimetics

4. MAO inhibitors

5. Nimodipine, quinidine

DIET
Avoid high-salt foods.

ALCOHOL AND TOBACCO
Avoid both.

PREGNANCY
Avoid drug.

BREAST-FEEDING
Avoid drug or avoid nursing.

because

1. Increase antihypertensive effect or heighten beta-blocker activity.

2. Beta-blockers increase their effects.

3. Beta-blockers decrease their effect.

4. If MAO inhibitors are discontinued suddenly, blood pressure will increase.

5. Will cause heartbeat problems.

Will increase fluid retention.

Alcohol will cause steep blood pressure drop. Tobacco could cause heart rhythm problems.

Drug has caused pregnancy problems in animal experiments. There have been reports of problems in humans, including respiratory distress, low blood pressure, and slow heartbeat in newborns.

Medications will migrate into breast milk and some could affect child. Discuss with your doctor.

AGE FACTOR

1. Administer to children only under close medical supervision.

2. Adults over 60 should use cautiously.

1. May lower blood sugar.

2. Beta-blockers could increase sensitivity to cold. Generally, older adults react more strongly to these medications.

MISSED DOSE

Take when you remember. Take next dose three hours later, but do not double amount taken. Then return to schedule.

OVERDOSE

Get emergency medical help immediately if patient has convulsions, severe blood pressure drop, breathing difficulties, or weak pulse.

STOPPING DRUG

Do not stop taking even if you feel better because generally hypertension is a symptomless disease. Discuss with your doctor.

OTHERS

Do not drive or operate machinery until you have determined how this medication affects you.

Beta-blockers are also used for heart disease and may decrease the angina usually associated with increased exercise or stress. Do not increase your activities without first consulting your doctor.

Beta-blockers may mask the symptoms of hypoglycemia. If you are diabetic, discuss drug with your doctor.

Some beta-blockers may reduce the effectiveness of some asthma medications.

drug or category:

CALCIUM CHANNEL BLOCKERS

condition:
HIGH BLOOD PRESSURE (HYPERTENSION), ANGINA, CARDIAC ARRHYTHMIAS

warning

Tell your doctor if you have or have had:
- an allergic reaction to this medication, or to any preservatives or foods
- diabetes
- kidney or liver disease

Tell your doctor if you are taking any other heart or blood pressure medication or if you have done so in the past.

Do not take if you have low blood pressure or liver disease.

drugs

GENERIC	BRAND	RX
diltiazem	Cardizem	Yes
nifedipine	Procardia	
verapamil	Calan, others	
nicardipine	Cardene	
isradipine	DynaCirc	

form/usage

TABLETS, CAPSULES (INCLUDING EXTENDED-RELEASE VERSIONS IN BOTH FORMS), INJECTIONS: All formulations may be taken with food to reduce stomach irritation.

Extended-release capsules and tablets must be taken whole. If you have a hard time swallowing a whole tablet, ask your doctor if you can break it in half.

Regular tablets must also be taken whole, without crushing or crumbling.

when

Ask your doctor for schedule, then follow every day. The drug is usually taken in the early morning to prevent night urination.

side effects and adverse reactions

Slow or fast heartbeat, coughing, mood and behavior changes, jaundice, breathing difficulties

Inability to sleep or unusual dreams, minor headaches, gastrointestinal problems, fatigue, swollen extremities, urination difficulties

Gum problems, including bleeding and swelling

what to do

Stop taking. Get in touch with doctor immediately.

Continue taking, but discuss with your physician.

Discuss with your dentist. Massaging gums and flossing could help.

special precautions

DRUG INTERACTIONS
1. Anticoagulants, antiarrhythmia drugs, hydantoin, carbamazepine, digitalis, propafenone, quinidine, theophylline

2. ACE inhibitors

3. Other high blood pressure medications, diuretics, nimodipine

4. Beta-blockers, disopyramide

5. Calcium supplements, rifampin, phenytoin, vitamin D

6. Encainide

DIET
Follow low-salt diet.

ALCOHOL AND TOBACCO
Avoid both.

PREGNANCY
Avoid drug.

because

1. Increase effect and toxicity of these drugs.

2. May increase potassium levels in blood.

3. May cause excessive blood pressure drop.

4. Heartbeat irregularities.

5. Decrease effectiveness of calcium blockers.

6. Calcium blocker may enhance toxicity of encainide to heart muscle.

High salt levels in body promote water retention.

Alcohol could induce severe blood pressure drops. Nicotine will increase heart rate.

Drug has caused fetal abnormalities in animal experiments. The compounds have not been studied in women.

(continued)

BREAST-FEEDING

Discuss with your doctor.

Medication will migrate into milk and could affect child, but there are no reports of problems in infants as a result.

AGE FACTOR

1. Children react to medication in same way as adults.

2. Patients over 60 years of age should use cautiously.

2. The elderly are more likely to have side effects.

MISSED DOSE

Take missed dose as soon as possible, up to two hours before next dose. If it is almost time for your next dose, wait to take that one, but don't double dose. Resume regular schedule.

OVERDOSE

Get emergency medical help immediately if patient has cardiac arrest or severe changes in heart rhythm, or loses consciousness.

STOPPING DRUG

Do not stop taking even if you feel better because high blood pressure can be present without symptoms. If your doctor decides you can stop the medicine, it will have to be discontinued gradually.

OTHERS

Do not drive or operate machinery until you have determined how medication affects you.

Getting up from a sitting or lying position may make you dizzy. Rise slowly from bed or chair. Check with your doctor if condition does not improve after a few days.

Drug also alleviates signs of heart disease. If these symptoms abate, do not increase your activities or exercise without checking with your physician.

May cause changes in menstruation.

Drug may make you more sensitive to heat. Be careful in hot environments and ask your doctor for guidance on taking hot showers or baths.

Periodic laboratory tests might be necessary to check heart, liver, and kidney functions.

CENTRAL ALPHA-BLOCKERS (CLONIDINE)

condition:
HIGH BLOOD PRESSURE (HYPERTENSION)

warning

Tell your doctor if you have or have had:
- an allergic reaction to this medication, or to any preservatives or foods
- heart disease or circulatory problems in the brain
- serious depression

Tell your doctor if you are taking sedatives or sleep medication, or are planning to have surgery.

drugs

GENERIC	BRAND	RX
clonidine	*Catapres*, others	Yes

form/usage

TABLETS, PATCHES: Tablets may be taken with or without food and may be crushed.

when

Tablet dosage is usually twice a day.

Patches are changed weekly.

side effects and adverse reactions

what to do

side effects and adverse reactions	what to do
Skin symptoms, changes in heart rhythm, swollen feet or legs, depression, pinpoint eye pupils, unusual fatigue or tiredness	Stop taking. Get in touch with doctor immediately.
Inability to sleep, gastrointestinal problems, lessened sexual desire, nightmares, drowsiness, fatigue, inability to ejaculate, male breast enlargement	Continue taking, but discuss with your physician.
With patches: Darkening of skin around patch; decreased libido, dizziness, fainting, loss of appetite, lightheadedness or fainting on getting up from chair or bed, nervousness	Continue taking, but discuss with your physician.

(continued)

side effects and adverse reactions	**what to do**
Dry mouth	Try sugarless candy or gum. If condition persists, discuss with your doctor or dentist.

special precautions	**because**
DRUG INTERACTIONS	
1. Tricyclic antidepressants	1. Decrease effect of clonidine.
2. Other high blood pressure medications, carteolol, diuretics, fenfluramine, nicardipine, nimodipine, nitrates, sotalol	2. May cause sudden blood pressure drop or longer-lasting increase in antihypertension effect.
3. ACE inhibitors	3. May increase blood potassium levels.
4. Clozapine, nabilone	4. Adverse impact on central nervous system.
5. Ethinamate	5. Clonidine increases its effects.
6. Terazosin	6. Clonidine decreases its effects.
7. Methyprylon	7. Clonidine heightens its effects.
DIET	
1. Avoid caffeine (coffee, cola drinks, etc.).	1. Decreases effect of drug.
2. Observe low-salt diet.	2. Salt increases retention of fluids in body.
ALCOHOL AND TOBACCO Avoid alcohol. No problems expected with tobacco.	Drug increases alcohol's sedative effects. Could also cause blood pressure to fall excessively.
PREGNANCY Avoid drug.	Manufacturer recommends that it not be taken by pregnant women. Drug may affect embryo.
BREAST-FEEDING Avoid drug or avoid nursing.	Medication will migrate into breast milk and could affect child. Discuss with your doctor. If you do take clonidine, keep a close eye on baby for any possible side effects. Drug may also hamper milk production.

AGE FACTOR

1. Avoid giving to children under 12.

2. People over 60 should use cautiously.

1. Safety and effectiveness in children under 12 not determined.

2. Adverse and side effects may be worse in older people, including dizziness and balance problems when getting up from bed or chair. May also cause severe emotional and mental disturbances.

MISSED DOSE

If you miss a dose, take it as soon as you remember, but do not double dose. Then go back to regular schedule. If you miss sveral doses, get in touch with doctor.

OVERDOSE

Get emergency medical help immediately in case of coma, breathing difficulties, sluggish reflexes, extreme fatigue, or vomiting.

STOPPING DRUG

Do not stop taking even if you feel better until you have talked with your doctor. You may have to come off drug slowly.

OTHERS

Do not drive or operate machinery until you have determined how this medication affects you.

Getting up from a sitting or lying position may make you dizzy. Rise slowly from bed or chair. Check with your doctor if condition does not improve after a few days.

Drug may make you more sensitive to heat. Be careful in hot environments and ask your doctor for guidance on taking hot showers or baths.

Drug may also cause extreme sensitivity to cold, including numbness of extremities.

You should have periodic checkups to make sure drug is working properly and to assess other body functions it may affect.

drug or category:

CENTRAL ALPHA-BLOCKERS (GUANFACINE)

condition:
HIGH BLOOD PRESSURE (HYPERTENSION)

warning

Tell your doctor if you have or have had:
- an allergic reaction to this medication, or to preservatives or food additives
- brain circulation problems or other cardiovascular disorders
- you are taking sleeping pills or antidepressants

Tell your doctor if you are likely to have surgery with general anesthesia within a short period of time.

drugs

GENERIC	BRAND	RX
guanfacine	Tenex	Yes

form/usage

TABLETS: Can be taken with or without food or liquid. Tablets may be crushed.

when

Usually taken at bedtime, but your doctor may recommend you take two doses a day.

side effects and adverse reactions

what to do

side effects and adverse reactions	what to do
If you discontinue drug suddenly and you have chest pains or irregular heartbeat, sleep disturbances, or unexplained sweating	Get emergency medical help immediately.
Confusion, balance problems, constipation, slower heartbeat	Stop taking. Get in touch with doctor immediately.
Sexual problems, depression, fatigue, headache, mild gastrointestinal problems	Continue taking, but discuss with your physician.
Dry mouth	Try candy or sugarless gum. If problem persists, discuss with your doctor or dentist.

special precautions	because
DRUG INTERACTIONS	
1. Other high blood pressure medications, carteolol, lisinopril, nicardipine, nimodipine, propafenone, sotalol	1. May cause sudden blood pressure drop or longer-lasting increase in antihypertension effect.
2. Central nervous system depressants, fluoxetine, nabilone	2. Increase depressant effect, including heightened depression of central nervous system.
3. Estrogens, nonsteroidal anti-inflammatory drugs, sympathomimetics	3. Can decrease effect of guanfacine.
4. Ethinamate	4. Ethinamate's effect will be increased.
5. Leucovorin	5. Has high alcoholic content. Could cause adverse effects, including sudden drop in blood pressure.
6. Methyprylon	6. Will greatly increase its sedative effect.
DIET	
Avoid high-salt foods.	Salt promotes retention of water in body.
ALCOHOL AND TOBACCO	
Avoid alcohol.	Alcohol can lead to excessive drops in blood pressure.
No interactions with tobacco.	
PREGNANCY	
No negative interactions reported, but do discuss with your doctor to make sure it is safe for you.	
BREAST-FEEDING	
Avoid drug or avoid nursing.	Drug migrates into breast milk.
AGE FACTOR	
1. Do not administer to children under 12.	1. Safety and effectiveness not established in children under 12.
2. People over 60 should use with caution.	2. Adverse and side effects may be worse in older people and may cause severe mood and behavioral changes.

(continued)

MISSED DOSE

You can take a missed dose up to two hours after scheduled time. Otherwise, wait for next dose but do not double the amount taken.

OVERDOSE

Get emergency medical help immediately if patient loses consciousness, suffers breathing difficulties, or had an exceedingly slow heartbeat.

STOPPING DRUG

Hypertension can cause damage even when it produces no symptoms. Do not stop taking even if you feel better until you have talked with your doctor. You may have to come off drug slowly.

OTHERS

Do not drive or operate machinery until you have determined how medication affects you.

Getting up from a sitting or lying position may make you dizzy. Rise slowly from bed or chair. Check with your doctor if condition does not improve after a few days.

Drug may make you more sensitive to heat. Be careful in hot environments and ask your doctor for guidance on taking hot showers or baths.

drug or category:

THIAZIDE DIURETICS

condition:

HIGH BLOOD PRESSURE (HYPERTENSION)

warning

Tell your doctor if you have or have had:
- an allergic reaction to this medication or to sulfa drugs, or to any preservatives, dyes, or foods
- diabetes, gout, lupus erythematosus, pancreatitis
- heart, blood vessel, kidney, or liver disease

Tell all doctors and dentists with whom you consult that you are taking this drug.

drugs

GENERIC	BRAND	RX
chlorothiazide	*Diuril*	Yes
chlorthalidone	*Hygroton, Thalitone*	
hydrochlorothiazide	*Esidrix, HydroDIURIL,* others	

form/usage

TABLETS, LIQUID: Swallow with beverage. Tablet may be crumbled and taken with food.

when

Your doctor will suggest a schedule. Take at same time every day.

side effects and adverse reactions

Skin reactions

Joint pain, tarry stools, vision problems, severe gastrointestinal problems, changes in heart rhythm, jaundice, weak pulse

Sore throat, mild headaches, fatigue, decrease in sexual desire, mild gastrointestinal problems

what to do

Get emergency medical help immediately.

Stop taking. Get in touch with doctor immediately.

Continue taking, but discuss with your physician.

(continued)

special precautions

because

DRUG INTERACTIONS

1. Tricyclic antidepressants, ACE inhibitors, other antihypertensives and diuretics, barbiturates, beta-blockers, carteolol, MAO inhibitors, nicardipine, nimodipine, nitrates, pentoxifylline, sotalol

1. Increase blood pressure fall or cause sudden drop in blood pressure.

2. Cholestyramine, colestipol, indomethacin

2. Decrease antihypertensive effect.

3. Amphotericin B

3. Increases potassium levels.

4. Steroids, digitalis

4. Decrease potassium levels.

5. Oral antidiabetics

5. Thiazides work against them.

6. Calcium supplements

6. Higher calcium concentrations in blood.

7. Lithium, probenecid, terazosin

7. Their effects are increased.

DIET

Your doctor may recommend a high-potassium diet or a potassium supplement. Observe carefully.

Diuretics may cause excessive loss of potassium and lead to possible disturbances in body's nervous system, especially in the heart.

ALCOHOL AND TOBACCO

Avoid alcohol.
No interactions with tobacco reported.

Alcohol could cause sharp drop in blood pressure.

PREGNANCY

Avoid drug.

Drug has caused jaundice, blood disorders, and low potassium levels in newborns.

BREAST-FEEDING

Avoid drug during first month of nursing.

Medication reduces the amount of milk.

AGE FACTOR

1. Avoid use in infants with jaundice.

1. Medication may make jaundice worse in infants who have the condition.

2. People over 60 should use cautiously.

2. Adverse and side effects may be worse in older people, especially dehydration and loss of body potassium.

MISSED DOSE

You can take a missed dose up to two hours after scheduled time. Otherwise, wait for next dose but do not double the amount taken.

OVERDOSE

Get emergency medical help immediately if patient falls into coma, feels weak, or has cramps or weak pulse.

STOPPING DRUG

Do not stop taking until you have talked with your doctor.

OTHERS

Do not drive or operate machinery until you have determined how medication affects you.

Getting up from a sitting or lying position may make you dizzy. Rise slowly from bed or chair. Check with your doctor if condition does not improve after a few days.

Some diuretics may make you more sensitive to side effects of digoxin. Make sure your doctor or pharmacist knows if you are taking digoxin.

May increase sensitivity to sun. If you go outdoors between 10 A.M. and 3 P.M., wear protective clothing and/ or sunblock.

Drug may make you more sensitive to heat. Be careful in hot environments and ask your doctor for guidance on taking hot showers or baths.

Periodic laboratory tests might be necessary to check kidney function and blood sugar and electrolyte levels.

drug or category:

INDOLINES (INDAPAMIDE)

condition:
HIGH BLOOD PRESSURE (HYPERTENSION), CONGESTIVE HEART FAILURE

warning

Tell your doctor if you have or have had:
- an allergic reaction to this medication or to sulfonamide drugs, or to any preservatives or food additives
- diabetes
- gout, kidney, or liver disease

Tell your doctor if you are scheduled for surgery soon or if you are taking lithium or digitalis.

Avoid asthma, hay fever, diet, or sinus pills, if possible, since they could cause an increase in blood pressure.

drugs

GENERIC	BRAND	RX
indapamide	*Lozol*	Yes

form/usage

TABLETS: May be taken with food to avoid irritating stomach.

when

Follow schedule set by your doctor for you.

side effects and adverse reactions

Weak pulse, skin reactions, changes in heart rhythm, muscle cramps, extreme fatigue

Increase in urination, inability to sleep, gastrointestinal problems, mild headache, dizziness on rising from bed or chair

Dry mouth

what to do

Stop taking. Get in touch with doctor immediately.

Continue taking, but discuss with your physician. Balance problems can be mitigated by rising slowly from bed or chair.

Try sugarless candy or gum. If condition persists, discuss with your doctor or dentist.

special precautions	because
DRUG INTERACTIONS	
1. Beta-blockers, barbiturates, MAO inhibitors	1. Increase effect of indapamide.
2. Cholestyramine, colestipol, indomethacin	2. Decrease effect of indapamide.
3. Calcium supplements, thiazide diuretics, sotalol	3. Indapamide increases their effect.
4. Allopurinol, probenecid, terazosin	4. Indapamide decreases their effect.
5. Lithium	5. Increases toxicity.
6. ACE inhibitors, tricyclic antidepressants, nicardipine, nimodipine	6. Decrease blood pressure; drop in blood pressure may be sudden.
7. Amphotericin B	7. Increases potassium.
8. Cortisone, digitalis	8. Decrease potassium.
DIET Your doctor may recommend a high-potassium diet or a potassium supplement. Observe carefully.	Diuretics may cause excessive loss of potassium and lead to possible disturbances in body's nervous system, especially in the heart.
ALCOHOL AND TOBACCO Avoid both.	Alcohol may cause severe drop in blood pressure. Tobacco interferes with indapamide.
PREGNANCY No negative interactions reported, but should not be taken to reduce fluid retention that comes with pregnancy.	Safety and effectiveness not established. No sufficient well-controlled studies have been done.
BREAST-FEEDING No problems reported.	
AGE FACTOR 1. Use in children only under medical supervision.	1. Safety and effectiveness not established.
2. People over 60 should use cautiously.	2. Adverse and side effects may be worse in older people.

(continued)

MISSED DOSE
You can take a missed dose up to three hours after scheduled time. Otherwise, wait for next dose but do not double the amount taken.

OVERDOSE
Get emergency medical help immediately if patient has severe gastrointestinal problems, experiences great thirst, has weak pulse or rapid heartbeat, or complains of excessive fatigue.

STOPPING DRUG
Do not stop taking even if you feel better until you have talked with your doctor. You may have to come off drug slowly.

OTHERS
Do not drive or operate machinery until you have determined how medication affects you.

Getting up from a sitting or lying position may make you dizzy. Rise slowly from bed or chair. Check with your doctor if condition does not improve after a few days.

You should have periodic checkups to make sure drug is working properly and to assess sodium, potassium, chloride, sugar, and uric acid levels.

drug or category:

LOOP DIURETICS

condition:

HIGH BLOOD PRESSURE (HYPERTENSION), CONGESTIVE HEART FAILURE

warning

Tell your doctor if you have or have had:
- an allergic reaction to this medication, sulfa drugs, or thiazide diuretics, or to any preservatives or foods
- diabetes
- diarrhea, gout, hearing difficulties, or pancreatitis
- heart disease, kidney or liver disease, or systemic lupus erythematosus

You may want to carry an emergency alert card or bracelet to alert medical personnel attending you that you take this medication.

drugs

GENERIC	BRAND	RX
bumetanide	*Bumex*	Yes
furosemide	*Lasix*	
others		

form/usage

TABLETS, ORAL SOLUTION, INJECTIONS: May be taken with food or milk.

Tablet may be crumbled.

when

Follow schedule set by your doctor.

side effects and adverse reactions

Skin reactions, vision changes, hearing loss or ringing in ears, gastrointestinal problems, unexplained bleeding or bruising, pain in joints, numbness or tingling in hands and feet, changes in heart rhythm, excessive drop in blood pressure

what to do

Stop taking. Get in touch with doctor immediately.

(continued)

special precautions	because

DRUG INTERACTIONS

1. ACE inhibitors

2. Steroids, digitalis, amphotericin B, laxatives, excessive amounts of vitamin D, antidiabetics, potassium supplements

3. Tricyclic antidepressants, barbiturates, other antihypertensives, beta-blockers, nimodipine, nitrates

4. Allopurinol, insulin, lithium, probenecid

5. Other diuretics, sedatives

6. Nonsteroidal anti-inflammatory agents, phenytoin

7. Amiodarone
8. Anticoagulants

9. Aspirin and similar drugs

DIET
Your doctor may recommend a high-potassium diet or a potassium supplement. Observe carefully.

ALCOHOL AND TOBACCO
Avoid both.

PREGNANCY
Avoid these drugs.

BREAST-FEEDING
Discuss with your doctor.

AGE FACTOR
1. Should be used in children only under close medical supervision.

---

1. Excessive potassium buildup.

2. Decrease potassium in blood or interfere with potassium absorption.

3. Decrease blood pressure; may cause sudden drop.

4. Their effectiveness is decreased.

5. Increase in diuretic effect.

6. Decrease in diuretic effect.

7. Possible heart rhythm disturbances.
8. Blood clotting problems.

9. Will accumulate in body.

Diuretics may cause excessive loss of potassium and lead to possible disturbances in body's nervous system, especially in the heart.

Alcohol can cause severe blood pressure drop. Tobacco decreases effect of medication.

Have caused fetal abnormalities in animal experiments.

Medications will migrate into breast milk.

1. Safety and effectiveness in children under age 10 have not been established.

AGE FACTOR

2. People over 60 should use cautiously.

2. Greater risk of adverse and side effects, including excessive loss of potassium. Excessive dehydration may occur.

MISSED DOSE

If you are taking one dose a day, you can take it up to 12 hours late. Beyond 12 hours, wait for next dose. Do not double dose.

If you are taking several doses a day, you can take a missed dose up to two hours after scheduled time. Otherwise, wait for next dose but do not double the amount taken.

OVERDOSE

Get emergency medical help immediately in case of cardiac arrest, inability to rouse patient from sleep, weak pulse, severe gastrointestinal problems, muscle cramps, lethargy, or confusion.

STOPPING DRUG

Do not stop taking even if you feel better until you have talked with your doctor. You may have to come off drug slowly.

OTHERS

Furosemide may increase sensitivity to sun. If you go outdoors between 10 A.M. and 3 P.M. wear protective clothing and/or sun block.

Getting up from a sitting or lying position may make you dizzy. Rise slowly from bed or chair. Check with your doctor if condition does not improve after a few days.

Periodic laboratory tests might be necessary to check sodium, potassium, chloride, sugar, and uric acid levels.

drug or category:

DIURETIC COMBINATIONS (TRIAMTERENE AND HYDROCHLOROTHIAZIDE)

condition:

HIGH BLOOD PRESSURE (HYPERTENSION)

warning

Tell your doctor if you have or have had:
- an allergic reaction to this medication or sulfa drugs, or to any preservatives or foods
- diabetes or kidney or liver disease
- gout, kidney stones, lupus erythematosus, or menstrual problems

Tell your doctor if you are taking cortisone, digitalis, or any antidiabetic.

These drugs may cause an increase in blood sugar levels. Monitor urine or blood levels closely and discuss changes in antidiabetic medication with your doctor.

Tell any doctor you consult that you are taking this medication. You may want to carry an emergency alert card or bracelet indicating that you are taking these drugs.

Avoid asthma, hay fever, diet, or sinus pills, since they could cause an increase in blood pressure.

drugs

GENERIC	BRAND	RX
triamterene and hydrochloro-thiazide	*Dyazide, Maxzide*, others	Yes

form/usage

SOLUTION, TABLETS: Take with or without food. Can be taken following meals to avoid stomach irritation.

when

Usually in the morning, though your doctor may establish another schedule for you.

side effects and adverse reactions

Changes in heart rhythm, breathing difficulties, signs of extreme allergic reaction (anaphylactic shock), including severe skin reactions and fainting

what to do

Get emergency medical help immediately.

side effects and adverse reactions	what to do
Cramps in muscles, changes in mood, vision problems, kidney stones, tarry stools, excessive dryness of mouth, jaundice, pain in muscles or joints, unexplained bleeding	Stop taking. Get in touch with doctor immediately.
Mild moodiness, constipation, diminished sex drive, mild headache, fatigue, unexplained loss or gain of weight	Continue taking, but discuss with your physician.

special precautions	because
DRUG INTERACTIONS	
1. ACE inhibitors, antidepressants, beta-blockers, lisinopril, nicardipine, nimodipine, nitrates	1. Sudden drop in blood pressure, increased long-term antihypertensive effects.
2. Amiloride, amphotericin B, potassium supplements, spironolactone	2. May increase levels of potassium, or lead to increased potassium retention.
3. Lithium	3. Increases effect of lithium.
4. Allopurinol, probenecid	4. Decreases effects of these drugs.
5. Barbiturates, cholestyramine, MAO inhibitors	5. May increase excretion of salts.
6. Other thiazide diuretics	6. Will increase their effect.
DIET	
1. No restrictions.	
2. Do not limit intake of salt unless told to do so by your doctor.	
3. Ask your doctor for advice on potassium in your diet.	3. Medication can cause you either to lose potassium or to accumulate it in your body.
ALCOHOL AND TOBACCO Avoid both.	Alcohol can lead to an excessive drop in blood pressure. Tobacco can reduce effectiveness of medication.

(continued)

PREGNANCY
Avoid drug.

Drug has caused jaundice, low potassium blood levels, and some blood problems in newborns.

BREAST-FEEDING
Discuss with your doctor.

Medication will migrate into breast milk, but no effects on babies have been reported.

AGE FACTOR
1. Monitor children carefully.

2. People over 60 should use cautiously.

1. May cause dehydration and potassium loss.

2. Adverse and side effects may be worse in older people, including potassium loss, impaired thought processes, and increased possibility of blood clots because blood is thickened as a result of fluid loss.

MISSED DOSE
You can take a missed dose up to six hours after scheduled time. Otherwise, wait for the next dose but do not double the amount taken.

OVERDOSE
Get emergency medical help immediately if patient falls into coma, is lethargic, has heart rhythm disturbances, or has severe gastrointestinal problems.

STOPPING DRUG
Do not stop taking until you have talked with your doctor. You may have to come off drug slowly.

OTHERS
May increase sensitivity to sun. If you go outdoors between 10 A.M. and 3 P.M., wear protective clothing and/or sun block.

Some diuretics may make you more sensitive to the side effects of digoxin. If you are taking digoxin, make sure your doctor or pharmacist knows this.

May cause decreased sexual desire and impotence.

Drug may make you more sensitive to heat. Be careful in hot environments and ask your doctor for guidance on taking hot showers and baths.

OTHERS

Do not drive or operate machinery until you have determined how medication affects you.

Getting up from a sitting or lying position may make you dizzy. Rise slowly from bed or chair. Check with your doctor if condition does not improve after a few days.

Periodic laboratory tests might be necessary to check kidney function, blood count, and blood sodium, potassium, and chloride levels.

drug or category:

POTASSIUM SUPPLEMENTS

condition:

POTASSIUM DEPLETION

warning

Tell your doctor if you have or have had:
- an allergic reaction to this medication, or to preservatives or food additives
- adrenal gland disease
- heart or kidney disease
- gastrointestinal problems like diarrhea, blockages, or ulcers

drugs

GENERIC	BRAND	RX
potassium chloride	K-Tab, K-Dur, Klor-Con, Slow-K	Yes

form/usage

EXTENDED-RELEASE TABLETS AND CAPSULES, SOLUTION, POWDER: Liquid, soluble tablet, and powder forms should be diluted in 4 ounces of cold water. Wait until bubbling or fizzing action has stopped before swallowing.

Extended-release tablets and capsules must be taken whole. If you cannot do so, discuss with your doctor or pharmacist.

when

Take right after meals or with food to lessen stomach irritation and decrease chances of diarrhea.

side effects and adverse reactions

Black or tarry stool, changes in heart rhythm, bleeding, severe pain in esophagus, breathing problems

Mild to moderate gastrointestinal or skin problems, tingling in arms and legs

what to do

Stop taking. Get in touch with doctor immediately.

Continue taking, but discuss with your physician.

special precautions	because
DRUG INTERACTIONS Potassium supplements can interact, affect, or be affected by almost three dozen medications including ACE inhibitors, digitalis, cortisone, and vitamin B_{12}. Discuss with your doctor or pharmacist any medication you are taking before using these supplements.	
DIET If possible, plan an appropriate diet with the help of a registered nutritionist, preferably one recommended by your doctor or by a social worker at a community hospital.	It is better to get potassium from foods. It is available in acorn and butternut squash, potatoes, spinach, kidney and navy beans, watermelon, bananas, collard greens, broccoli, and zucchini.
ALCOHOL AND TOBACCO No interactions reported.	
PREGNANCY No negative interactions reported.	
BREAST-FEEDING No problems reported, but discuss with your doctor.	Medication does pass into breast milk.
AGE FACTOR 1. Give to children only under medical supervision. 2. Adults over 60 must use supplements very carefully and with strict adherence to suggested doses and scheduling.	1. Safety and effectiveness not established. 2. Potassium imbalances can have critical effects, particularly on heart function.

MISSED DOSE
You can take a missed dose up to two hours after scheduled time. Otherwise, wait for next dose but do not double the amount taken.

OVERDOSE
Get emergency medical help immediately if patient falls into coma, has an irregular heart rhythm, or suffers cardiac arrest, convulsions, extreme blood pressure drop, or paralysis of limbs.

(continued)

STOPPING DRUG

Do not stop taking even if you feel better until you have talked with your doctor. You may have to come off drug slowly.

OTHERS

You should have periodic checkups to make sure supplements are working properly and to assess other body functions they may affect.

a

SORBITRATE Sublingual 5 mg Zeneca *760*	ISORDIL Sublingual 5 mg Wyeth-Ayerst	LEVOTHROID 112 µg Forest *LJ*	LEVOTHROID 200 µg Forest *LR*	ZAROXOLYN 2.5 mg Fisons Pharmaceuticals	

b

NORLUTATE 5 mg Parke-Davis *918*	DELTASONE 2.5 mg Upjohn *32*	METHERGINE 0.2 mg Sandoz Pharmaceuticals *78-54*	ADALAT CC 30 mg Miles Pharmaceutical *884*	DARICON-PB SmithKline Beecham *146*	SYNTHROID 200 µg Boots Pharmaceuticals

c

DICUMAROL 50 mg Abbott *AO*	HALODRIN Upjohn *38*	ESIDRIX 25 mg CIBA *22*	THYROLAR-1 Forest *YE*	ETRAFON 2-25 Schering *598 or ANC*	ESTINYL 0.05 mg Schering *070*

d

DIUTENSEN-R Wallace *274*	ISORDIL Oral Titradose 5 mg Wyeth-Ayerst *4152*	OREXIN Roberts		CELESTONE 0.6 mg Schering *011 or BDA*	MICRONASE 2.5 mg Upjohn

e

MESANTOIN 100 mg Sandoz Pharmaceuticals *78-52*	ANASPAZ PB Ascher *225/300*		TRIAMINICOL Sandoz Consumer	NOLAMINE Carnrick *86204*	PROCARDIA XL 30 mg Pratt

f

COUMADIN 1 mg Du Pont	SER-AP-ES CIBA *71*	PARNATE 10 mg SmithKline Beecham	ST. JOSEPH Aspirin-Free Children's 80 mg Schering-Plough *fruit-flavored*	ADALAT CC 60 mg Miles Pharmaceuticals *885*	CORRECTOL Schering-Plough

g

SPARINE 100 mg Wyeth-Ayerst *200*	NALDECON Apothecon *N1*		DIUPRES-250 Merck & Co. *230*	PHENERGAN 50 mg Wyeth-Ayerst *227*	METAHYDRIN 2 mg Marion Merrell Dow *62*

h

	LARODOPA 250 mg Roche		DIMETANE 8 mg Robins *1868*	Children's TYLENOL 80 mg McNeil Consumer *fruit flavored*	BUTISOL Sodium 100 mg Wallace *37-115*

i

	PROCARDIA XL 60 mg Pratt	Without Drowsiness SINUTAB Warner-Wellcome	Extra Gentle EX-LAX Sandoz Consumer	SKELAXIN 400 mg Carnrick *86-62*	URECHOLINE 10 mg Merck & Co. *412*

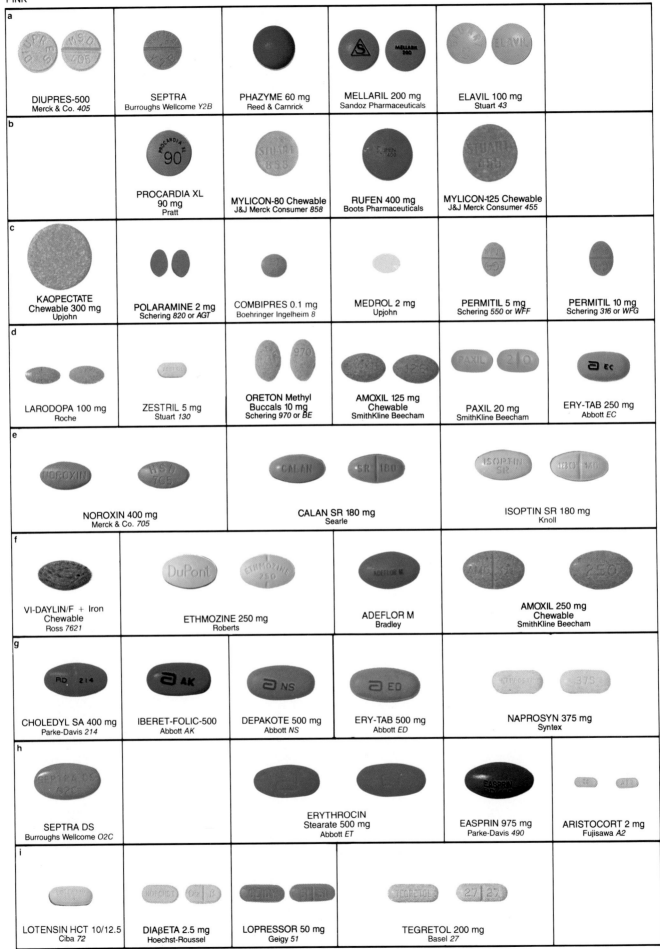

a

DIUPRES-500
Merck & Co. *405*

SEPTRA
Burroughs Wellcome *Y2B*

PHAZYME 60 mg
Reed & Carnrick

MELLARIL 200 mg
Sandoz Pharmaceuticals

ELAVIL 100 mg
Stuart *43*

b

PROCARDIA XL
90 mg
Pratt

MYLICON-80 Chewable
J&J Merck Consumer *858*

RUFEN 400 mg
Boots Pharmaceuticals

MYLICON-125 Chewable
J&J Merck Consumer *455*

c

KAOPECTATE
Chewable 300 mg
Upjohn

POLARAMINE 2 mg
Schering *820* or *AGT*

COMBIPRES 0.1 mg
Boehringer Ingelheim *8*

MEDROL 2 mg
Upjohn

PERMITIL 5 mg
Schering *550* or *WFF*

PERMITIL 10 mg
Schering *316* or *WFG*

d

LARODOPA 100 mg
Roche

ZESTRIL 5 mg
Stuart *130*

ORETON Methyl
Buccals 10 mg
Schering *970* or *BE*

AMOXIL 125 mg
Chewable
SmithKline Beecham

PAXIL 20 mg
SmithKline Beecham

ERY-TAB 250 mg
Abbott *EC*

e

NOROXIN 400 mg
Merck & Co. *705*

CALAN SR 180 mg
Searle

ISOPTIN SR 180 mg
Knoll

f

VI-DAYLIN/F + Iron
Chewable
Ross *7621*

ETHMOZINE 250 mg
Roberts

ADEFLOR M
Bradley

AMOXIL 250 mg
Chewable
SmithKline Beecham

g

CHOLEDYL SA 400 mg
Parke-Davis *214*

IBERET-FOLIC-500
Abbott *AK*

DEPAKOTE 500 mg
Abbott *NS*

ERY-TAB 500 mg
Abbott *ED*

NAPROSYN 375 mg
Syntex

h

SEPTRA DS
Burroughs Wellcome *O2C*

ERYTHROCIN
Stearate 500 mg
Abbott *ET*

EASPRIN 975 mg
Parke-Davis *490*

ARISTOCORT 2 mg
Fujisawa *A2*

i

LOTENSIN HCT 10/12.5
Ciba *72*

DIAβETA 2.5 mg
Hoechst-Roussel

LOPRESSOR 50 mg
Geigy *51*

TEGRETOL 200 mg
Basel *27*

a

LOPRESSOR-HCT 100/25
Geigy *53*

SUMYCIN 250 mg
Apothecon *663*

MENEST 2.5 mg
SmithKline Beecham *128*

MAGAN 545 mg
Savage *412*

b

TRENTAL 400 mg
Hoechst-Roussel

PMB 400
Wyeth-Ayerst *881*

Non-Drowsy Formula
CONTAC SINUS
SmithKline Beecham
Consumer

LARODOPA 500 mg
Roche

c

SUMYCIN 500 mg
Apothecon *603*

VIGRAN Plus
Apothecon

KANULASE
Sandoz Consumer

THERAGRAN
Hematinic
Apothecon *535*

FILIBON
Lederle *F4*

d

FILIBON F.A.
Lederle *F5*

FILIBON Forte
Lederle *F6*

CARAFATE 1 g
Marion Merrell Dow
1712

e

VEPESID 50 mg
Bristol-Myers Oncology *3091*

BENADRYL 25 mg
Warner-Wellcome *471*

BENADRYL 50 mg
Parke-Davis *373*

SERAX 10 mg
Wyeth-Ayerst *51*

DARVON 65 mg
Lilly *H03*

f

DILATRATE-SR 40 mg
Reed & Carnrick *0920*

SINEQUAN 75 mg
Roerig *539*

LARODOPA 250 mg
Roche

CARDENE SR 30 mg
Syntex *2440*

MINIPRESS 2 mg
Pfizer *437*

g

APRESAZIDE 50/50
CIBA *149*

SINEQUAN 50 mg
Roerig *536*

SUMYCIN 250 mg
Apothecon *655*

APRESAZIDE 100/50
CIBA *159*

DYNACIRC 5 mg
Sandoz Pharmaceuticals

h

CONVERZYME
Ascher

LARODOPA 500 mg
Roche

PANCREASE MT-10
McNeil Pharmaceutical

SUMYCIN 500 mg
Apothecon *763*

i

PANCREASE MT-16
McNeil Pharmaceutical

ACTIGALL 300 mg
Summit

LIVITAMIN
SmithKline Beecham *121*

DECADRON 1.5 mg
Merck & Co. *95*

PROSOM 2 mg
Abbott *UD*

NAQUA 2 mg
Schering *822 or AHG*

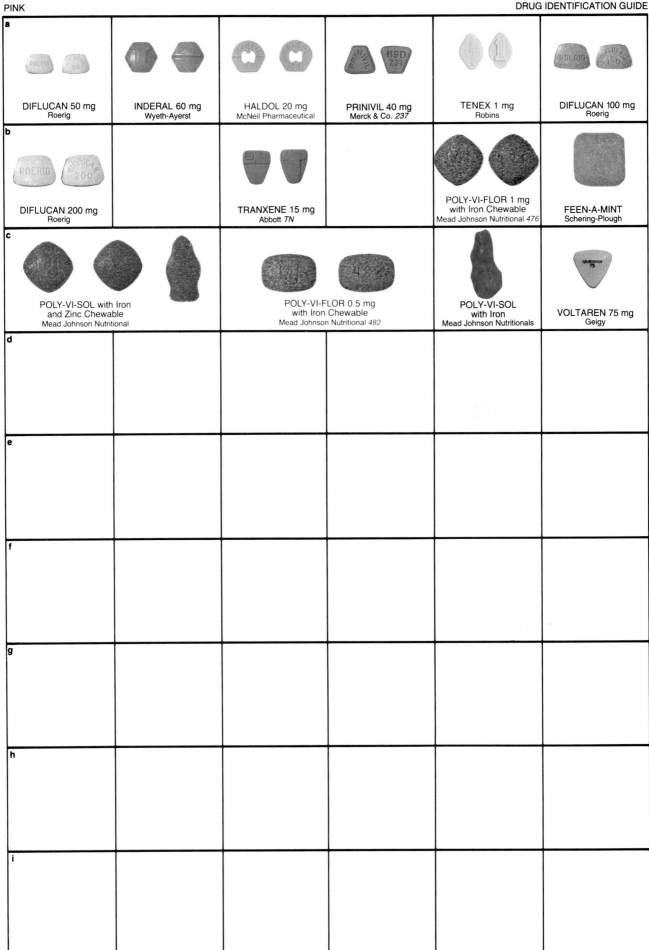

a

DIFLUCAN 50 mg
Roerig

INDERAL 60 mg
Wyeth-Ayerst

HALDOL 20 mg
McNeil Pharmaceutical

PRINIVIL 40 mg
Merck & Co. 237

TENEX 1 mg
Robins

DIFLUCAN 100 mg
Roerig

b

DIFLUCAN 200 mg
Roerig

TRANXENE 15 mg
Abbott TN

POLY-VI-FLOR 1 mg
with Iron Chewable
Mead Johnson Nutritional 476

FEEN-A-MINT
Schering-Plough

c

POLY-VI-SOL with Iron
and Zinc Chewable
Mead Johnson Nutritional

POLY-VI-FLOR 0.5 mg
with Iron Chewable
Mead Johnson Nutritional 482

POLY-VI-SOL
with Iron
Mead Johnson Nutritionals

VOLTAREN 75 mg
Geigy

d

e

f

g

h

i

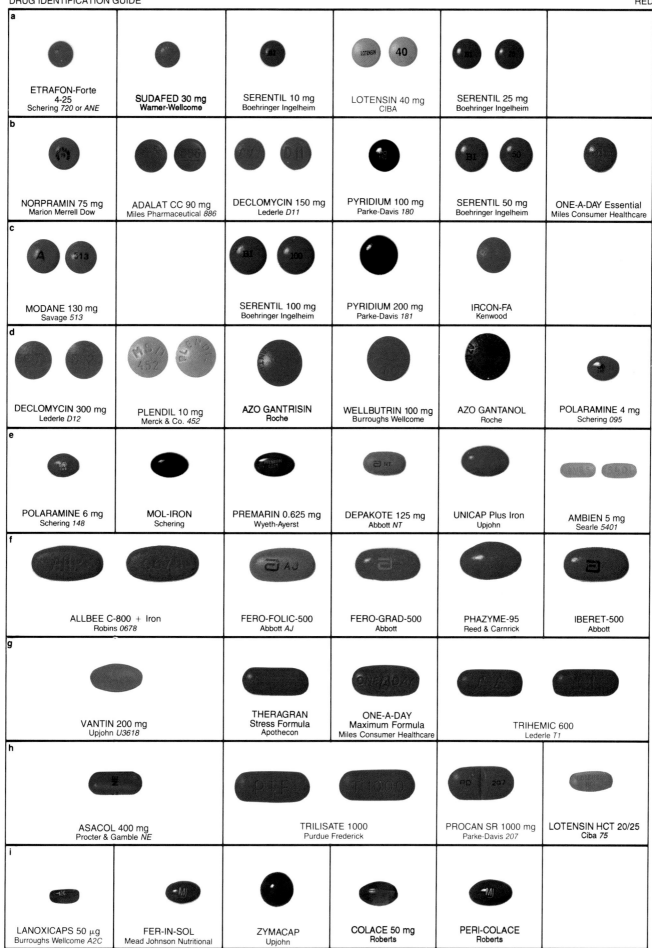

a

ETRAFON-Forte
4-25
Schering *720* or *ANE*

SUDAFED 30 mg
Warner-Wellcome

SERENTIL 10 mg
Boehringer Ingelheim

LOTENSIN 40 mg
CIBA

SERENTIL 25 mg
Boehringer Ingelheim

b

NORPRAMIN 75 mg
Marion Merrell Dow

ADALAT CC 90 mg
Miles Pharmaceutical *886*

DECLOMYCIN 150 mg
Lederle *D11*

PYRIDIUM 100 mg
Parke-Davis *180*

SERENTIL 50 mg
Boehringer Ingelheim

ONE-A-DAY Essential
Miles Consumer Healthcare

c

MODANE 130 mg
Savage *513*

SERENTIL 100 mg
Boehringer Ingelheim

PYRIDIUM 200 mg
Parke-Davis *181*

IRCON-FA
Kenwood

d

DECLOMYCIN 300 mg
Lederle *D12*

PLENDIL 10 mg
Merck & Co. *452*

AZO GANTRISIN
Roche

WELLBUTRIN 100 mg
Burroughs Wellcome

AZO GANTANOL
Roche

POLARAMINE 4 mg
Schering *095*

e

POLARAMINE 6 mg
Schering *148*

MOL-IRON
Schering

PREMARIN 0.625 mg
Wyeth-Ayerst

DEPAKOTE 125 mg
Abbott *NT*

UNICAP Plus Iron
Upjohn

AMBIEN 5 mg
Searle *5401*

f

ALLBEE C-800 + Iron
Robins *0678*

FERO-FOLIC-500
Abbott *AJ*

FERO-GRAD-500
Abbott

PHAZYME-95
Reed & Carnrick

IBERET-500
Abbott

g

VANTIN 200 mg
Upjohn *U3618*

THERAGRAN
Stress Formula
Apothecon

ONE-A-DAY
Maximum Formula
Miles Consumer Healthcare

TRIHEMIC 600
Lederle *T1*

h

ASACOL 400 mg
Procter & Gamble *NE*

TRILISATE 1000
Purdue Frederick

PROCAN SR 1000 mg
Parke-Davis *207*

LOTENSIN HCT 20/25
Ciba *75*

i

LANOXICAPS 50 µg
Burroughs Wellcome *A2C*

FER-IN-SOL
Mead Johnson Nutritional

ZYMACAP
Upjohn

COLACE 50 mg
Roberts

PERI-COLACE
Roberts

a					
COLACE 100 mg Roberts	ACCUTANE 20 mg Roche Dermatologics	PHAZYME-125 Reed & Carnrick	CHROMAGEN OB Savage 0763	SYMMETREL 100 mg Du Pont	DOXIDAN Upjohn

b					
SINEQUAN 10 mg Roerig 534		ALTACE 5 mg Hoechst-Roussel	DYRENIUM 50 mg SmithKline Beecham	SERAX 15 mg Wyeth-Ayerst 6	LARODOPA 100 mg Roche

c					
SERAX 30 mg Wyeth-Ayerst 52	RESTORIL 15 mg Sandoz Pharmaceuticals	RESTORIL 30 mg Sandoz Pharmaceuticals	DIBENZYLINE 10 mg SmithKline Beecham E33	DYRENIUM 100 mg SmithKline Beecham	

d					
FELDENE 20 mg Pfizer/Pratt 323			FELDENE 10 mg Pfizer/Pratt 322	MEXITIL 150 mg Boehringer Ingelheim 66	

e					
DALMANE 30 mg Roche	FEOSOL SmithKline Beecham Consumer	ALBAMYCIN 250 mg Upjohn	CONTROL Thompson	RIFADIN 300 mg Marion Merrell Dow	CLEOCIN HCl 150 mg Upjohn

f					
RIMACTANE 300 mg CIBA 154	MEPERGAN Fortis Wyeth-Ayerst 261		MEXITIL 200 mg Boehringer Ingelheim 67		DURICEF 500 mg Princeton 784

g					
DIALUME 500 mg Rhone-Poulenc Rorer Pharmaceuticals RD		TYLENOL Gelcaps 500 mg McNeil Consumer	MEXITIL 250 mg Boehringer Ingelheim 68	COGNEX 30 mg Parke-Davis	Extra Strength Aspirin-Free SINE-OFF SmithKline Beecham Consumer

h					
DEXATRIM Extra Strength with Vitamin C Thompson	MIDRIN Carnrick 86120		SURFAK 240 mg Upjohn	ZITHROMAX 250 mg Pfizer 305	TYLOX McNeil Pharmaceutical

i					
CLEOCIN HCl 300 mg Upjohn		BASALJEL Wyeth-Ayerst 472	CHROMAGEN Savage 4285	VASERETIC Merck & Co. 720	

a				
ASPERGUM Schering-Plough *cherry flavored*		SPEC-T Anesthetic Lozenges Apothecon	THERAGRAN Apothecon *842*	ZOCOR 40 mg Merck & Co. *749*
b				
c				
d				
e				
f				
g				
h				
i				

a

| ESTRACE 1 mg Bristol-Myers Squibb 755 | LEVOTHROID 125 µg Forest LH | | MELLARIL 15 mg Sandoz Pharmaceuticals 78-8 | BUTISOL Sodium 15 mg Wallace 37-112 | SYNTHROID 75 µg Boots Pharmaceuticals |

b

| THYROLAR-¼ Forest YC | CHLORTHALIDONE 50 mg Abbott AB | PBZ-SR 100 mg Geigy 48 | MS CONTIN 30 mg Purdue Frederick M30 | MOBAN 10 mg Gate | URISED Webcon Uriceuticals W-2183 |

c

| COUMADIN 2 mg Du Pont | METATENSIN No. 4 Marion Merrell Dow 65 | Children's TYLENOL 80 mg McNeil Consumer grape flavored | TEMPRA Chewable 80 mg Mead Johnson Nutritional | Children's Chewable TYLENOL Cold McNeil Consumer | PHRENILIN Carnrick 8650 |

d

| LOTENSIN HCT 20/12.5 Ciba 74 | | | ISOPTIN SR 120 mg Knoll | CALAN SR 120 mg Searle | PREMARIN 2.5 mg Wyeth-Ayerst |

e

| PRAMILET FA Ross 121 | MANDELAMINE 1 g Parke-Davis 167 | TEMPRA Chewable 160 mg Mead Johnson Nutritional grape flavored | | | |

f

| CECLOR 250 mg Lilly 3061 | SECTRAL 200 mg Wyeth-Ayerst 4177 | PATHOCIL 250 mg Wyeth-Ayerst 360 | OMNIPEN 250 mg Wyeth-Ayerst 53 | ACHROMYCIN V 250 mg Lederle A3 | COGNEX 40 mg Parke-Davis |

g

| | AMOXIL 250 mg SmithKline Beecham | SLO-PHYLLIN 250 mg Rhone-Poulenc Rorer Pharmaceuticals 1356 | OMNIPEN 500 mg Wyeth-Ayerst 309 | PATHOCIL 500 mg Wyeth-Ayerst 593 | PHRENILIN Forte Carnrick 8656 |

h

| CECLOR 500 mg Lilly 3062 | ACHROMYCIN V 500 mg Lederle A5 | AMOXIL 500 mg SmithKline Beecham | HALDOL 2 mg McNeil Pharmaceutical | | ORTHO-EST 1.25 1.5 mg Ortho 1800 |

i

| | | | | | |

a

NORPRAMIN 10 mg
Marion Merrell Dow
68-7

ELAVIL 10 mg
Stuart 40

ORTHO-CYCLEN and
ORTHO TRI-CYCLEN
Ortho 250

LEVOTHROID 150 µg
Forest LN

CYSTOSPAZ 0.15 mg
Webcon Uriceuticals
2225

BLOCADREN 5 mg
Merck & Co. 59

b

ZAROXOLYN 5 mg
Fisons Pharmaceuticals

ORTHO TRI-CYCLEN
Ortho 215

BREVICON or
TRI-NORINYL
Syntex 110

RITALIN 10 mg
CIBA 3

STELAZINE 1 mg
SmithKline Beecham S03

LEVOTHROID 137 µg
Forest LC

c

TRANXENE-SD
11.25 mg
Abbott TX

ESTROVIS 100 µg
Parke-Davis 437

SYNTHROID 150 µg
Boots Pharmaceuticals

BENTYL 20 mg
Marion Merrell Dow

ISOPTIN 40 mg
Knoll

STELAZINE 2 mg
SmithKline Beecham S04

d

MICRONASE 5 mg
Upjohn

COUMADIN 4 mg
Du Pont

BLOCADREN 10 mg
Merck & Co. 136

DITROPAN 5 mg
Marion Merrell Dow 1375

CHLOR-TRIMETON
Decongestant
Schering-Plough 901

MOBAN 50 mg
Gate

e

KLONOPIN 1 mg
Roche

APRESOLINE 25 mg
CIBA 39

ISORDIL Titradose
30 mg
Wyeth-Ayerst 4159

CORGARD 20 mg
Bristol Laboratories 232

DILOR 200 mg
Savage 1115

FLAGYL 250 mg
Searle 1831

f

STELAZINE 5 mg
SmithKline Beecham S06

DEMAZIN
Schering 751

APRESOLINE 50 mg
CIBA 73

METAHYDRIN 4 mg
Marion Merrell Dow 63

ESIDRIX 100 mg
CIBA 192

DIMETAPP
Robins 2254

g

LIMBITROL
Roche

STELAZINE 10 mg
SmithKline Beecham S07

CORGARD 40 mg
Bristol Laboratories 207

FIORICET
Sandoz Pharmaceuticals

CORGARD 80 mg
Bristol Laboratories 241

h

DIMETAPP
Extentabs
Robins

DRIXORAL
Non-Drowsy
Extended Release
Schering-Plough

NORMODYNE 300 mg
Schering 438

i

COMBIPRES 0.2 mg
Boehringer Ingelheim 9

HALCION 0.25 mg
Upjohn

BETAPACE 80 mg
Berlex

SORBITRATE Oral
40 mg
Zeneca 774

SORBITRATE Oral
20 mg
Zeneca 820

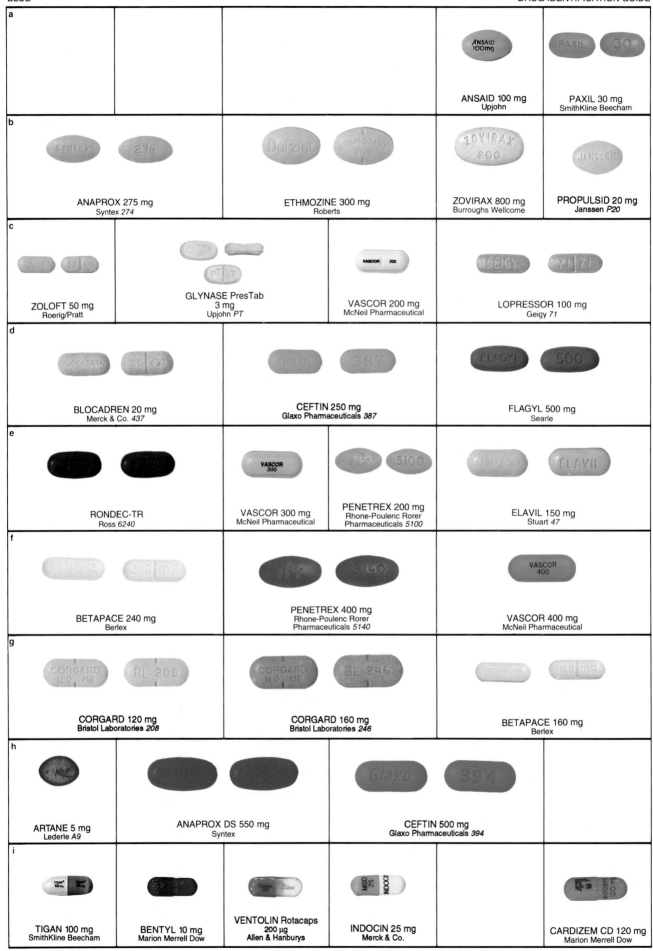

a

ANSAID 100 mg
Upjohn

PAXIL 30 mg
SmithKline Beecham

b

ANAPROX 275 mg
Syntex *274*

ETHMOZINE 300 mg
Roberts

ZOVIRAX 800 mg
Burroughs Wellcome

PROPULSID 20 mg
Janssen *P20*

c

ZOLOFT 50 mg
Roerig/Pratt

GLYNASE PresTab
3 mg
Upjohn *PT*

VASCOR 200 mg
McNeil Pharmaceutical

LOPRESSOR 100 mg
Geigy *71*

d

BLOCADREN 20 mg
Merck & Co. *437*

CEFTIN 250 mg
Glaxo Pharmaceuticals *387*

FLAGYL 500 mg
Searle

e

RONDEC-TR
Ross *6240*

VASCOR 300 mg
McNeil Pharmaceutical

PENETREX 200 mg
Rhone-Poulenc Rorer
Pharmaceuticals *5100*

ELAVIL 150 mg
Stuart *47*

f

BETAPACE 240 mg
Berlex

PENETREX 400 mg
Rhone-Poulenc Rorer
Pharmaceuticals *5140*

VASCOR 400 mg
McNeil Pharmaceutical

g

CORGARD 120 mg
Bristol Laboratories *208*

CORGARD 160 mg
Bristol Laboratories *246*

BETAPACE 160 mg
Berlex

h

ARTANE 5 mg
Lederle *A9*

ANAPROX DS 550 mg
Syntex

CEFTIN 500 mg
Glaxo Pharmaceuticals *394*

i

TIGAN 100 mg
SmithKline Beecham

BENTYL 10 mg
Marion Merrell Dow

VENTOLIN Rotacaps
200 µg
Allen & Hanburys

INDOCIN 25 mg
Merck & Co.

CARDIZEM CD 120 mg
Marion Merrell Dow

a

SINEQUAN 25 mg Roerig 535	APRESAZIDE 25/25 CIBA 139	VIBRAMYCIN 50 mg Pfizer 094	ALTACE 10 mg Hoechst-Roussel	CYSTOSPAZ-M 375 µg Webcon Uriceuticals W-2260	DYNAPEN 250 mg Apothecon 7893

b

SINEQUAN 100 mg Roerig 538	FASTIN 30 mg SmithKline Beecham	CARDENE 30 mg Syntex 2438	VELOSEF 250 mg Apothecon 113	INDOCIN SR 75 mg Merck & Co. 693	

c

VALRELEASE 15 mg Roche	SURMONTIL 25 mg Wyeth-Ayerst 4132	RESTORIL 7.5 mg Sandoz Pharmaceuticals	DORYX 100 mg Parke-Davis		INDERAL LA 120 mg Wyeth-Ayerst

d

INDERAL LA 160 mg Wyeth-Ayerst	TIGAN 250 mg SmithKline Beecham	TUSS-ORNADE SmithKline Beecham	INDOCIN 50 mg Merck & Co. 50	ZOVIRAX 200 mg Burroughs Wellcome	CLEOCIN 300 mg Upjohn

e

ISORDIL Tembids 40 mg Wyeth-Ayerst 4140	NAVANE 20 mg Roerig 577	SYNALGOS-DC Wyeth-Ayerst 4191	DYCILL 250 mg SmithKline Beecham 165	DEPAKOTE Sprinkle 125 mg Abbott	ANAFRANIL 50 mg Basel

f

VIBRAMYCIN 100 mg Pfizer 095	CARDENE SR 45 mg Syntex 2441	CARDENE SR 60 mg Syntex 2442	LORABID 200 mg Lilly 3170	CARDIZEM CD 180 mg Marion Merrell Dow	SPORANOX 100 mg Janssen

g

MINIPRESS 5 mg Pfizer 438	HYDROCET Carnrick 8657	SINEQUAN 150 mg Roerig 537	VELOSEF 500 mg Apothecon 114	THEOBID 260 mg Whitby 268	FIORINAL with Codeine No. 3 Sandoz Pharmaceuticals 78-107

h

COGNEX 20 mg Parke-Davis	LINCOCIN 500 mg Upjohn	NICOBID 500 mg Rhone-Poulenc Rorer Pharmaceuticals	VERELAN 240 mg Lederle V9	CARDIZEM CD 240 mg Marion Merrell Dow	CLEOCIN 150 mg Upjohn

i

CARDIZEM CD 300 mg Marion Merrell Dow	PENTASA 250 mg Marion Merrell Dow	INDERAL 20 mg Wyeth-Ayerst	DECADRON 0.75 mg Merck & Co. 63	DIABINESE 100 mg Pfizer 393	LEVSIN/SL Sublingual 0.125 mg Schwarz Pharma Kremers Urban 532

11

a					
HYGROTON 50 mg Rhone-Poulenc Rorer Pharmaceuticals *20*	**TIMOLIDE 10-25** Merck & Co. *67*	**ASENDIN 100 mg** Lederle *A17*	**MEVACOR 20 mg** Merck & Co. *731*	**TRIAVIL 2-10** Merck & Co. *914*	**VALIUM 10 mg** Roche
b					
HALDOL 10 mg McNeil Pharmaceutical	**DIABINESE 250 mg** Pfizer *394*	**TRANXENE 3.75 mg** Abbott *TL*	**PROSCAR 5 mg** Merck & Co. *72*		
c					
d					
e					
f					
g					
h					
i					

a MELLARIL 10 mg Sandoz Pharmaceuticals 78-2	ESTRACE 2 mg Bristol-Myers Squibb 756	LOESTRIN 21 1.5/30 Parke-Davis 916	LEVOTHROID 88 µg Forest LA	SYNTHROID 88 µg Boots Pharmaceuticals	LIBRITABS 5 mg Roche
b NORINYL 1 + 35 or TRI-NORINYL Syntex 111	HYDROPRES 25 Merck & Co. 53	MICRONOR 0.35 mg Ortho	LEVOTHROID 175 µg Forest LP		
c HYTRIN 10 mg Abbott DI			BUTISOL Sodium 30 mg Wallace 37-113	SYNTHROID 300 µg Boots Pharmaceuticals	LIBRITABS 10 mg Roche
d LANOXIN 500 µg Burroughs Wellcome T9A	NORPRAMIN 50 mg Marion Merrell Dow	NITRONG 2.6 mg Rhone-Poulenc Rorer Pharmaceuticals 411	HYDROPRES 50 Merck & Co. 127		CARDIZEM 30 mg Marion Merrell Dow 1771
e DONNATAL No. 2 Robins 4264	DESOGEN Placebo Organon KH 2	ISORDIL Oral Titradose 20 mg Wyeth-Ayerst 4154	LIBRITABS 25 mg Roche	COMPAZINE 5 mg SmithKline Beecham C66	SORBITRATE 5 mg Chewable Zeneca 810
f SALUTENSIN Roberts S1	ATROCHOLIN Allen & Hanburys	MELLARIL 100 mg Sandoz Pharmaceuticals		BONTRIL PDM 35 mg Carnrick 8648	COMPAZINE 10 mg SmithKline Beecham C67
g DONNATAL Extentabs Robins		COMPAZINE 25 mg SmithKline Beecham C69	COUMADIN 2.5 mg Du Pont Pharmaceuticals	ISORDIL Oral Titradose 40 mg Wyeth-Ayerst 4192	TAGAMET 300 mg SmithKline Beecham
h FUROXONE 100 mg Roberts 072	ENDECON Du Pont	P-A-C Upjohn	ASBRON G Sandoz Pharmaceuticals 78-202	CHLOR-TRIMETON Decongestant Schering-Plough LA CTM D	
i DRIXORAL Schering-Plough	DONNAZYME Robins 4650	GANTANOL 0.5 g Roche			

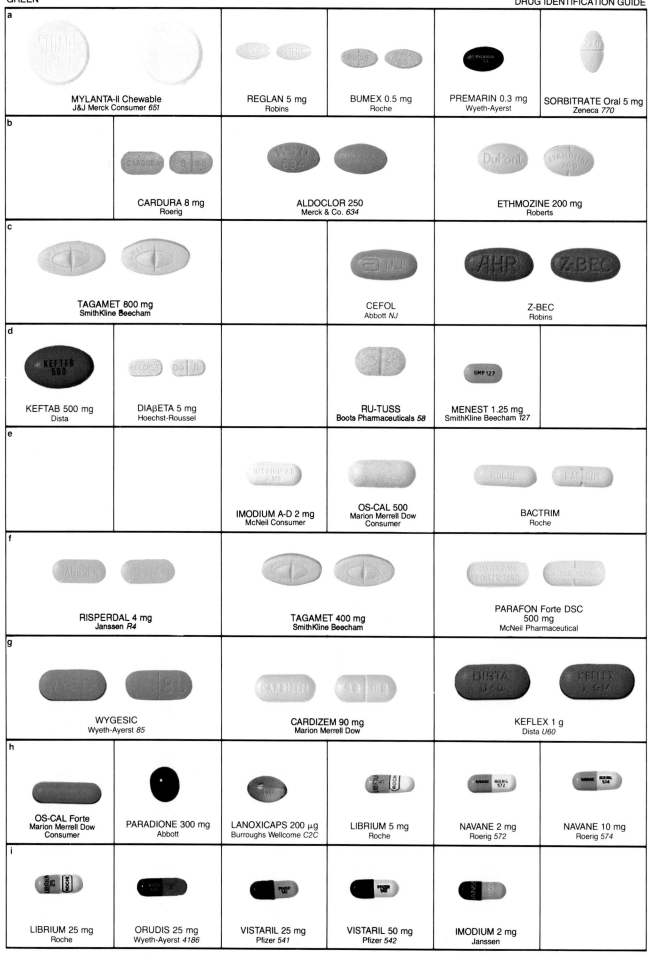

a

MYLANTA-II Chewable
J&J Merck Consumer *651*

REGLAN 5 mg
Robins

BUMEX 0.5 mg
Roche

PREMARIN 0.3 mg
Wyeth-Ayerst

SORBITRATE Oral 5 mg
Zeneca *770*

b

CARDURA 8 mg
Roerig

ALDOCLOR 250
Merck & Co. *634*

ETHMOZINE 200 mg
Roberts

c

TAGAMET 800 mg
SmithKline Beecham

CEFOL
Abbott *NJ*

Z-BEC
Robins

d

KEFTAB 500 mg
Dista

DIAβETA 5 mg
Hoechst-Roussel

RU-TUSS
Boots Pharmaceuticals *58*

MENEST 1.25 mg
SmithKline Beecham *127*

e

IMODIUM A-D 2 mg
McNeil Consumer

OS-CAL 500
Marion Merrell Dow
Consumer

BACTRIM
Roche

f

RISPERDAL 4 mg
Janssen *R4*

TAGAMET 400 mg
SmithKline Beecham

PARAFON Forte DSC
500 mg
McNeil Pharmaceutical

g

WYGESIC
Wyeth-Ayerst *85*

CARDIZEM 90 mg
Marion Merrell Dow

KEFLEX 1 g
Dista *U60*

h

OS-CAL Forte
Marion Merrell Dow
Consumer

PARADIONE 300 mg
Abbott

LANOXICAPS 200 μg
Burroughs Wellcome *C2C*

LIBRIUM 5 mg
Roche

NAVANE 2 mg
Roerig *572*

NAVANE 10 mg
Roerig *574*

i

LIBRIUM 25 mg
Roche

ORUDIS 25 mg
Wyeth-Ayerst *4186*

VISTARIL 25 mg
Pfizer *541*

VISTARIL 50 mg
Pfizer *542*

IMODIUM 2 mg
Janssen

a

DOPAR 100 mg Roberts	DONNATAL Robins *4207*	LIBRAX Roche	PROZAC 20 mg Dista *3105*

b

VISTARIL 100 mg Pfizer *543*		NORPACE CR 100 mg Searle *2732*	CINOBAC 250 mg Oclassen *55*	MINIZIDE 2 Pfizer *432*

MINIZIDE 1
Pfizer *430*

c

MINOCIN 100 mg Lederle *M46*		ORUDIS 75 mg Wyeth-Ayerst *4187*	ANCOBON 250 mg Roche	ORUDIS 50 mg Wyeth-Ayerst *4181*

LOXITANE 5 mg
Lederle *L1*

d

LOXITANE 10 mg Lederle *L2*	TRIMOX 250 mg Apothecon *230*	DUADACIN Bradley	LOXITANE 25 mg Lederle *L3*	PRELU-2 105 mg Boehringer Ingelheim *64*

e

LOXITANE 50 mg Lederle *L4*	DOPAR 250 mg Roberts	BONTRIL 105 mg Carnrick *8647*	CeeNU 100 mg Bristol-Myers Oncology *3032*	ANTURANE 200 mg CIBA *168*

PROZAC 10 mg
Dista *3104*

f

CLEOCIN 75 mg Upjohn	MINIZIDE 5 Pfizer *436*	COGNEX 10 mg Parke-Davis	DOPAR 500 mg Roberts	FIORINAL Sandoz Pharmaceuticals *78-103*

g

	NICOBID 250 mg Rhone-Poulenc Rorer Pharmaceuticals	PHENAPHEN with Codeine No. 4 Robins *6274*	KEFLEX 250 mg Dista *H69*	TACE 25 mg Marion Merrell Dow *691*

h

COTAZYM 25 mg Organon *381*	SOLATENE 30 mg Roche	TRIMOX 500 mg Apothecon *231*	UNIPEN 250 mg Wyeth-Ayerst *57*	PANMYCIN 250 mg Upjohn

i

CINOBAC 500 mg Oclassen *56*	KEFLEX 500 mg Dista *H71*	TACE 12 mg Marion Merrell Dow *690*	ATARAX 25 mg Roerig	FEOSOL SmithKline Beecham Consumer	DECADRON 6 mg Merck & Co. *147*

a

MEVACOR 40 mg Merck & Co. *732*	NAQUA 4 mg Schering *547* or *ÀHH*	MAXZIDE 25 Lederle *M9*	HALDOL 5 mg McNeil Pharmaceutical	INDERAL 40 mg Wyeth-Ayerst	

b

SPEC-T Decongestant Lozenges Apothecon					

c

d

ISORDIL Sublingual 2.5 mg Wyeth-Ayerst	OVRETTE 0.075 mg Wyeth-Ayerst *62*	TRIPHASIL Wyeth-Ayerst *643*	ANTROCOL Poythress *9540*	TRI-LEVLEN Berlex *97*	SANSERT 2 mg Sandoz Pharmaceuticals *78-58*

e

DULCOLAX 5 mg Upjohn *12*	SORBITRATE Sublingual 10 mg Zeneca *761*	DILAUDID 4 mg Knoll	OVCON-50 Bristol-Myers Squibb *584*		

f

INVERSINE 2.5 mg Merck & Co. *52*	LANOXIN 125 µg Burroughs Wellcome *Y3B*	MEPHYTON 5 mg Merck & Co. *43*	RITALIN 5 mg CIBA *7*		CANTIL 25 mg Marion Merrell Dow *37*

g

LEVOTHROID 100 µg Forest *LM*	ORTHO-NOVUM 1/50 Ortho *150*	ZAROXOLYN 10 mg Fisons Pharmaceuticals	TORECAN 10 mg Roxane *28*		

h

SPARINE 25 mg Wyeth-Ayerst *29*	SYNTHROID 100 µg Boots Pharmaceuticals	PLEGINE 35 mg Wyeth-Ayerst	RHEUMATREX 2.5 mg Lederle *M1*	ELAVIL 25 mg Stuart *45*	THYROLAR-3 Forest *YH*

i

ETRAFON 2-10 Schering *287* or *ANA*	RITALIN 20 mg CIBA *34*	HEXADROL 0.5 mg Organon *792*	APRESOLINE 10 mg CIBA *37*		

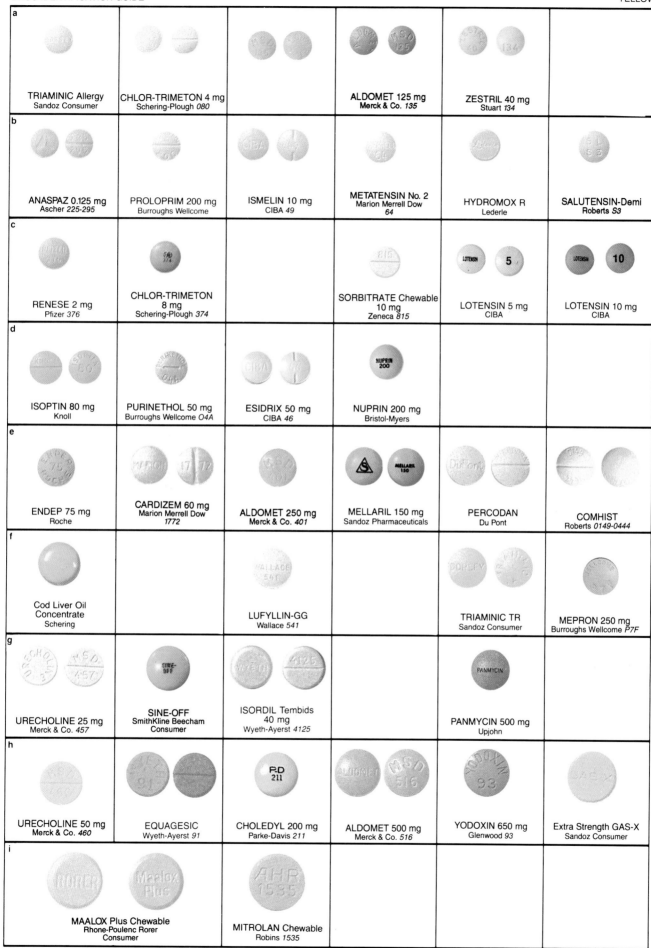

a

TRIAMINIC Allergy Sandoz Consumer	CHLOR-TRIMETON 4 mg Schering-Plough *080*		ALDOMET 125 mg Merck & Co. *135*	ZESTRIL 40 mg Stuart *134*	

b

ANASPAZ 0.125 mg Ascher *225-295*	PROLOPRIM 200 mg Burroughs Wellcome	ISMELIN 10 mg CIBA *49*	METATENSIN No. 2 Marion Merrell Dow *64*	HYDROMOX R Lederle	SALUTENSIN-Demi Roberts *S3*

c

RENESE 2 mg Pfizer *376*	CHLOR-TRIMETON 8 mg Schering-Plough *374*		SORBITRATE Chewable 10 mg Zeneca *815*	LOTENSIN 5 mg CIBA	LOTENSIN 10 mg CIBA

d

ISOPTIN 80 mg Knoll	PURINETHOL 50 mg Burroughs Wellcome *O4A*	ESIDRIX 50 mg CIBA *46*	NUPRIN 200 mg Bristol-Myers

e

ENDEP 75 mg Roche	CARDIZEM 60 mg Marion Merrell Dow *1772*	ALDOMET 250 mg Merck & Co. *401*	MELLARIL 150 mg Sandoz Pharmaceuticals	PERCODAN Du Pont	COMHIST Roberts *0149-0444*

f

Cod Liver Oil Concentrate Schering		LUFYLLIN-GG Wallace *541*		TRIAMINIC TR Sandoz Consumer	MEPRON 250 mg Burroughs Wellcome *P7F*

g

URECHOLINE 25 mg Merck & Co. *457*	SINE-OFF SmithKline Beecham Consumer	ISORDIL Tembids 40 mg Wyeth-Ayerst *4125*	PANMYCIN 500 mg Upjohn	

h

URECHOLINE 50 mg Merck & Co. *460*	EQUAGESIC Wyeth-Ayerst *91*	CHOLEDYL 200 mg Parke-Davis *211*	ALDOMET 500 mg Merck & Co. *516*	YODOXIN 650 mg Glenwood *93*	Extra Strength GAS-X Sandoz Consumer

i

MAALOX Plus Chewable Rhone-Poulenc Rorer Consumer	MITROLAN Chewable Robins *1535*	

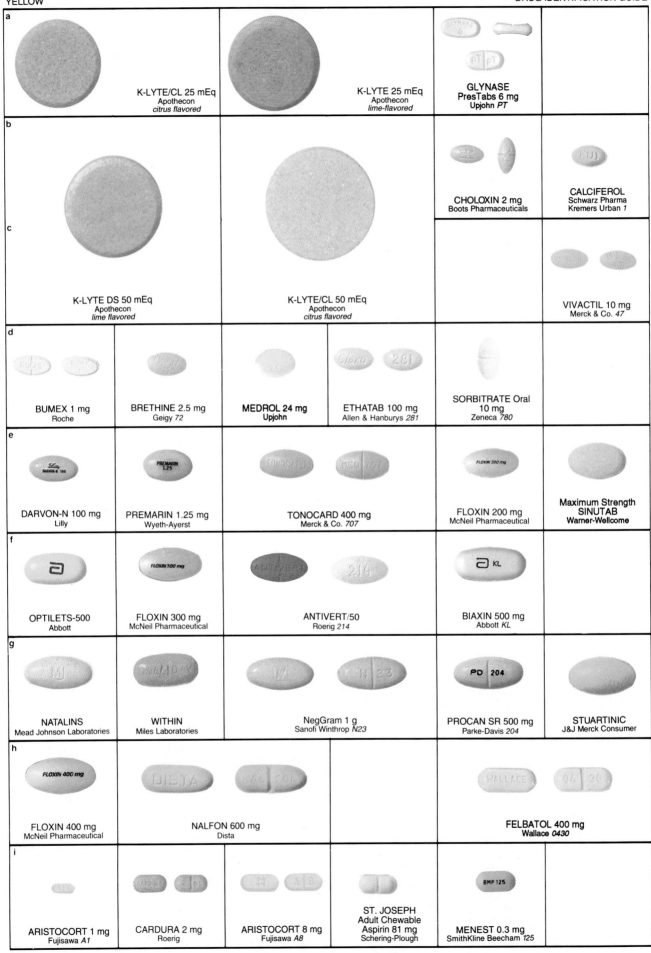

a

K-LYTE/CL 25 mEq
Apothecon
citrus flavored

K-LYTE 25 mEq
Apothecon
lime-flavored

GLYNASE
PresTabs 6 mg
Upjohn *PT*

b

CHOLOXIN 2 mg
Boots Pharmaceuticals

CALCIFEROL
Schwarz Pharma
Kremers Urban *1*

c

K-LYTE DS 50 mEq
Apothecon
lime flavored

K-LYTE/CL 50 mEq
Apothecon
citrus flavored

VIVACTIL 10 mg
Merck & Co. *47*

d

BUMEX 1 mg
Roche

BRETHINE 2.5 mg
Geigy *72*

MEDROL 24 mg
Upjohn

ETHATAB 100 mg
Allen & Hanburys *281*

SORBITRATE Oral
10 mg
Zeneca *780*

e

DARVON-N 100 mg
Lilly

PREMARIN 1.25 mg
Wyeth-Ayerst

TONOCARD 400 mg
Merck & Co. *707*

FLOXIN 200 mg
McNeil Pharmaceutical

Maximum Strength
SINUTAB
Warner-Wellcome

f

OPTILETS-500
Abbott

FLOXIN 300 mg
McNeil Pharmaceutical

ANTIVERT/50
Roerig *214*

BIAXIN 500 mg
Abbott *KL*

g

NATALINS
Mead Johnson Laboratories

WITHIN
Miles Laboratories

NegGram 1 g
Sanofi Winthrop *N23*

PROCAN SR 500 mg
Parke-Davis *204*

STUARTINIC
J&J Merck Consumer

h

FLOXIN 400 mg
McNeil Pharmaceutical

NALFON 600 mg
Dista

FELBATOL 400 mg
Wallace *0430*

i

ARISTOCORT 1 mg
Fujisawa *A1*

CARDURA 2 mg
Roerig

ARISTOCORT 8 mg
Fujisawa *A8*

ST. JOSEPH
Adult Chewable
Aspirin 81 mg
Schering-Plough

MENEST 0.3 mg
SmithKline Beecham *125*

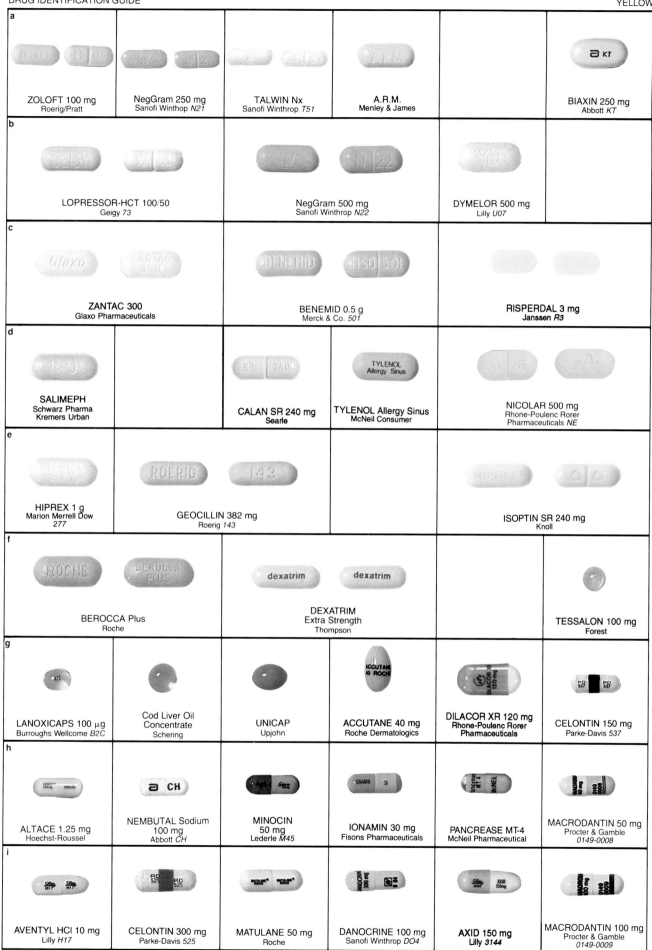

a

ZOLOFT 100 mg
Roerig/Pratt

NegGram 250 mg
Sanofi Winthop *N21*

TALWIN Nx
Sanofi Winthrop *T51*

A.R.M.
Menley & James

BIAXIN 250 mg
Abbott *KT*

b

LOPRESSOR-HCT 100/50
Geigy *73*

NegGram 500 mg
Sanofi Winthrop *N22*

DYMELOR 500 mg
Lilly *U07*

c

ZANTAC 300
Glaxo Pharmaceuticals

BENEMID 0.5 g
Merck & Co. *501*

RISPERDAL 3 mg
Janssen *R3*

d

SALIMEPH
Schwarz Pharma
Kremers Urban

CALAN SR 240 mg
Searle

TYLENOL Allergy Sinus
McNeil Consumer

NICOLAR 500 mg
Rhone-Poulenc Rorer
Pharmaceuticals *NE*

e

HIPREX 1 g
Marion Merrell Dow
277

GEOCILLIN 382 mg
Roerig *143*

ISOPTIN SR 240 mg
Knoll

f

BEROCCA Plus
Roche

DEXATRIM
Extra Strength
Thompson

TESSALON 100 mg
Forest

g

LANOXICAPS 100 µg
Burroughs Wellcome *B2C*

Cod Liver Oil
Concentrate
Schering

UNICAP
Upjohn

ACCUTANE 40 mg
Roche Dermatologics

DILACOR XR 120 mg
Rhone-Poulenc Rorer
Pharmaceuticals

CELONTIN 150 mg
Parke-Davis *537*

h

ALTACE 1.25 mg
Hoechst-Roussel

NEMBUTAL Sodium
100 mg
Abbott *CH*

MINOCIN
50 mg
Lederle *M45*

IONAMIN 30 mg
Fisons Pharmaceuticals

PANCREASE MT-4
McNeil Pharmaceutical

MACRODANTIN 50 mg
Procter & Gamble
0149-0008

i

AVENTYL HCl 10 mg
Lilly *H17*

CELONTIN 300 mg
Parke-Davis *525*

MATULANE 50 mg
Roche

DANOCRINE 100 mg
Sanofi Winthrop *DO4*

AXID 150 mg
Lilly *3144*

MACRODANTIN 100 mg
Procter & Gamble
0149-0009

a

VERELAN
120 mg
Lederle V8

CUPRIMINE 250 mg
Merck & Co. 602

PONSTEL 250 mg
Parke-Davis 540

COMHIST LA
Roberts 0149-0446

KU-ZYME
Schwarz Pharma
Kremers Urban 522

ANAFRANIL 75 mg
Basel

b

AVENTYL HCI 25 mg
Lilly H19

NEURONTIN 300 mg
Parke-Davis

UROBIOTIC-250
Roerig 092

GRISACTIN 250 mg
Wyeth-Ayerst

TERRAMYCIN 250 mg
Pfizer 073

c

DECADRON 0.5 mg
Merck & Co. 41

VASOTEC 2.5 mg
Merck & Co. 14

VOLTAREN 25 mg
Geigy

d

ZOCOR 5 mg
Merck & Co. 726

HALDOL 1 mg
McNeil Pharmaceutical

ENDURONYL
Abbott LS

ATARAX 50 mg
Roerig

SERAX 15 mg
Wyeth-Ayerst 317

FLEXERIL 10 mg
Merck & Co. 931

e

PRINZIDE 20–12.5
Merck & Co. 140

PRINIVIL 20 mg
Merck & Co. 207

TRIAVIL 4-25
Merck & Co. 946

TENEX 2 mg
Robins

VALIUM 5 mg
Roche

INDERAL 80 mg
Wyeth-Ayerst

f

CLINORIL 150 mg
Merck & Co. 941

DILANTIN Infatabs
50 mg
Parke-Davis 007

MYSOLINE 250 mg
Wyeth-Ayerst

CLINORIL 200 mg
Merck & Co. 942

IMURAN 50 mg
Burroughs Wellcome

KENACORT 8 mg
Apothecon 518

g

PRINIVIL 10 mg
Merck & Co. 106

MAXZIDE
Lederle M8

DESYREL 300 mg
Apothecon 796

SPEC-T Cough
Suppressant Lozenges
Apothecon

h

TONOCARD 600 mg
Merck & Co. 709

CLOZARIL 25 mg
Sandoz Pharmaceuticals

CLOZARIL 100 mg
Sandoz Pharmaceuticals

i

a

PERSANTINE 25 mg Boehringer Ingelheim *17*	NORDETTE Wyeth-Ayerst *75*	ERGOSTAT Sublingual 2 mg Parke-Davis *111*	DILAUDID 2 mg Knoll	ORTHO-CEPT Ortho *D150*	

b

LEVOTHROID 25 µg Forest *LK*	ENDEP 10 mg Roche	LUDIOMIL 50 mg CIBA *26*	VONTROL 25 mg SmithKline Beecham		PERSANTINE 50 mg Boehringer Ingelheim *18*

c

THYROLAR-½ Forest *YD*	MOBAN 5 mg Gate	PONDIMIN 20 mg Robins *6447*	HEXADROL 1.5 mg Organon *790*	KLONOPIN 0.5 mg Roche	

d

TRIAMINIC Cold Tablets Sandoz Consumer			LODOSYN Merck & Co. *129*	ENDEP 25 mg Roche	

e

PHENERGAN 12.5 mg Wyeth-Ayerst *19*		MARPLAN 10 mg Roche	PAXIPAM 20 mg Schering *251*	PERSANTINE 75 mg Boehringer Ingelheim *19*	CHLOR-TRIMETON 12 mg Schering-Plough *009*

f

SPARINE 50 mg Wyeth-Ayerst *28*	NORPRAMIN 25 mg Marion Merrell Dow	PREMARIN with Methyl- testosterone 1.25/10 Wyeth-Ayerst *879*			

g

	NARDIL 15 mg Parke-Davis *270*		SENOKOT-S Purdue Frederick	ST. JOSEPH Cold for Children Schering-Plough	

h

	GENTLAX S Purdue Frederick	TREXAN 50 mg Du Pont Pharmaceuticals	ENDEP 50 mg Roche	TOFRANIL 50 mg Geigy *136*	ECOTRIN 325 mg SmithKline Beecham Consumer

i

	NORPRAMIN 100 mg Marion Merrell Dow	ENDEP 150 mg Roche	MODANE Plus Savage *515*	TRINALIN Key *703*	ELAVIL 75 mg Stuart *42*

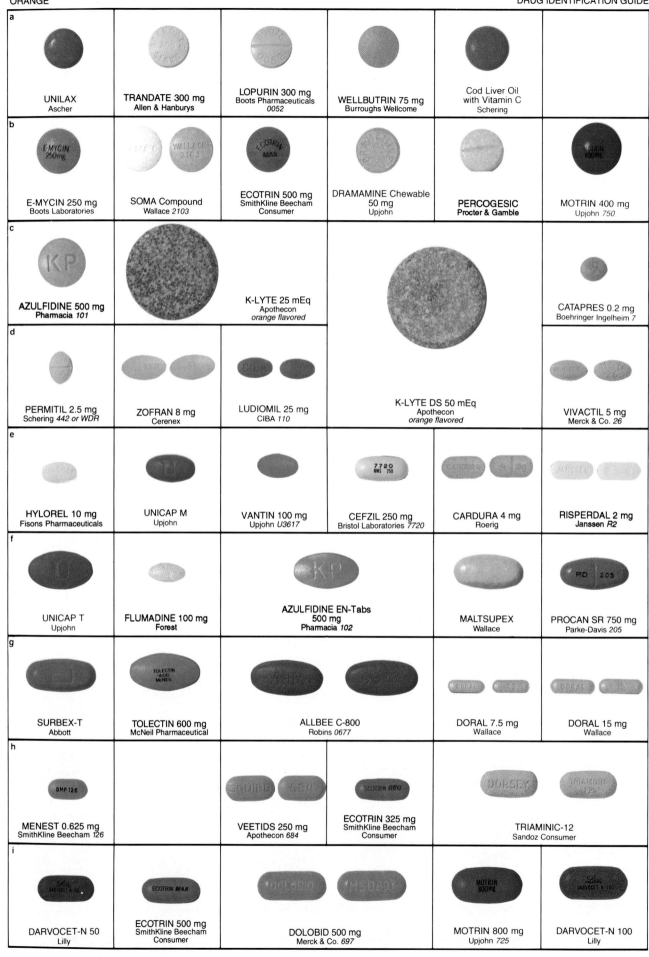

a

UNILAX
Ascher

TRANDATE 300 mg
Allen & Hanburys

LOPURIN 300 mg
Boots Pharmaceuticals
0052

WELLBUTRIN 75 mg
Burroughs Wellcome

Cod Liver Oil
with Vitamin C
Schering

b

E-MYCIN 250 mg
Boots Laboratories

SOMA Compound
Wallace *2103*

ECOTRIN 500 mg
SmithKline Beecham
Consumer

DRAMAMINE Chewable
50 mg
Upjohn

PERCOGESIC
Procter & Gamble

MOTRIN 400 mg
Upjohn *750*

c

AZULFIDINE 500 mg
Pharmacia *101*

K-LYTE 25 mEq
Apothecon
orange flavored

CATAPRES 0.2 mg
Boehringer Ingelheim *7*

d

PERMITIL 2.5 mg
Schering *442 or WDR*

ZOFRAN 8 mg
Cerenex

LUDIOMIL 25 mg
CIBA *110*

K-LYTE DS 50 mEq
Apothecon
orange flavored

VIVACTIL 5 mg
Merck & Co. *26*

e

HYLOREL 10 mg
Fisons Pharmaceuticals

UNICAP M
Upjohn

VANTIN 100 mg
Upjohn *U3617*

CEFZIL 250 mg
Bristol Laboratories *7720*

CARDURA 4 mg
Roerig

RISPERDAL 2 mg
Janssen *R2*

f

UNICAP T
Upjohn

FLUMADINE 100 mg
Forest

AZULFIDINE EN-Tabs
500 mg
Pharmacia *102*

MALTSUPEX
Wallace

PROCAN SR 750 mg
Parke-Davis *205*

g

SURBEX-T
Abbott

TOLECTIN 600 mg
McNeil Pharmaceutical

ALLBEE C-800
Robins *0677*

DORAL 7.5 mg
Wallace

DORAL 15 mg
Wallace

h

MENEST 0.625 mg
SmithKline Beecham *126*

VEETIDS 250 mg
Apothecon *684*

ECOTRIN 325 mg
SmithKline Beecham
Consumer

TRIAMINIC-12
Sandoz Consumer

i

DARVOCET-N 50
Lilly

ECOTRIN 500 mg
SmithKline Beecham
Consumer

DOLOBID 500 mg
Merck & Co. *697*

MOTRIN 800 mg
Upjohn *725*

DARVOCET-N 100
Lilly

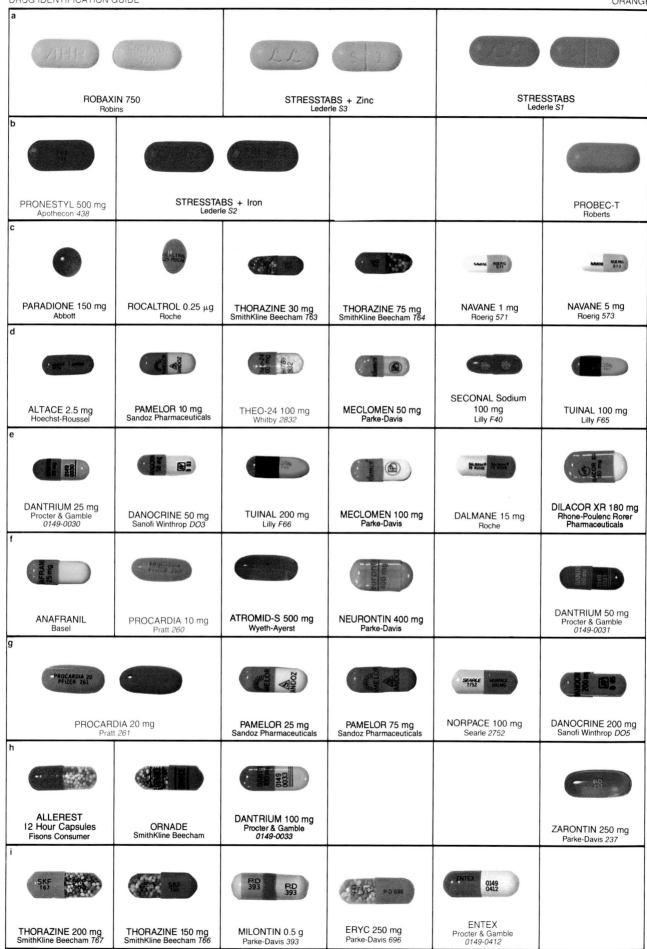

a

ROBAXIN 750
Robins

STRESSTABS + Zinc
Lederle *S3*

STRESSTABS
Lederle *S1*

b

PRONESTYL 500 mg
Apothecon *438*

STRESSTABS + Iron
Lederle *S2*

PROBEC-T
Roberts

c

PARADIONE 150 mg
Abbott

ROCALTROL 0.25 µg
Roche

THORAZINE 30 mg
SmithKline Beecham *T63*

THORAZINE 75 mg
SmithKline Beecham *T64*

NAVANE 1 mg
Roerig *571*

NAVANE 5 mg
Roerig *573*

d

ALTACE 2.5 mg
Hoechst-Roussel

PAMELOR 10 mg
Sandoz Pharmaceuticals

THEO-24 100 mg
Whitby *2832*

MECLOMEN 50 mg
Parke-Davis

SECONAL Sodium
100 mg
Lilly *F40*

TUINAL 100 mg
Lilly *F65*

e

DANTRIUM 25 mg
Procter & Gamble
0149-0030

DANOCRINE 50 mg
Sanofi Winthrop *DO3*

TUINAL 200 mg
Lilly *F66*

MECLOMEN 100 mg
Parke-Davis

DALMANE 15 mg
Roche

DILACOR XR 180 mg
Rhone-Poulenc Rorer
Pharmaceuticals

f

ANAFRANIL
Basel

PROCARDIA 10 mg
Pratt *260*

ATROMID-S 500 mg
Wyeth-Ayerst

NEURONTIN 400 mg
Parke-Davis

DANTRIUM 50 mg
Procter & Gamble
0149-0031

g

PROCARDIA 20 mg
Pratt *261*

PAMELOR 25 mg
Sandoz Pharmaceuticals

PAMELOR 75 mg
Sandoz Pharmaceuticals

NORPACE 100 mg
Searle *2752*

DANOCRINE 200 mg
Sanofi Winthrop *DO5*

h

ALLEREST
12 Hour Capsules
Fisons Consumer

ORNADE
SmithKline Beecham

DANTRIUM 100 mg
Procter & Gamble
0149-0033

ZARONTIN 250 mg
Parke-Davis *237*

i

THORAZINE 200 mg
SmithKline Beecham *T67*

THORAZINE 150 mg
SmithKline Beecham *T66*

MILONTIN 0.5 g
Parke-Davis *393*

ERYC 250 mg
Parke-Davis *696*

ENTEX
Procter & Gamble
0149-0412

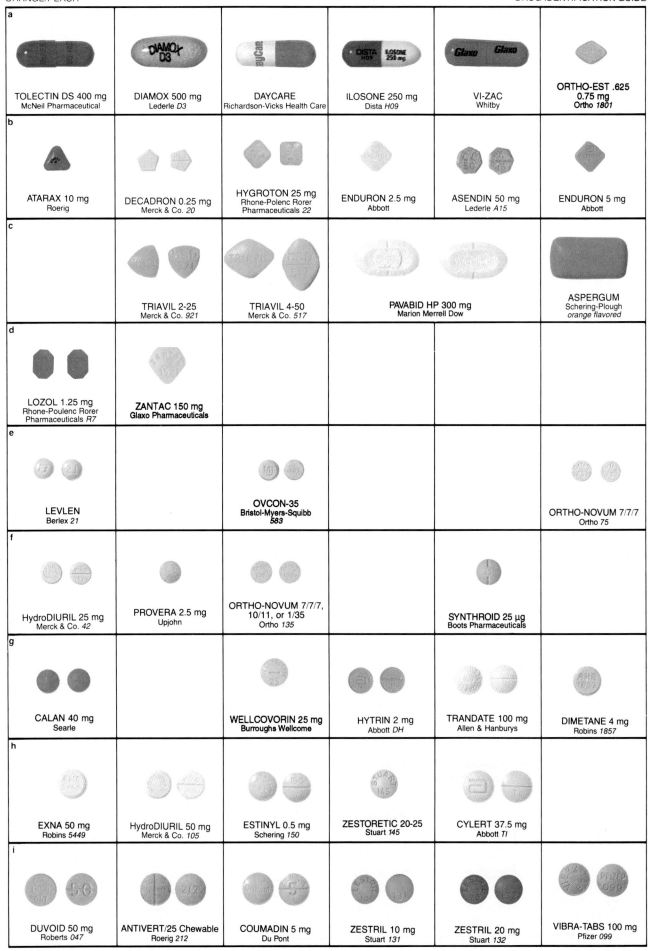

a

TOLECTIN DS 400 mg
McNeil Pharmaceutical

DIAMOX 500 mg
Lederle *D3*

DAYCARE
Richardson-Vicks Health Care

ILOSONE 250 mg
Dista *H09*

VI-ZAC
Whitby

ORTHO-EST .625
0.75 mg
Ortho *1801*

b

ATARAX 10 mg
Roerig

DECADRON 0.25 mg
Merck & Co. *20*

HYGROTON 25 mg
Rhone-Polenc Rorer
Pharmaceuticals *22*

ENDURON 2.5 mg
Abbott

ASENDIN 50 mg
Lederle *A15*

ENDURON 5 mg
Abbott

c

TRIAVIL 2-25
Merck & Co. *921*

TRIAVIL 4-50
Merck & Co. *517*

PAVABID HP 300 mg
Marion Merrell Dow

ASPERGUM
Schering-Plough
orange flavored

d

LOZOL 1.25 mg
Rhone-Poulenc Rorer
Pharmaceuticals *R7*

ZANTAC 150 mg
Glaxo Pharmaceuticals

e

LEVLEN
Berlex *21*

OVCON-35
Bristol-Myers-Squibb
583

ORTHO-NOVUM 7/7/7
Ortho *75*

f

HydroDIURIL 25 mg
Merck & Co. *42*

PROVERA 2.5 mg
Upjohn

ORTHO-NOVUM 7/7/7,
10/11, or 1/35
Ortho *135*

SYNTHROID 25 µg
Boots Pharmaceuticals

g

CALAN 40 mg
Searle

WELLCOVORIN 25 mg
Burroughs Wellcome

HYTRIN 2 mg
Abbott *DH*

TRANDATE 100 mg
Allen & Hanburys

DIMETANE 4 mg
Robins *1857*

h

EXNA 50 mg
Robins *5449*

HydroDIURIL 50 mg
Merck & Co. *105*

ESTINYL 0.5 mg
Schering *150*

ZESTORETIC 20-25
Stuart *145*

CYLERT 37.5 mg
Abbott *TI*

i

DUVOID 50 mg
Roberts *047*

ANTIVERT/25 Chewable
Roerig *212*

COUMADIN 5 mg
Du Pont

ZESTRIL 10 mg
Stuart *131*

ZESTRIL 20 mg
Stuart *132*

VIBRA-TABS 100 mg
Pfizer *099*

a

DIMETANE 12 mg
Robins *1843*

ORGANIDIN
Wallace *4224*

DUVOID 10 mg
Roberts *045*

HydroDIURIL 100 mg
Merck & Co. *410*

b

DELTASONE 20 mg
Upjohn

ORETON Methyl 25 mg
Schering *499 or JE*

ENDEP 100 mg
Roche

APRESOLINE 100 mg
CIBA *101*

ZYLOPRIM 300 mg
Burroughs Wellcome

c

ALDORIL 15
Merck & Co. *423*

VERMOX 100 mg
Janssen

GRISACTIN 500 mg
Wyeth-Ayerst

SUDAFED Sinus
Warner-Wellcome

ROBAXIN 500 mg
Robins

d

PLENDIL 5 mg
Merck & Co. *451*

SINULIN
Carnrick *8666*

ERYTHROCIN
Stearate 250 mg
Abbott *ES*

CATAPRES 0.3 mg
Boehringer Ingelheim *11*

XANAX 0.5 mg
Upjohn

CHOLOXIN 1 mg
Boots Pharmaceuticals

e

MEDROL 8 mg
Upjohn

MEDROL 32 mg
Upjohn

FELBATOL 600 mg
Wallace *0431*

CAPOZIDE 50/25
Squibb

SINEMET CR 50/200
Du Pont Pharmaceuticals
521

f

BUMEX 2 mg
Roche

DEPAKOTE 250 mg
Abbott *NR*

Maximum Strength
Without Drowsiness
SINUTAB
Warner-Wellcome

ALDORIL D30
Merck & Co. *694*

g

MOTRIN 600 mg
Upjohn *742*

PARAFLEX 250 mg
McNeil Pharmaceutical

DOLOBID 250 mg
Merck & Co. *675*

h

TRILISATE 500
Purdue Frederick

CENTRUM
Lederle *C1*

i

ACCUTANE 10 mg
Roche Dermatologics

AXID 300 mg
Lilly *3145*

MICRO-K Extencaps
600 mg
Robins *5720*

MICRO-K 10 Extencaps
750 mg
Robins *5730*

WYTENSIN 4 mg
Wyeth-Ayerst *73*

INDERAL 10 mg
Wyeth-Ayerst

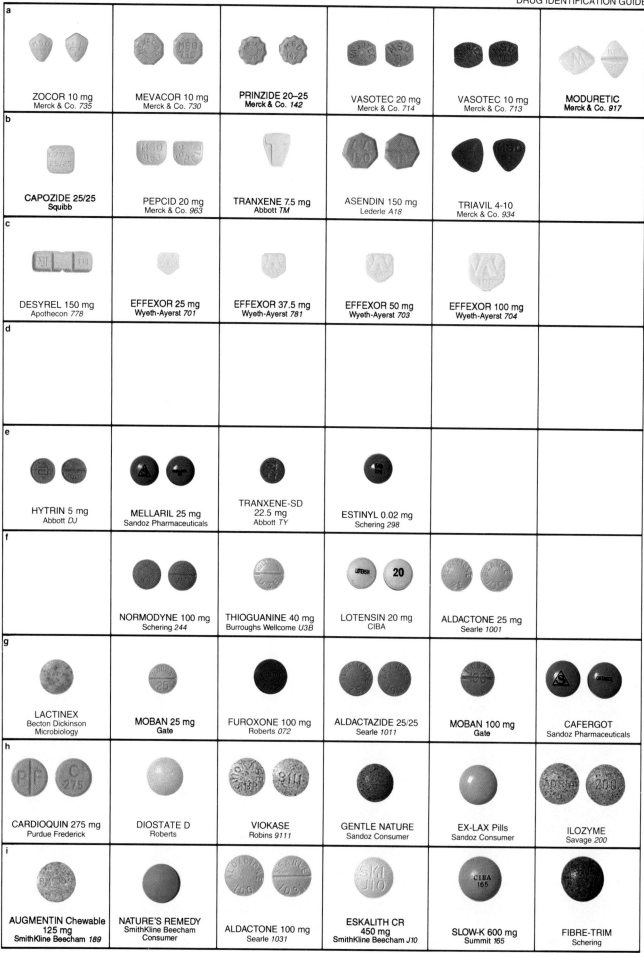

a

ZOCOR 10 mg
Merck & Co. *735*

MEVACOR 10 mg
Merck & Co. *730*

PRINZIDE 20–25
Merck & Co. *142*

VASOTEC 20 mg
Merck & Co. *714*

VASOTEC 10 mg
Merck & Co. *713*

MODURETIC
Merck & Co. *917*

b

CAPOZIDE 25/25
Squibb

PEPCID 20 mg
Merck & Co. *963*

TRANXENE 7.5 mg
Abbott *TM*

ASENDIN 150 mg
Lederle *A18*

TRIAVIL 4-10
Merck & Co. *934*

c

DESYREL 150 mg
Apothecon *778*

EFFEXOR 25 mg
Wyeth-Ayerst *701*

EFFEXOR 37.5 mg
Wyeth-Ayerst *781*

EFFEXOR 50 mg
Wyeth-Ayerst *703*

EFFEXOR 100 mg
Wyeth-Ayerst *704*

d

e

HYTRIN 5 mg
Abbott *DJ*

MELLARIL 25 mg
Sandoz Pharmaceuticals

TRANXENE-SD
22.5 mg
Abbott *TY*

ESTINYL 0.02 mg
Schering *298*

f

NORMODYNE 100 mg
Schering *244*

THIOGUANINE 40 mg
Burroughs Wellcome *U3B*

LOTENSIN 20 mg
CIBA

ALDACTONE 25 mg
Searle *1001*

g

LACTINEX
Becton Dickinson
Microbiology

MOBAN 25 mg
Gate

FUROXONE 100 mg
Roberts *072*

ALDACTAZIDE 25/25
Searle *1011*

MOBAN 100 mg
Gate

CAFERGOT
Sandoz Pharmaceuticals

h

CARDIOQUIN 275 mg
Purdue Frederick

DIOSTATE D
Roberts

VIOKASE
Robins *9111*

GENTLE NATURE
Sandoz Consumer

EX-LAX Pills
Sandoz Consumer

ILOZYME
Savage *200*

i

AUGMENTIN Chewable
125 mg
SmithKline Beecham *189*

NATURE'S REMEDY
SmithKline Beecham
Consumer

ALDACTONE 100 mg
Searle *1031*

ESKALITH CR
450 mg
SmithKline Beecham *J10*

SLOW-K 600 mg
Summit *165*

FIBRE-TRIM
Schering

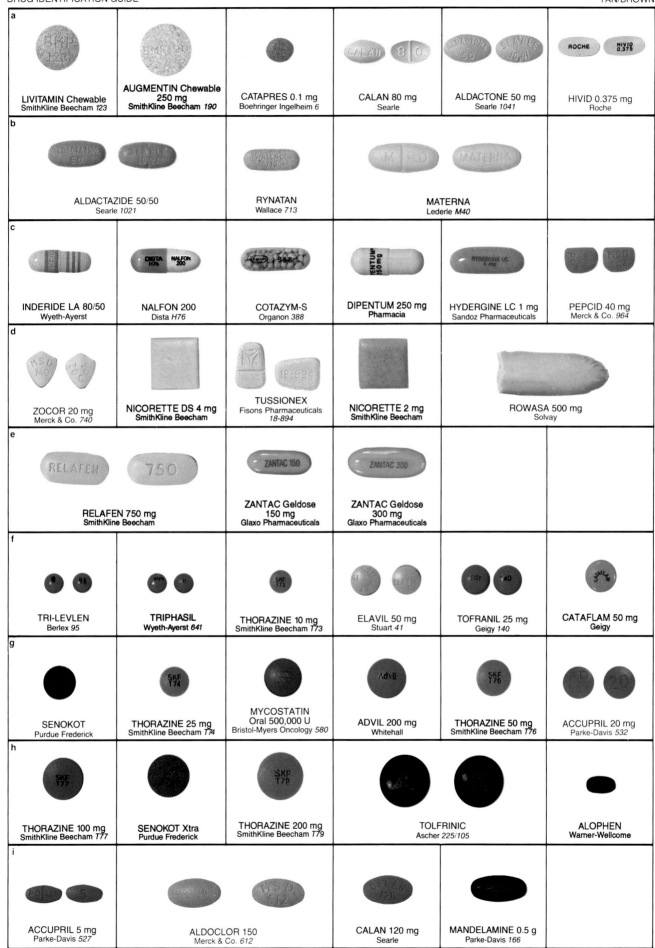

a

LIVITAMIN Chewable
SmithKline Beecham *123*

AUGMENTIN Chewable
250 mg
SmithKline Beecham *190*

CATAPRES 0.1 mg
Boehringer Ingelheim *6*

CALAN 80 mg
Searle

ALDACTONE 50 mg
Searle *1041*

HIVID 0.375 mg
Roche

b

ALDACTAZIDE 50/50
Searle *1021*

RYNATAN
Wallace *713*

MATERNA
Lederle *M40*

c

INDERIDE LA 80/50
Wyeth-Ayerst

NALFON 200
Dista *H76*

COTAZYM-S
Organon *388*

DIPENTUM 250 mg
Pharmacia

HYDERGINE LC 1 mg
Sandoz Pharmaceuticals

PEPCID 40 mg
Merck & Co. *964*

d

ZOCOR 20 mg
Merck & Co. *740*

NICORETTE DS 4 mg
SmithKline Beecham

TUSSIONEX
Fisons Pharmaceuticals
18-894

NICORETTE 2 mg
SmithKline Beecham

ROWASA 500 mg
Solvay

e

RELAFEN 750 mg
SmithKline Beecham

ZANTAC Geldose
150 mg
Glaxo Pharmaceuticals

ZANTAC Geldose
300 mg
Glaxo Pharmaceuticals

f

TRI-LEVLEN
Berlex *95*

TRIPHASIL
Wyeth-Ayerst *641*

THORAZINE 10 mg
SmithKline Beecham *T73*

ELAVIL 50 mg
Stuart *41*

TOFRANIL 25 mg
Geigy *140*

CATAFLAM 50 mg
Geigy

g

SENOKOT
Purdue Frederick

THORAZINE 25 mg
SmithKline Beecham *T74*

MYCOSTATIN
Oral 500,000 U
Bristol-Myers Oncology *580*

ADVIL 200 mg
Whitehall

THORAZINE 50 mg
SmithKline Beecham *T76*

ACCUPRIL 20 mg
Parke-Davis *532*

h

THORAZINE 100 mg
SmithKline Beecham *T77*

SENOKOT Xtra
Purdue Frederick

THORAZINE 200 mg
SmithKline Beecham *T79*

TOLFRINIC
Ascher *225/105*

ALOPHEN
Warner-Wellcome

i

ACCUPRIL 5 mg
Parke-Davis *527*

ALDOCLOR 150
Merck & Co. *612*

CALAN 120 mg
Searle

MANDELAMINE 0.5 g
Parke-Davis *166*

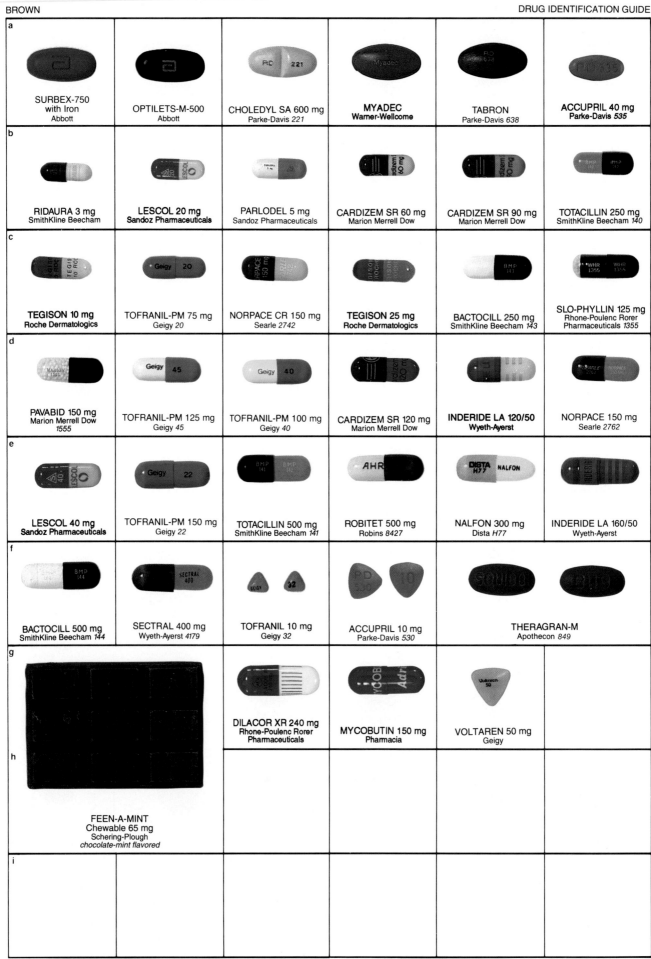

a

SURBEX-750
with Iron
Abbott

OPTILETS-M-500
Abbott

CHOLEDYL SA 600 mg
Parke-Davis *221*

MYADEC
Warner-Wellcome

TABRON
Parke-Davis *638*

ACCUPRIL 40 mg
Parke-Davis *535*

b

RIDAURA 3 mg
SmithKline Beecham

LESCOL 20 mg
Sandoz Pharmaceuticals

PARLODEL 5 mg
Sandoz Pharmaceuticals

CARDIZEM SR 60 mg
Marion Merrell Dow

CARDIZEM SR 90 mg
Marion Merrell Dow

TOTACILLIN 250 mg
SmithKline Beecham *140*

c

TEGISON 10 mg
Roche Dermatologics

TOFRANIL-PM 75 mg
Geigy *20*

NORPACE CR 150 mg
Searle *2742*

TEGISON 25 mg
Roche Dermatologics

BACTOCILL 250 mg
SmithKline Beecham *143*

SLO-PHYLLIN 125 mg
Rhone-Poulenc Rorer
Pharmaceuticals *1355*

d

PAVABID 150 mg
Marion Merrell Dow
1555

TOFRANIL-PM 125 mg
Geigy *45*

TOFRANIL-PM 100 mg
Geigy *40*

CARDIZEM SR 120 mg
Marion Merrell Dow

INDERIDE LA 120/50
Wyeth-Ayerst

NORPACE 150 mg
Searle *2762*

e

LESCOL 40 mg
Sandoz Pharmaceuticals

TOFRANIL-PM 150 mg
Geigy *22*

TOTACILLIN 500 mg
SmithKline Beecham *141*

ROBITET 500 mg
Robins *8427*

NALFON 300 mg
Dista *H77*

INDERIDE LA 160/50
Wyeth-Ayerst

f

BACTOCILL 500 mg
SmithKline Beecham *144*

SECTRAL 400 mg
Wyeth-Ayerst *4179*

TOFRANIL 10 mg
Geigy *32*

ACCUPRIL 10 mg
Parke-Davis *530*

THERAGRAN-M
Apothecon *849*

g

DILACOR XR 240 mg
Rhone-Poulenc Rorer
Pharmaceuticals

MYCOBUTIN 150 mg
Pharmacia

VOLTAREN 50 mg
Geigy

h

FEEN-A-MINT
Chewable 65 mg
Schering-Plough
chocolate-mint flavored

i

a

LEVOTHROID 75 µg
Forest *LT*

TRILAFON 2 mg
Schering *705* or *ADH*

b

TRILAFON 4 mg
Schering *940* or *ADK*

TEMARIL 2.5 mg
Allergan Herbert *HL T41*

TRILAFON 8 mg
Schering *313* or *ADJ*

TRILAFON 16 mg
Schering *077* or *ADM*

ESKALITH 300 mg
SmithKline Beecham *J09*

RYNATUSS
Wallace *717*

c

TEMARIL 5 mg
Allergan Herbert *HL T50*

CUPRIMINE 125 mg
Merck & Co. *672*

IONAMIN 15 mg
Fisons Pharmaceuticals

WYMOX 250 mg
Wyeth-Ayerst *559*

PRINCIPEN 250 mg
Apothecon *971*

ESKALITH 300 mg
SmithKline Beecham

d

ANCOBON 500 mg
Roche

LODINE 200 mg
Wyeth-Ayerst

LODINE 300 mg
Wyeth-Ayerst

PRINCIPEN 500 mg
Apothecon *974*

e

WYMOX 500 mg
Wyeth-Ayerst *560*

VERELAN 180 mg
Lederle

ENDURONYL Forte
Abbott *LT*

HIVID 0.75 mg
Roche

f

g

LIBRIUM 10 mg
Roche

COMPAZINE 10 mg
SmithKline Beecham *C44*

COMPAZINE 15 mg
SmithKline Beecham *C46*

TEGOPEN 250 mg
Apothecon *7935*

NICOBID 125 mg
Rhone-Poulenc Rorer
Pharmaceuticals

h

DEXATRIM
Regular Strength
Thompson

PHENAPHEN
with Codeine No. 3
Robins *6257*

PHENAPHEN
with Codeine No. 2
Robins *6242*

i

TEGOPEN 500 mg
Apothecon *7496*

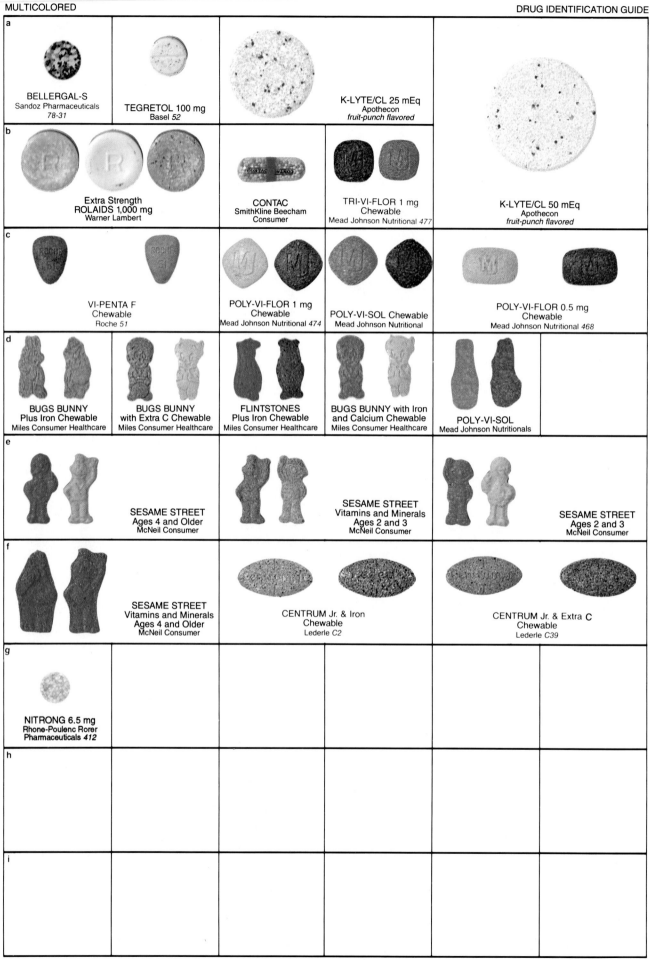

a

BELLERGAL-S
Sandoz Pharmaceuticals
78-31

TEGRETOL 100 mg
Basel *52*

K-LYTE/CL 25 mEq
Apothecon
fruit-punch flavored

b

Extra Strength
ROLAIDS 1,000 mg
Warner Lambert

CONTAC
SmithKline Beecham
Consumer

TRI-VI-FLOR 1 mg
Chewable
Mead Johnson Nutritional *477*

K-LYTE/CL 50 mEq
Apothecon
fruit-punch flavored

c

VI-PENTA F
Chewable
Roche *51*

POLY-VI-FLOR 1 mg
Chewable
Mead Johnson Nutritional *474*

POLY-VI-SOL Chewable
Mead Johnson Nutritional

POLY-VI-FLOR 0.5 mg
Chewable
Mead Johnson Nutritional *468*

d

BUGS BUNNY
Plus Iron Chewable
Miles Consumer Healthcare

BUGS BUNNY
with Extra C Chewable
Miles Consumer Healthcare

FLINTSTONES
Plus Iron Chewable
Miles Consumer Healthcare

BUGS BUNNY with Iron
and Calcium Chewable
Miles Consumer Healthcare

POLY-VI-SOL
Mead Johnson Nutritionals

e

SESAME STREET
Ages 4 and Older
McNeil Consumer

SESAME STREET
Vitamins and Minerals
Ages 2 and 3
McNeil Consumer

SESAME STREET
Ages 2 and 3
McNeil Consumer

f

SESAME STREET
Vitamins and Minerals
Ages 4 and Older
McNeil Consumer

CENTRUM Jr. & Iron
Chewable
Lederle *C2*

CENTRUM Jr. & Extra C
Chewable
Lederle *C39*

g

NITRONG 6.5 mg
Rhone-Poulenc Rorer
Pharmaceuticals *412*

h

i

a

SORBITRATE 2.5 mg
Sublingual
Zeneca *853*

NITROGARD
Transmucosal 1 mg
Forest

NORINYL 1 + 50
Syntex *1*

DESOGEN
Organon *TR 5*

NITROSTAT Sublingual
0.3 mg
Parke-Davis

NITROSTAT Sublingual
0.4 mg
Parke-Davis

b

NITROGARD
Transmucosal 2 mg
Forest

TRI-LEVLEN
Berlex *96*

ISORDIL 10 mg
Sublingual
Wyeth-Ayerst

NITROGARD
Transmucosal 3 mg
Forest

LO/OVRAL
Wyeth-Ayerst *78*

CYTOMEL 5 µg
SmithKline Beecham *D14*

c

ARMOUR Thyroid
30 mg
Forest *TD*

LOMOTIL
Searle *61*

NITROSTAT 0.6 mg
Parke-Davis

TRIPHASIL
Wyeth-Ayerst *642*

TENORMIN 25 mg
Zeneca *107*

d

TAMBOCOR 50 mg
3M Pharmaceuticals *TR*

CLARITIN 10 mg
Schering *458*

MAZANOR 1 mg
Wyeth-Ayerst *71*

ORTHO TRI-CYCLEN
Ortho *180*

MYKROX ½ mg
Fisons Pharmaceuticals

e

COGENTIN 0.5 mg
Merck & Co. *21*

DEMULEN 1/50
Searle *71*

PROVENTIL 2 mg
Schering *252*

LEVOTHROID 50 µg
Forest *LL*

DEMEROL 50 mg
Sanofi Winthrop *D35*

MODICON,
ORTHO-NOVUM 7/7/7,
or ORTHO-NOVUM 10/11
Ortho *535*

f

DELTASONE 5 mg
Upjohn

OVRAL
Wyeth-Ayerst *56*

MYLERAN 2 mg
Burroughs Wellcome *K2A*

VENTOLIN 2 mg
Allen & Hanburys

MEBARAL 32 mg
Sanofi Winthrop *M31*

DEMULEN 1/35
Searle *151*

g

LOESTRIN Fe 1/20
Parke-Davis *915*

TAPAZOLE 5 mg
Lilly *J94*

PARLODEL 2½ mg
Sandoz Pharmaceuticals

TAVIST 2.68 mg
Sandoz Pharmaceuticals
78-72

PBZ 25 mg
Geigy *111*

LEUKERAN 2 mg
Burroughs Wellcome *635*

h

KEMADRIN 5 mg
Burroughs Wellcome *S3A*

PERIACTIN 4 mg
Merck & Co. *62*

CYTOMEL 25 µg
SmithKline Beecham *D16*

HYTRIN 1 mg
Abbott *DF*

i

HISMANAL 10 mg
Janssen *AST/10*

CURRETAB 10 mg
Solvay *1007*

RENESE 1 mg
Pfizer *375*

COGENTIN 2 mg
Merck & Co. *60*

ANADROL-50
Syntex *2902*

LONITEN 10 mg
Upjohn *137*

a

SYNTHROID 50 µg
Boots Pharmaceuticals

LONITEN 2.5 mg
Upjohn *121*

PROVERA 10 mg
Upjohn

CYLERT 18.75 mg
Abbott *TH*

SUDAFED Plus
Warner-Wellcome

b

LANOXIN 250 µg
Burroughs Wellcome *X3A*

ARMOUR Thyroid
60 mg
Forest *TE*

DARAPRIM 25 mg
Burroughs Wellcome *A3A*

TENORMIN 50 mg
Zeneca *105*

NEPTAZANE 50 mg
Storz *N1*

MAREZINE 50 mg
Himmel *T4A*

c

ACTIFED
Warner-Wellcome *M2A*

ALKERAN 2 mg
Burroughs Wellcome *A2A*

KERLONE 10 mg
Searle

SYNKAVITE 5 mg
Roche

SALURON 50 mg
Roberts *S2*

d

HEXADROL 0.75 mg
Organon *791*

HYDERGINE 1 mg
Sandoz Pharmaceuticals

ALUPENT 10 mg
Boehringer Ingelheim *74*

TENORETIC 50/25
Zeneca *115*

DEMEROL 100 mg
Sanofi Winthrop *D37*

LEUCOVORIN
Calcium 5 mg
Lederle *C33*

e

LASIX 40 mg
Hoechst-Roussel

LEVSIN 0.125 mg
Schwarz Pharma
Kremers Urban *531*

BRETHINE 5 mg
Geigy *105*

SLOW FE 50 mg
Ciba Consumer *NR*

WELLCOVORIN 5 mg
Burroughs Wellcome

ORETIC 50 mg
Abbott

f

MEBARAL 100 mg
Sanofi Winthrop *M33*

PBZ 50 mg
Geigy *117*

DONNATAL
Robins *4250*

KLONOPIN 2 mg
Roche

g

METAPREL 10 mg
Sandoz Pharmaceuticals
78-212

CYTOTEC 100 µg
Searle *1451*

SLO-PHYLLIN 100 mg
Rhone-Poulenc Rorer
Pharmaceuticals *351*

PHENERGAN 25 mg
Wyeth-Ayerst *27*

SLO-PHYLLIN 200 mg
Rhone-Poulenc Rorer
Pharmaceuticals *352*

h

CYTOMEL 50 µg
SmithKline Beecham *D17*

MYAMBUTOL 100 mg
Lederle *M6*

CORTEF 5 mg
Upjohn

PAXIPAM 40 mg
Schering *538*

NOLVADEX 10 mg
Zeneca *600*

i

ZESTORETIC 20-12.5
Stuart *142*

ISORDIL Oral
Titradose 10 mg
Wyeth-Ayerst *4153*

SANOREX 2 mg
Sandoz Pharmaceuticals
78-66

MICRONASE 1.25 mg
Upjohn

ARTANE 2 mg
Lederle *A11*

SEROPHENE 50 mg
Serono *11*

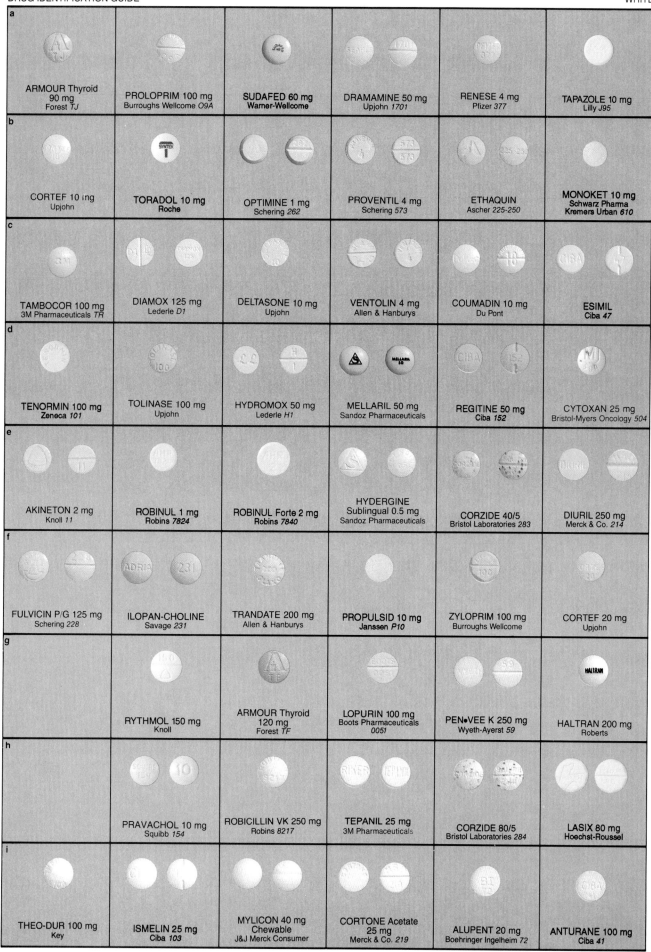

a

ARMOUR Thyroid
90 mg
Forest *TJ*

PROLOPRIM 100 mg
Burroughs Wellcome *O9A*

SUDAFED 60 mg
Warner-Wellcome

DRAMAMINE 50 mg
Upjohn *1701*

RENESE 4 mg
Pfizer *377*

TAPAZOLE 10 mg
Lilly *J95*

b

CORTEF 10 mg
Upjohn

TORADOL 10 mg
Roche

OPTIMINE 1 mg
Schering *262*

PROVENTIL 4 mg
Schering *573*

ETHAQUIN
Ascher *225-250*

MONOKET 10 mg
Schwarz Pharma
Kremers Urban *610*

c

TAMBOCOR 100 mg
3M Pharmaceuticals *TR*

DIAMOX 125 mg
Lederle *D1*

DELTASONE 10 mg
Upjohn

VENTOLIN 4 mg
Allen & Hanburys

COUMADIN 10 mg
Du Pont

ESIMIL
Ciba *47*

d

TENORMIN 100 mg
Zeneca *101*

TOLINASE 100 mg
Upjohn

HYDROMOX 50 mg
Lederle *H1*

MELLARIL 50 mg
Sandoz Pharmaceuticals

REGITINE 50 mg
Ciba *152*

CYTOXAN 25 mg
Bristol-Myers Oncology *504*

e

AKINETON 2 mg
Knoll *11*

ROBINUL 1 mg
Robins *7824*

ROBINUL Forte 2 mg
Robins *7840*

HYDERGINE
Sublingual 0.5 mg
Sandoz Pharmaceuticals

CORZIDE 40/5
Bristol Laboratories *283*

DIURIL 250 mg
Merck & Co. *214*

f

FULVICIN P/G 125 mg
Schering *228*

ILOPAN-CHOLINE
Savage *231*

TRANDATE 200 mg
Allen & Hanburys

PROPULSID 10 mg
Janssen *P10*

ZYLOPRIM 100 mg
Burroughs Wellcome

CORTEF 20 mg
Upjohn

g

RYTHMOL 150 mg
Knoll

ARMOUR Thyroid
120 mg
Forest *TF*

LOPURIN 100 mg
Boots Pharmaceuticals
0051

PEN•VEE K 250 mg
Wyeth-Ayerst *59*

HALTRAN 200 mg
Roberts

h

PRAVACHOL 10 mg
Squibb *154*

ROBICILLIN VK 250 mg
Robins *8217*

TEPANIL 25 mg
3M Pharmaceuticals

CORZIDE 80/5
Bristol Laboratories *284*

LASIX 80 mg
Hoechst-Roussel

i

THEO-DUR 100 mg
Key

ISMELIN 25 mg
Ciba *103*

MYLICON 40 mg
Chewable
J&J Merck Consumer

CORTONE Acetate
25 mg
Merck & Co. *219*

ALUPENT 20 mg
Boehringer Ingelheim *72*

ANTURANE 100 mg
Ciba *41*

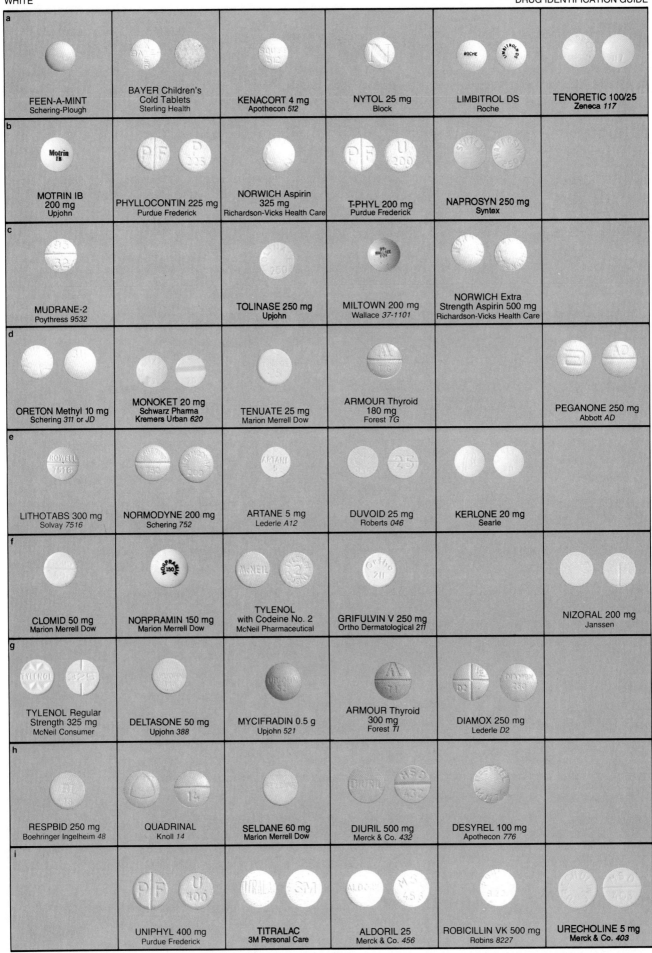

a

FEEN-A-MINT
Schering-Plough

BAYER Children's
Cold Tablets
Sterling Health

KENACORT 4 mg
Apothecon *512*

NYTOL 25 mg
Block

LIMBITROL DS
Roche

TENORETIC 100/25
Zeneca *117*

b

MOTRIN IB
200 mg
Upjohn

PHYLLOCONTIN 225 mg
Purdue Frederick

NORWICH Aspirin
325 mg
Richardson-Vicks Health Care

T-PHYL 200 mg
Purdue Frederick

NAPROSYN 250 mg
Syntex

c

MUDRANE-2
Poythress *9532*

TOLINASE 250 mg
Upjohn

MILTOWN 200 mg
Wallace *37-1101*

NORWICH Extra
Strength Aspirin 500 mg
Richardson-Vicks Health Care

d

ORETON Methyl 10 mg
Schering *311 or JD*

MONOKET 20 mg
Schwarz Pharma
Kremers Urban *620*

TENUATE 25 mg
Marion Merrell Dow

ARMOUR Thyroid
180 mg
Forest *TG*

PEGANONE 250 mg
Abbott *AD*

e

LITHOTABS 300 mg
Solvay *7516*

NORMODYNE 200 mg
Schering *752*

ARTANE 5 mg
Lederle *A12*

DUVOID 25 mg
Roberts *046*

KERLONE 20 mg
Searle

f

CLOMID 50 mg
Marion Merrell Dow

NORPRAMIN 150 mg
Marion Merrell Dow

TYLENOL
with Codeine No. 2
McNeil Pharmaceutical

GRIFULVIN V 250 mg
Ortho Dermatological *211*

NIZORAL 200 mg
Janssen

g

TYLENOL Regular
Strength 325 mg
McNeil Consumer

DELTASONE 50 mg
Upjohn *388*

MYCIFRADIN 0.5 g
Upjohn *521*

ARMOUR Thyroid
300 mg
Forest *71*

DIAMOX 250 mg
Lederle *D2*

h

RESPBID 250 mg
Boehringer Ingelheim *48*

QUADRINAL
Knoll *14*

SELDANE 60 mg
Marion Merrell Dow

DIURIL 500 mg
Merck & Co. *432*

DESYREL 100 mg
Apothecon *776*

i

UNIPHYL 400 mg
Purdue Frederick

TITRALAC
3M Personal Care

ALDORIL 25
Merck & Co. *456*

ROBICILLIN VK 500 mg
Robins *8227*

URECHOLINE 5 mg
Merck & Co. *403*

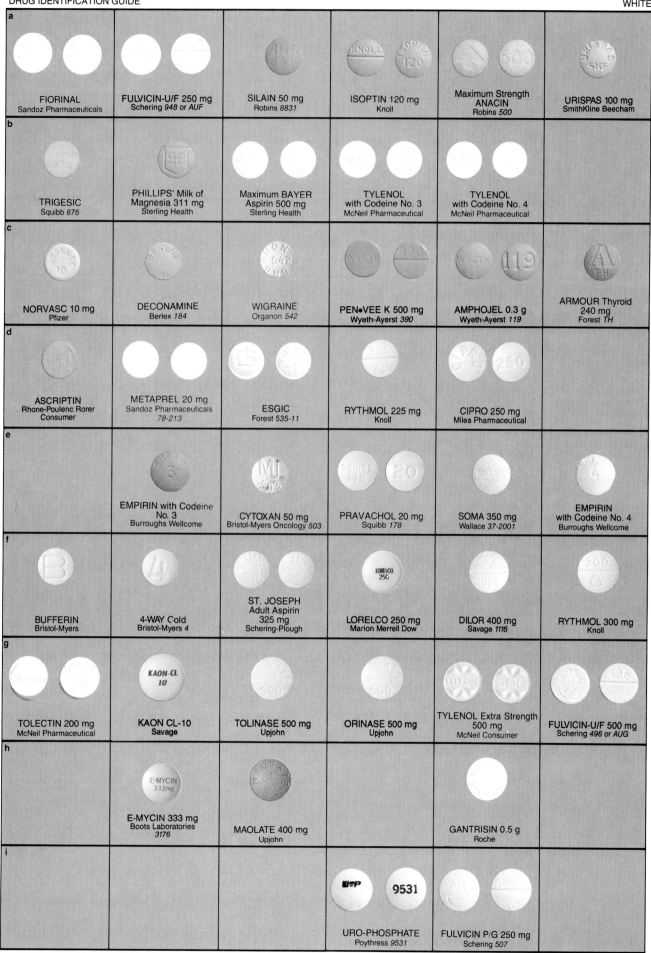

a

FIORINAL
Sandoz Pharmaceuticals

FULVICIN-U/F 250 mg
Schering *948* or *AUF*

SILAIN 50 mg
Robins *8831*

ISOPTIN 120 mg
Knoll

Maximum Strength
ANACIN
Robins *500*

URISPAS 100 mg
SmithKline Beecham

b

TRIGESIC
Squibb *876*

PHILLIPS' Milk of
Magnesia 311 mg
Sterling Health

Maximum BAYER
Aspirin 500 mg
Sterling Health

TYLENOL
with Codeine No. 3
McNeil Pharmaceutical

TYLENOL
with Codeine No. 4
McNeil Pharmaceutical

c

NORVASC 10 mg
Pfizer

DECONAMINE
Berlex *184*

WIGRAINE
Organon *542*

PEN•VEE K 500 mg
Wyeth-Ayerst *390*

AMPHOJEL 0.3 g
Wyeth-Ayerst *119*

ARMOUR Thyroid
240 mg
Forest *TH*

d

ASCRIPTIN
Rhone-Poulenc Rorer
Consumer

METAPREL 20 mg
Sandoz Pharmaceuticals
78-213

ESGIC
Forest *535-11*

RYTHMOL 225 mg
Knoll

CIPRO 250 mg
Miles Pharmaceutical

e

EMPIRIN with Codeine
No. 3
Burroughs Wellcome

CYTOXAN 50 mg
Bristol-Myers Oncology *503*

PRAVACHOL 20 mg
Squibb *178*

SOMA 350 mg
Wallace *37-2001*

EMPIRIN
with Codeine No. 4
Burroughs Wellcome

f

BUFFERIN
Bristol-Myers

4-WAY Cold
Bristol-Myers *4*

ST. JOSEPH
Adult Aspirin
325 mg
Schering-Plough

LORELCO 250 mg
Marion Merrell Dow

DILOR 400 mg
Savage *1116*

RYTHMOL 300 mg
Knoll

g

TOLECTIN 200 mg
McNeil Pharmaceutical

KAON CL-10
Savage

TOLINASE 500 mg
Upjohn

ORINASE 500 mg
Upjohn

TYLENOL Extra Strength
500 mg
McNeil Consumer

FULVICIN-U/F 500 mg
Schering *496* or *AUG*

h

E-MYCIN 333 mg
Boots Laboratories
3176

MAOLATE 400 mg
Upjohn

GANTRISIN 0.5 g
Roche

i

URO-PHOSPHATE
Poythress *9531*

FULVICIN P/G 250 mg
Schering *507*

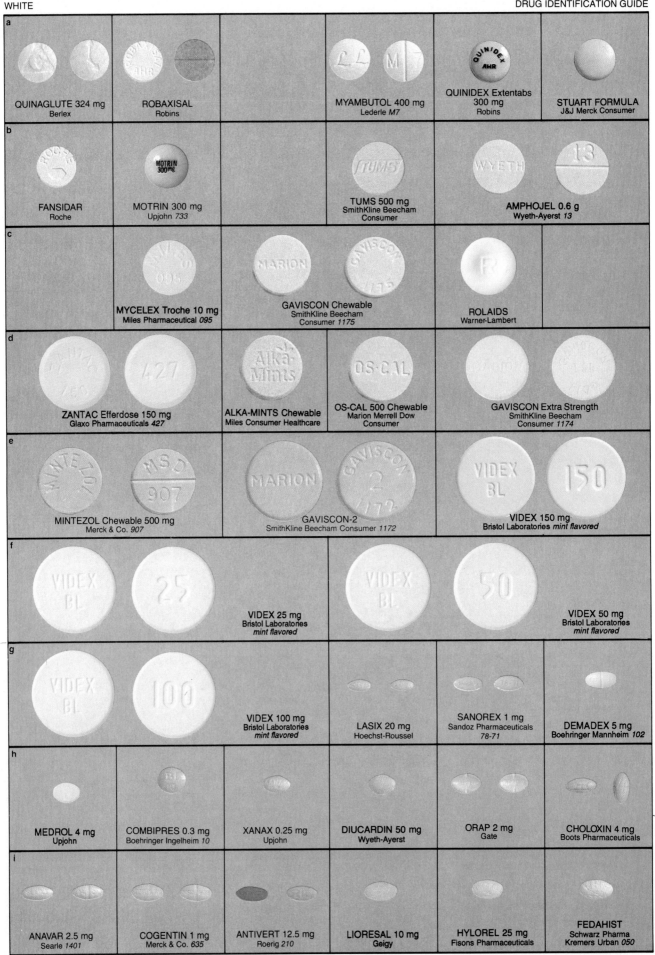

a

QUINAGLUTE 324 mg
Berlex

ROBAXISAL
Robins

MYAMBUTOL 400 mg
Lederle *M7*

QUINIDEX Extentabs
300 mg
Robins

STUART FORMULA
J&J Merck Consumer

b

FANSIDAR
Roche

MOTRIN 300 mg
Upjohn *733*

TUMS 500 mg
SmithKline Beecham
Consumer

AMPHOJEL 0.6 g
Wyeth-Ayerst *13*

c

MYCELEX Troche 10 mg
Miles Pharmaceutical *095*

GAVISCON Chewable
SmithKline Beecham
Consumer *1175*

ROLAIDS
Warner-Lambert

d

ZANTAC Efferdose 150 mg
Glaxo Pharmaceuticals *427*

ALKA-MINTS Chewable
Miles Consumer Healthcare

OS-CAL 500 Chewable
Marion Merrell Dow
Consumer

GAVISCON Extra Strength
SmithKline Beecham
Consumer *1174*

e

MINTEZOL Chewable 500 mg
Merck & Co. *907*

GAVISCON-2
SmithKline Beecham Consumer *1172*

VIDEX 150 mg
Bristol Laboratories *mint flavored*

f

VIDEX 25 mg
Bristol Laboratories
mint flavored

VIDEX 50 mg
Bristol Laboratories
mint flavored

g

VIDEX 100 mg
Bristol Laboratories
mint flavored

LASIX 20 mg
Hoechst-Roussel

SANOREX 1 mg
Sandoz Pharmaceuticals
78-71

DEMADEX 5 mg
Boehringer Mannheim *102*

h

MEDROL 4 mg
Upjohn

COMBIPRES 0.3 mg
Boehringer Ingelheim *10*

XANAX 0.25 mg
Upjohn

DIUCARDIN 50 mg
Wyeth-Ayerst

ORAP 2 mg
Gate

CHOLOXIN 4 mg
Boots Pharmaceuticals

i

ANAVAR 2.5 mg
Searle *1401*

COGENTIN 1 mg
Merck & Co. *635*

ANTIVERT 12.5 mg
Roerig *210*

LIORESAL 10 mg
Geigy

HYLOREL 25 mg
Fisons Pharmaceuticals

FEDAHIST
Schwarz Pharma
Kremers Urban *050*

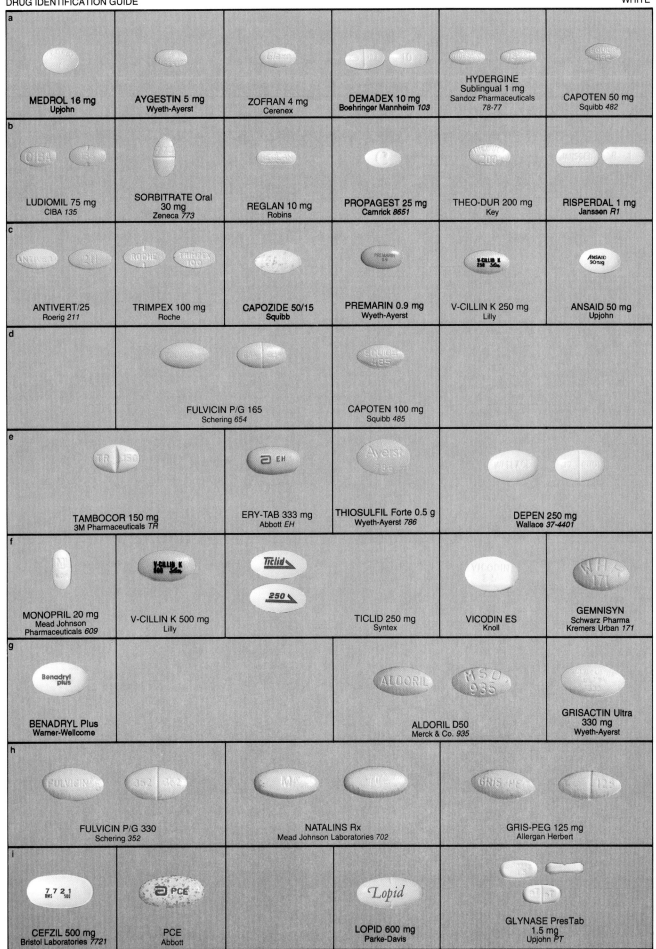

a

MEDROL 16 mg
Upjohn

AYGESTIN 5 mg
Wyeth-Ayerst

ZOFRAN 4 mg
Cerenex

DEMADEX 10 mg
Boehringer Mannheim *103*

HYDERGINE
Sublingual 1 mg
Sandoz Pharmaceuticals
78-77

CAPOTEN 50 mg
Squibb *482*

b

LUDIOMIL 75 mg
CIBA *135*

SORBITRATE Oral
30 mg
Zeneca *773*

REGLAN 10 mg
Robins

PROPAGEST 25 mg
Camrick *8651*

THEO-DUR 200 mg
Key

RISPERDAL 1 mg
Janssen *R1*

c

ANTIVERT/25
Roerig *211*

TRIMPEX 100 mg
Roche

CAPOZIDE 50/15
Squibb

PREMARIN 0.9 mg
Wyeth-Ayerst

V-CILLIN K 250 mg
Lilly

ANSAID 50 mg
Upjohn

d

FULVICIN P/G 165
Schering *654*

CAPOTEN 100 mg
Squibb *485*

e

TAMBOCOR 150 mg
3M Pharmaceuticals *TR*

ERY-TAB 333 mg
Abbott *EH*

THIOSULFIL Forte 0.5 g
Wyeth-Ayerst *786*

DEPEN 250 mg
Wallace *37-4401*

f

MONOPRIL 20 mg
Mead Johnson
Pharmaceuticals *609*

V-CILLIN K 500 mg
Lilly

TICLID 250 mg
Syntex

VICODIN ES
Knoll

GEMNISYN
Schwarz Pharma
Kremers Urban *171*

g

BENADRYL Plus
Warner-Wellcome

ALDORIL D50
Merck & Co. *935*

GRISACTIN Ultra
330 mg
Wyeth-Ayerst

h

FULVICIN P/G 330
Schering *352*

NATALINS Rx
Mead Johnson Laboratories *702*

GRIS-PEG 125 mg
Allergan Herbert

i

CEFZIL 500 mg
Bristol Laboratories *7721*

PCE
Abbott

LOPID 600 mg
Parke-Davis

GLYNASE PresTab
1.5 mg
Upjohn *PT*

a

CAPOTEN 12.5 mg
Squibb *450*

ARISTOCORT 4 mg
Fujisawa *A4*

EDECRIN 25 mg
Merck & Co. *65*

MSIR 30 mg
Purdue Frederick *MI30*

BUSPAR 5 mg
Mead Johnson
Pharmaceuticals

b

CARDURA 1 mg
Roerig

LOTENSIN HCT 5/6.25
Ciba *57*

DYMELOR 250 mg
Lilly *U03*

CEFTIN 125 mg
Glaxo Pharmaceuticals *395*

HISTALET Forte
Solvay *1039*

c

DIAβETA 1.25 mg
Hoechst-Roussel

AMBIEN 10 mg
Searle *5421*

BUSPAR 10 mg
Mead Johnson
Pharmaceuticals

PROTOSTAT 250 mg
Ortho *1570*

PANADOL
Junior Strength 160 mg
Sterling Health

THEO-DUR 300 mg
Key

d

DIDRONEL 400 mg
Procter & Gamble *406*

LOPRESSOR-HCT 50/25
Geigy *35*

LUFYLLIN-400
Wallace *731*

e

LIORESAL 20 mg
Geigy

GRIS-PEG 250 mg
Allergan Herbert

TYLENOL Regular
Strength 325 mg
McNeil Consumer

ANACIN
Robins

f

ESGIC-Plus
Forest *678*

MOTRIN IB
200 mg
Upjohn

VICODIN
Knoll

LACTAID 3,000 U
McNeil Consumer

g

RELAFEN 500 mg
SmithKline Beecham

TYLENOL Extra Strength
500 mg
McNeil Consumer

MAXAQUIN 400 mg
Searle/Wyeth-Ayerst

MILTOWN 600
Wallace *37-1601*

MIDOL
Sterling Health

h

DAYPRO 600 mg
Searle *1381*

NAPROSYN 500 mg
Syntex

SUPRAX 200 mg
Lederle

i

Extra Strength
BUFFERIN
Bristol-Myers

CoLBENEMID
Merck & Co. *614*

CHLOR-TRIMETON
Sinus
Schering-Plough *CTM*

AXOTAL
Savage *130*

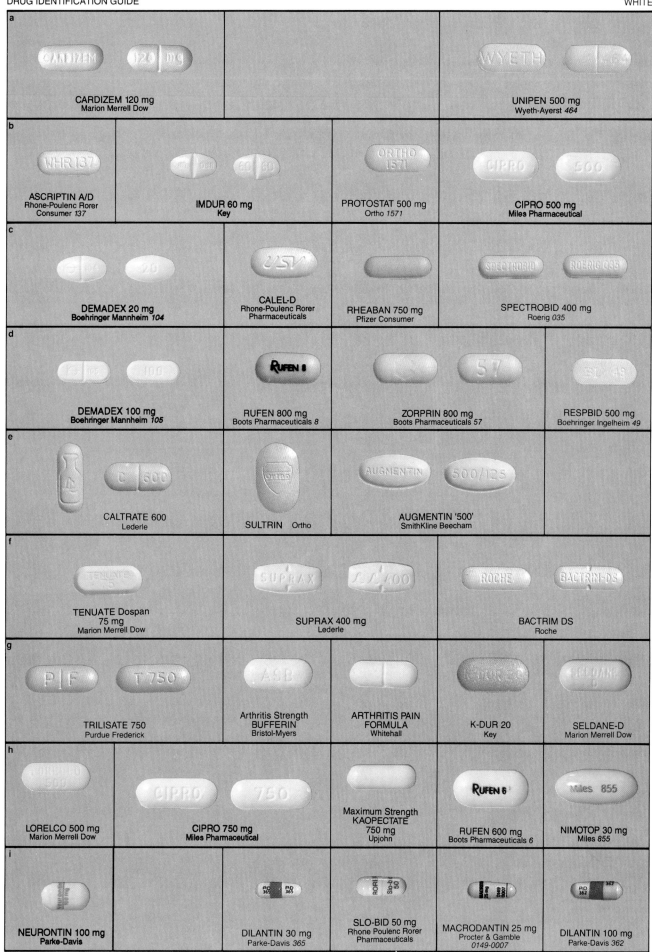

a

CARDIZEM 120 mg
Marion Merrell Dow

UNIPEN 500 mg
Wyeth-Ayerst *464*

b

ASCRIPTIN A/D
Rhone-Poulenc Rorer
Consumer *137*

IMDUR 60 mg
Key

PROTOSTAT 500 mg
Ortho *1571*

CIPRO 500 mg
Miles Pharmaceutical

c

DEMADEX 20 mg
Boehringer Mannheim *104*

CALEL-D
Rhone-Poulenc Rorer
Pharmaceuticals

RHEABAN 750 mg
Pfizer Consumer

SPECTROBID 400 mg
Roerig *035*

d

DEMADEX 100 mg
Boehringer Mannheim *105*

RUFEN 800 mg
Boots Pharmaceuticals *8*

ZORPRIN 800 mg
Boots Pharmaceuticals *57*

RESPBID 500 mg
Boehringer Ingelheim *49*

e

CALTRATE 600
Lederle

SULTRIN   Ortho

AUGMENTIN '500'
SmithKline Beecham

f

TENUATE Dospan
75 mg
Marion Merrell Dow

SUPRAX 400 mg
Lederle

BACTRIM DS
Roche

g

TRILISATE 750
Purdue Frederick

Arthritis Strength
BUFFERIN
Bristol-Myers

ARTHRITIS PAIN
FORMULA
Whitehall

K-DUR 20
Key

SELDANE-D
Marion Merrell Dow

h

LORELCO 500 mg
Marion Merrell Dow

CIPRO 750 mg
Miles Pharmaceutical

Maximum Strength
KAOPECTATE
750 mg
Upjohn

RUFEN 600 mg
Boots Pharmaceuticals *6*

NIMOTOP 30 mg
Miles *855*

i

NEURONTIN 100 mg
Parke-Davis

DILANTIN 30 mg
Parke-Davis *365*

SLO-BID 50 mg
Rhone Poulenc Rorer
Pharmaceuticals

MACRODANTIN 25 mg
Procter & Gamble
0149-0007

DILANTIN 100 mg
Parke-Davis *362*

a					
SLO-BID 75 mg Rhone Poulenc Rorer Pharmaceuticals	THEO-DUR Sprinkle 50 mg Key	RETROVIR 100 mg Burroughs Wellcome *Y9C*	SLO-PHYLLIN 60 mg Rhone-Poulenc Rorer Pharmaceuticals *1354*	CHLOROMYCETIN 250 mg Parke-Davis *379*	MINIPRESS 1 mg Pfizer *431*

b					
THEO-DUR Sprinkle 75 mg Key	INDERAL LA 60 mg Wyeth-Ayerst	CARDENE 20 mg Syntex *2437*	SLO-BID 100 mg Rhone Poulenc Rorer Pharmaceuticals	SLO-BID 125 mg Rhone Poulenc Rorer Pharmaceuticals	CeeNU 10 mg Bristol-Myers Oncology *3030*

c					
ESGIC Forest *535-12*	PAMELOR 50 mg Sandoz Pharmaceuticals	TRIDIONE 300 mg Abbott *AM*	THEO-DUR Sprinkle 125 mg Key	SLO-BID 200 mg Rhone Poulenc Rorer Pharmaceuticals	PANCREASE McNeil Pharmaceutical

d					
CeeNU 40 mg Bristol-Myers Oncology *3031*	DYNACIRC 2.5 mg Sandoz Pharmaceuticals	THEO-DUR Sprinkle 200 mg Key	SLO-BID 300 mg Rhone Poulenc Rorer Pharmaceuticals	LOZOL 2.5 mg Rhone-Poulenc Rorer Pharmaceuticals *R8*	EMCYT 140 mg Pharmacia *132*

e					
NORVASC 2.5 mg Pfizer	ATIVAN 0.5 mg Wyeth-Ayerst *81*	NEPTAZANE 25 mg Storz *N2*	ATIVAN 1 mg Wyeth-Ayerst *64*	PROVERA 5 mg Upjohn	ASENDIN 25 mg Lederle *A13*

f					
ATIVAN 2 mg Wyeth-Ayerst *65*	DECADRON 4 mg Merck & Co. *97*	VISKEN 5 mg Sandoz Pharmaceuticals	VISKEN 10 mg Sandoz Pharmaceuticals	NORVASC 5 mg Pfizer	HALDOL ½ mg McNeil Pharmaceutical

g					
PRINIVIL 5 mg Merck & Co. *19*	VALIUM 2 mg Roche	VASOTEC 5 mg Merck & Co. *712*	INDERIDE 40/25 Wyeth-Ayerst	INDERIDE 80/25 Wyeth-Ayerst	CYTOTEC 200 µg Searle *1461*

h					
GLUCOTROL 5 mg Pratt *411*	EQUANIL 200 mg Wyeth-Ayerst *2*	LUFYLLIN 200 mg Wallace *521*	CAPOTEN 25 mg Squibb *452*	CAPOZIDE 25/15 Squibb	CARDILATE 10 mg Burroughs Wellcome *X7A*

i					
MONOPRIL 10 mg Mead Johnson Pharmaceuticals *158*	GRISACTIN Ultra 250 mg Wyeth-Ayerst	DIDRONEL 200 mg Procter & Gamble *402*	PROSOM 1 mg Abbott *UC*	MARAX Roerig *254*	GLUCOTROL 10 mg Pratt *412*

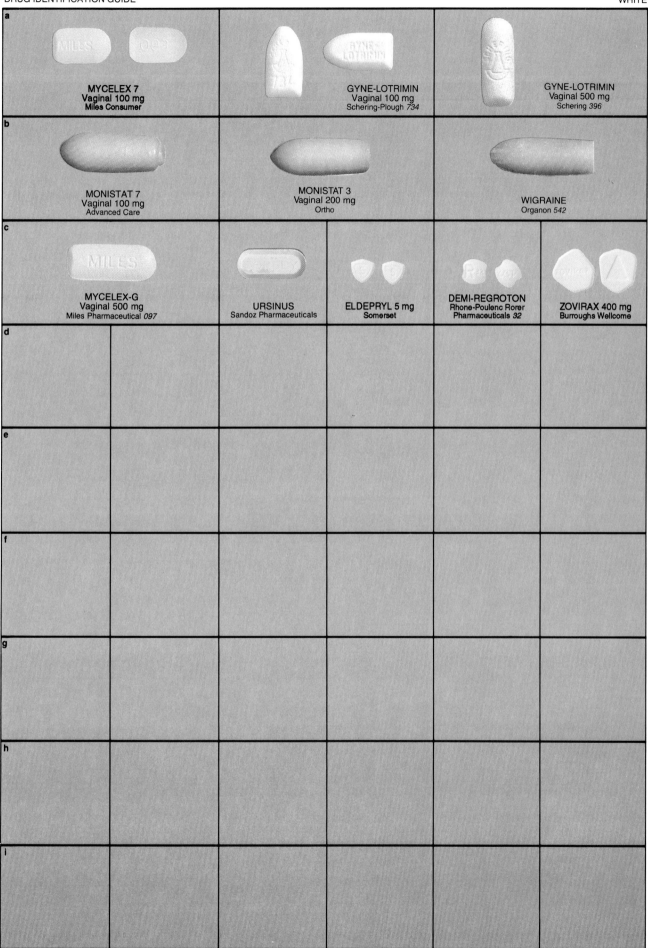

a

MYCELEX 7
Vaginal 100 mg
Miles Consumer

GYNE-LOTRIMIN
Vaginal 100 mg
Schering-Plough *734*

GYNE-LOTRIMIN
Vaginal 500 mg
Schering *396*

b

MONISTAT 7
Vaginal 100 mg
Advanced Care

MONISTAT 3
Vaginal 200 mg
Ortho

WIGRAINE
Organon *542*

c

MYCELEX-G
Vaginal 500 mg
Miles Pharmaceutical *097*

URSINUS
Sandoz Pharmaceuticals

ELDEPRYL 5 mg
Somerset

DEMI-REGROTON
Rhone-Poulenc Rorer
Pharmaceuticals *32*

ZOVIRAX 400 mg
Burroughs Wellcome

d

e

f

g

h

i

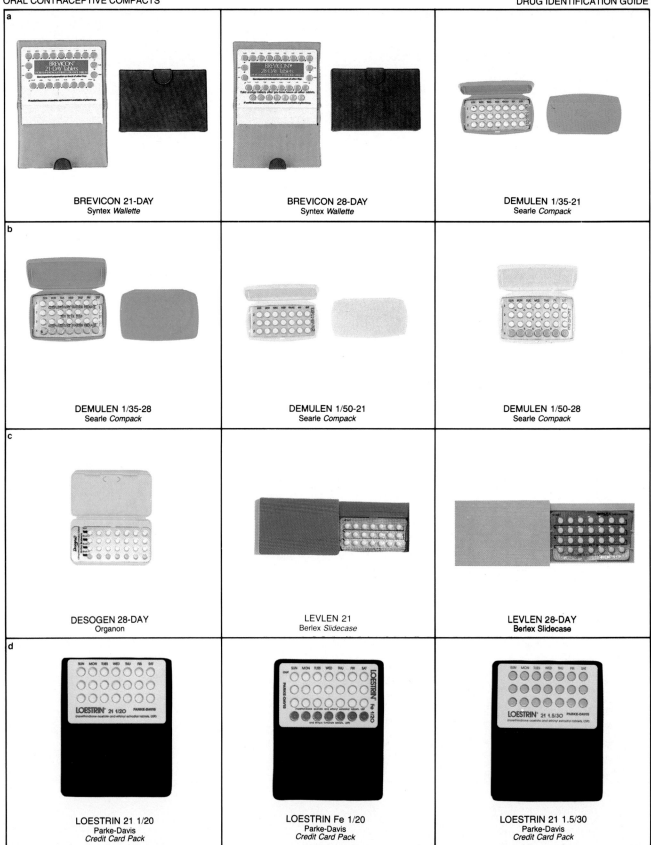

a

BREVICON 21-DAY
Syntex *Wallette*

BREVICON 28-DAY
Syntex *Wallette*

DEMULEN 1/35-21
Searle *Compack*

b

DEMULEN 1/35-28
Searle *Compack*

DEMULEN 1/50-21
Searle *Compack*

DEMULEN 1/50-28
Searle *Compack*

c

DESOGEN 28-DAY
Organon

LEVLEN 21
Berlex *Slidecase*

LEVLEN 28-DAY
Berlex Slidecase

d

LOESTRIN 21 1/20
Parke-Davis
Credit Card Pack

LOESTRIN Fe 1/20
Parke-Davis
Credit Card Pack

LOESTRIN 21 1.5/30
Parke-Davis
Credit Card Pack

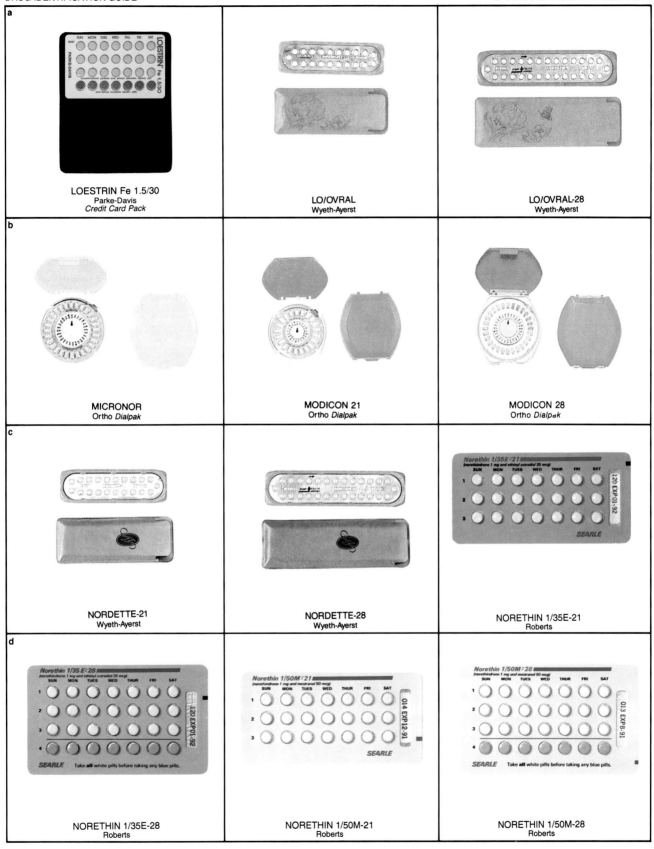

a

LOESTRIN Fe 1.5/30
Parke-Davis
Credit Card Pack

LO/OVRAL
Wyeth-Ayerst

LO/OVRAL-28
Wyeth-Ayerst

b

MICRONOR
Ortho *Dialpak*

MODICON 21
Ortho *Dialpak*

MODICON 28
Ortho *Dialpak*

c

NORDETTE-21
Wyeth-Ayerst

NORDETTE-28
Wyeth-Ayerst

NORETHIN 1/35E-21
Roberts

d

NORETHIN 1/35E-28
Roberts

NORETHIN 1/50M-21
Roberts

NORETHIN 1/50M-28
Roberts

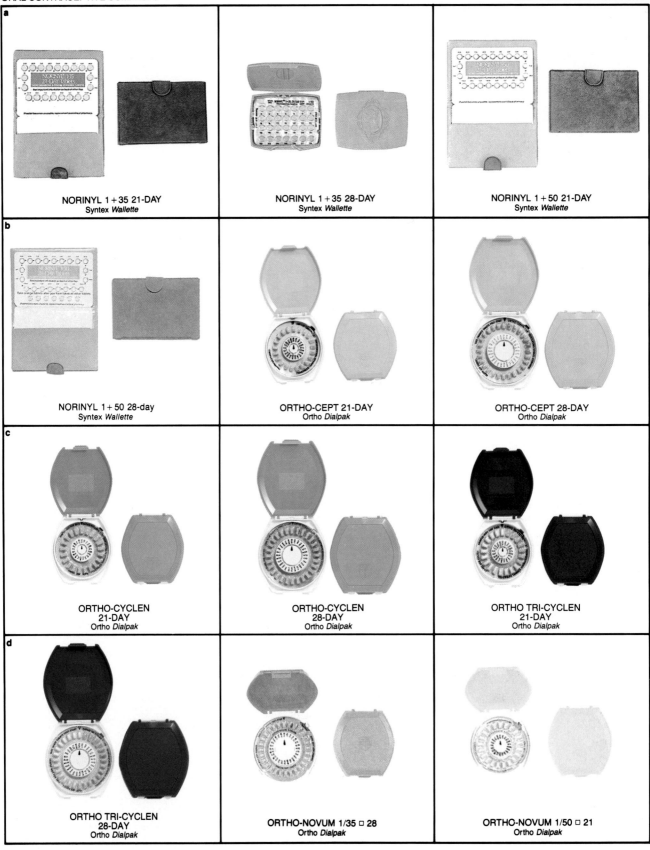

a

NORINYL 1 + 35 21-DAY
Syntex *Wallette*

NORINYL 1 + 35 28-DAY
Syntex *Wallette*

NORINYL 1 + 50 21-DAY
Syntex *Wallette*

b

NORINYL 1 + 50 28-day
Syntex *Wallette*

ORTHO-CEPT 21-DAY
Ortho *Dialpak*

ORTHO-CEPT 28-DAY
Ortho *Dialpak*

c

ORTHO-CYCLEN
21-DAY
Ortho *Dialpak*

ORTHO-CYCLEN
28-DAY
Ortho *Dialpak*

ORTHO TRI-CYCLEN
21-DAY
Ortho *Dialpak*

d

ORTHO TRI-CYCLEN
28-DAY
Ortho *Dialpak*

ORTHO-NOVUM 1/35 □ 28
Ortho *Dialpak*

ORTHO-NOVUM 1/50 □ 21
Ortho *Dialpak*

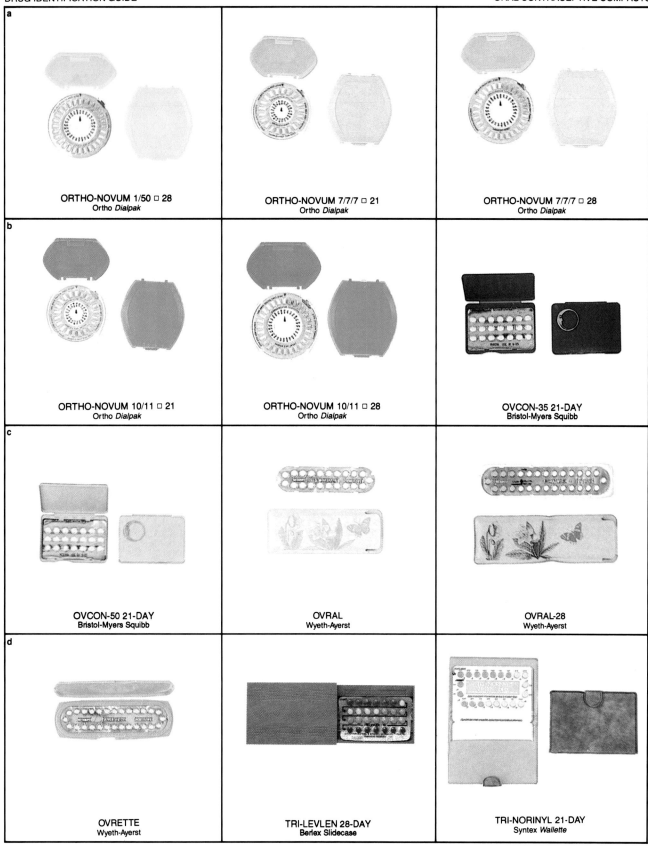

a

ORTHO-NOVUM 1/50 □ 28
Ortho *Dialpak*

ORTHO-NOVUM 7/7/7 □ 21
Ortho *Dialpak*

ORTHO-NOVUM 7/7/7 □ 28
Ortho *Dialpak*

b

ORTHO-NOVUM 10/11 □ 21
Ortho *Dialpak*

ORTHO-NOVUM 10/11 □ 28
Ortho *Dialpak*

OVCON-35 21-DAY
Bristol-Myers Squibb

c

OVCON-50 21-DAY
Bristol-Myers Squibb

OVRAL
Wyeth-Ayerst

OVRAL-28
Wyeth-Ayerst

d

OVRETTE
Wyeth-Ayerst

TRI-LEVLEN 28-DAY
Berlex Slidecase

TRI-NORINYL 21-DAY
Syntex *Wallette*

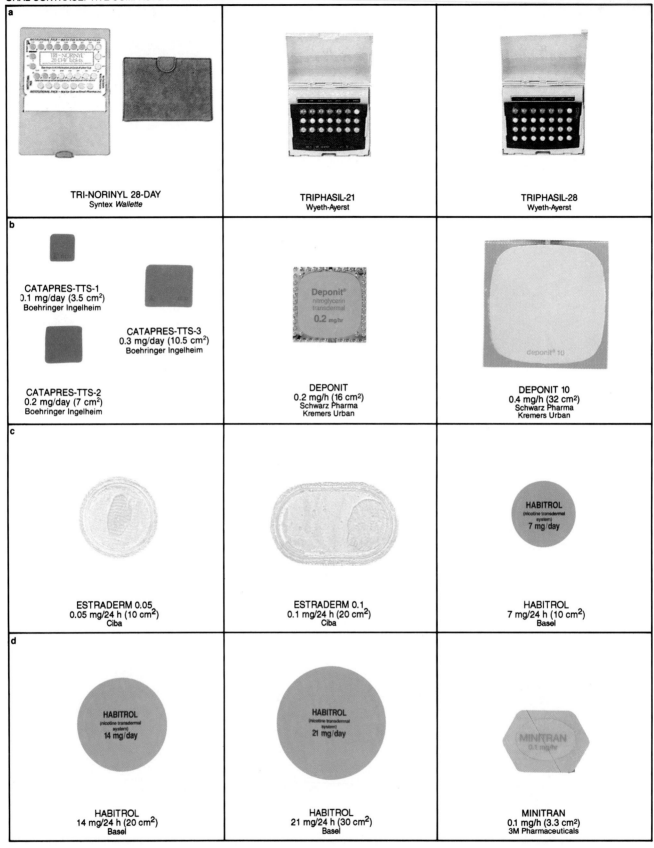

a

TRI-NORINYL 28-DAY
Syntex *Wallette*

TRIPHASIL-21
Wyeth-Ayerst

TRIPHASIL-28
Wyeth-Ayerst

b

CATAPRES-TTS-1
0.1 mg/day (3.5 cm^2)
Boehringer Ingelheim

CATAPRES-TTS-3
0.3 mg/day (10.5 cm^2)
Boehringer Ingelheim

CATAPRES-TTS-2
0.2 mg/day (7 cm^2)
Boehringer Ingelheim

DEPONIT
0.2 mg/h (16 cm^2)
Schwarz Pharma
Kremers Urban

DEPONIT 10
0.4 mg/h (32 cm^2)
Schwarz Pharma
Kremers Urban

c

ESTRADERM 0.05
0.05 mg/24 h (10 cm^2)
Ciba

ESTRADERM 0.1
0.1 mg/24 h (20 cm^2)
Ciba

HABITROL
7 mg/24 h (10 cm^2)
Basel

d

HABITROL
14 mg/24 h (20 cm^2)
Basel

HABITROL
21 mg/24 h (30 cm^2)
Basel

MINITRAN
0.1 mg/h (3.3 cm^2)
3M Pharmaceuticals

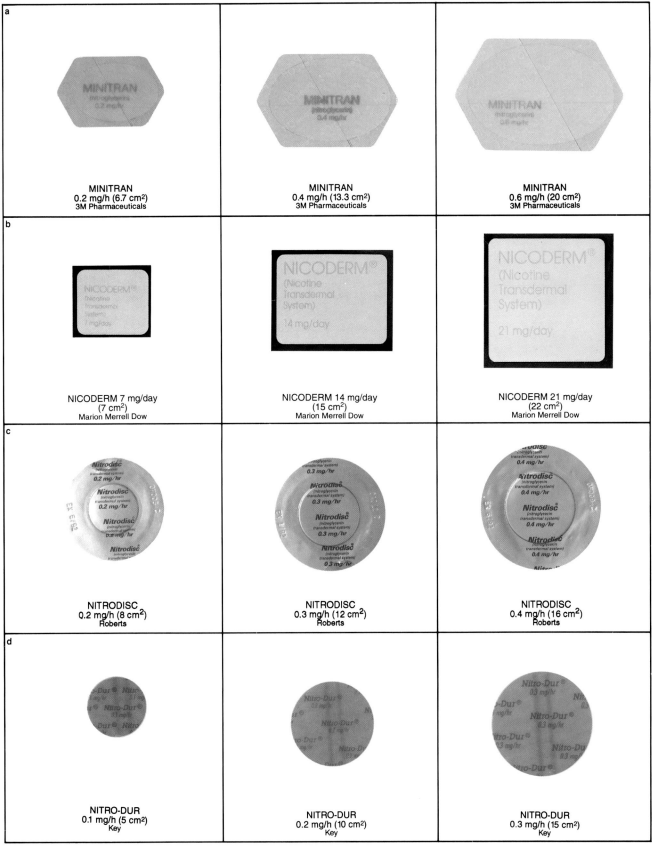

a

MINITRAN
0.2 mg/h (6.7 cm²)
3M Pharmaceuticals

MINITRAN
0.4 mg/h (13.3 cm²)
3M Pharmaceuticals

MINITRAN
0.6 mg/h (20 cm²)
3M Pharmaceuticals

b

NICODERM 7 mg/day
(7 cm²)
Marion Merrell Dow

NICODERM 14 mg/day
(15 cm²)
Marion Merrell Dow

NICODERM 21 mg/day
(22 cm²)
Marion Merrell Dow

c

NITRODISC
0.2 mg/h (8 cm²)
Roberts

NITRODISC
0.3 mg/h (12 cm²)
Roberts

NITRODISC
0.4 mg/h (16 cm²)
Roberts

d

NITRO-DUR
0.1 mg/h (5 cm²)
Key

NITRO-DUR
0.2 mg/h (10 cm²)
Key

NITRO-DUR
0.3 mg/h (15 cm²)
Key

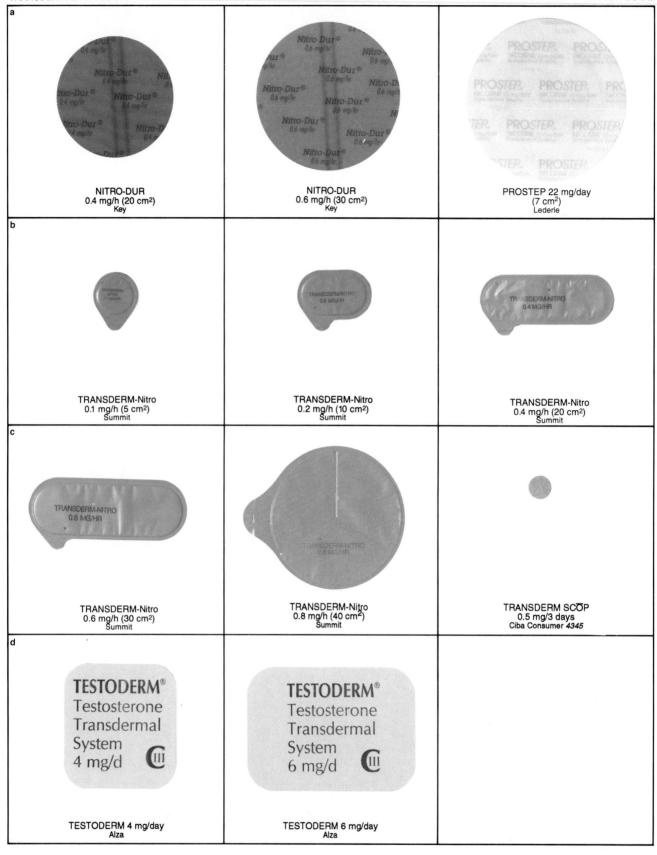

a

NITRO-DUR
0.4 mg/h (20 cm²)
Key

NITRO-DUR
0.6 mg/h (30 cm²)
Key

PROSTEP 22 mg/day
(7 cm²)
Lederle

b

TRANSDERM-Nitro
0.1 mg/h (5 cm²)
Summit

TRANSDERM-Nitro
0.2 mg/h (10 cm²)
Summit

TRANSDERM-Nitro
0.4 mg/h (20 cm²)
Summit

c

TRANSDERM-Nitro
0.6 mg/h (30 cm²)
Summit

TRANSDERM-Nitro
0.8 mg/h (40 cm²)
Summit

TRANSDERM SCOP
0.5 mg/3 days
Ciba Consumer 4345

d

TESTODERM 4 mg/day
Alza

TESTODERM 6 mg/day
Alza

-21-

ANTINAUSEA MEDICATIONS

NAUSEA AND VOMITING are unpleasant reactions that may signal a serious underlying disease or something as trivial as the sight or smell of blood. Although nausea and vomiting often occur together, they can strike independently because each arises in a different part of the body. Nausea, for example, can originate in the labyrinth part of the ear, the brain, or the gastrointestinal tract. In contrast, vomiting is a reflex controlled in part of the brain stem called the vomiting center. Thus, nausea and vomiting can be set off by unrelated events, including such diverse factors as poisoning, motion, pregnancy, or fear.

When nausea and vomiting are related to illness—everything from a minor viral infection to a heart attack—there are usually other symptoms such as fever, pain, rash, swelling, and so forth. In such cases, treatment varies depending upon the underlying cause.

Nausea and vomiting associated with motion sickness, vertigo, and chemotherapy can be prevented or minimized by a variety of antinausea drugs. Among them are:

- **Antihistamines** such as dimenhydrinate (*Dramamine* and others), and meclizine (*Antivert, Bonine*), which work by reducing the sensitivity of the brain's vomiting center.

These drugs, which are especially effective against motion sickness, are available as tablets, elixirs, syrups, and suppositories. Trimethobenzamide (*Tigan*), another antihistamine, is a stronger antinausea drug that is most often prescribed for surgery patients or those undergoing radiation treatments.

- **Scopolamine**, which comes in the form of a medicated patch that is worn behind the ear (*Transderm Scōp*) or in capsule or elixir form (*Donnatal*). It is most commonly used to control motion sickness, but it also may be prescribed to people undergoing cancer chemotherapy. It works by blocking some of the nerve impulses that result in vomiting.

- **Metoclopramide** (*Reglan*), which alleviates nausea and vomiting in two ways—it speeds emptying of the stomach by stimulating peristalsis, the wavelike muscle contractions that move food through the intestinal tract, and it also reduces the activity of the brain's vomiting center. It is prescribed for patients undergoing chemotherapy and radiation treatments as well as for premedication before surgery, in order to clear the digestive tract more rapidly.

- **Phenothiazines** (*Thorazine*) and **haloperidol** (*Haldol, Halperon, Peridol*) which also work by quelling the activity in the brain's vomiting center. Small doses of these drugs are often prescribed for chemotherapy and surgery patients (see Chapter 22).

Although specific side effects vary, most anti-nausea medications, especially antihistamines, cause drowsiness, dry mouth, and constipation. When used for nausea and vomiting, the phenothiazines and other antipsychotic drugs are prescribed in low doses and are unlikely to produce the movement disorders often associated with these medications. Scopolamine interacts with a number of drugs, and must be used with care if you are taking other medications.

drug or category:

DIMENHYDRINATE

condition:

NAUSEA

warning

Tell your doctor if you have or have had:

- an allergic reaction to this medication, or to any preservatives or foods
- asthma, glaucoma, or prostate or urinary tract problems
- ulcers or kidney disease

Tell your doctor if you are taking:

- any other medication to relieve spasms
- central nervous system depressants or MAO inhibitors

Tell your doctor if you are scheduled for surgery involving general or spinal anesthesia within two weeks.

drugs

GENERIC	BRAND	RX
dimenhydrinate	*Dramamine*	Some

form/usage

CAPSULES (REGULAR AND EXTENDED-RELEASE), TABLETS (REGULAR AND CHEWABLE), SYRUP, ELIXIR: May be taken with food or beverages.

Extended-release formulations must be taken whole.

when

Half an hour to an hour before boarding plane, train, boat, or automobile.

side effects and adverse reactions

Fatigue, weakness, confusion, unexplained bleeding, increased heartbeat, sore throat, vision problems, skin reactions

Decrease in appetite, urination problems, problems with contact lenses, drowsiness

Dry mouth, throat

what to do

Stop taking. Get in touch with doctor immediately.

Continue taking, but discuss with your physician.

Try sugarless candy or gum. If condition persists, discuss with your doctor or dentist.

(continued)

special precautions

because

DRUG INTERACTIONS

1. Anticholinergics, antidepressants, antihistamines, dronabinol, sleep medications, MAO inhibitors, molindone, nabilone, drugs containing narcotics, procarbazine, sedatives, sotalol, tranquilizers

2. Clozapine

3. Beta-blockers

1. Increase sedative and depressant effects.

2. Dangerous impact on central nervous system.

3. May diminish effectiveness of *Dramamine*.

DIET

No restrictions.

ALCOHOL AND TOBACCO

Avoid alcohol.
No problems reported with tobacco.

Alcohol may increase sedative effects.

PREGNANCY

Avoid drug during first three months of pregnancy.

Antihistamines like dimenhydrinate have been reported to cause fetal abnormalities in animal experiments.

BREAST-FEEDING

Avoid drug or avoid nursing.

Medication may migrate into breast milk and could affect child.

AGE FACTOR

1. Do not give to infants and use with caution in children.

2. People over 60 should use cautiously.

1. May cause convulsions in young children and irritability and behavior problems in older children.

2. Adverse and side effects may be worse in older people, including urination problems and increased impact on central nervous system functions.

MISSED DOSE

You can take a missed dose up to two hours after scheduled time. Otherwise, wait for next dose but do not double the amount taken.

OVERDOSE

Get emergency medical help immediately if patient falls into coma or has convulsions or hallucinations, or if patient's face turns bright red.

STOPPING DRUG

Discontinue when you feel no longer need medication.

OTHERS

Do not drive or operate machinery until you have determined how medication affects you.

May increase sensitivity to sun. Wear protective clothing and sunblock as well as sunglasses.

drug or category:

MECLIZINE

condition:

NAUSEA

warning

Tell your doctor if you have or have had:
- an allergic reaction to this medication, or to any preservatives or foods
- prostate disease, asthma, glaucoma, or intestinal or urinary tract blockage

Tell your doctor if you are in heart failure.

May affect skin tests for allergies.

drugs

GENERIC	BRAND	RX
meclizine	*Antivert, Bonine*, others	some

form/usage

TABLETS: May be taken with food or liquid.
Tablets may be crumbled.

when

Half an hour to an hour before boarding plane, train, boat, or automobile.

side effects and adverse reactions

Skin reactions

Loss of appetite, inability to sleep, mild gastrointestinal problems, restlessness, drowsiness, vision problems, headache

Dry mouth

what to do

Stop taking. Get in touch with doctor immediately.

Continue taking, but discuss with your physician.

Try sugarless gum or candy, or saliva substitutes. If condition persists, discuss with your doctor or dentist.

special precautions	**because**
DRUG INTERACTIONS	
1. Other anticholinergics, tricyclic antidepressants and tranquilizers, dronabinol, guanfacine, MAO inhibitors, methyprylon, narcotic drugs, pain relievers, sedatives, sleeping medication	1. Will increase effects of meclizine and lead to increased sedative effect.
2. Amphetamines	2. May decrease impact of meclizine.
3. Sotalol, ethinamate	3. Meclizine will increase sotalol effects.
4. Nabilone, clozapine	4. Increase impact on central nervous system.
5. Any medication containing alcohol	5. Alcohol increases sedative effect.
DIET	
No restrictions.	
ALCOHOL AND TOBACCO	
Avoid alcohol. No problems reported with tobacco.	Alcohol will increase sedative effect.
PREGNANCY	
Discuss with your doctor.	Drug has caused fetal abnormalities in animal experiments. There have been no reports of increased risk of fetal deformations in humans.
BREAST-FEEDING	
Discuss with your doctor.	Medication will migrate into breast milk. May also decrease milk production.
AGE FACTOR	
1. Use in children with caution.	1. Children may be more sensitive to drug's effects.
2. People over 60 should use cautiously.	2. Adverse and side effects may be worse in older people.
MISSED DOSE	
Take when you remember, but do not take next dose for four hours. Do not double dose.	

(continued)

OVERDOSE
Get emergency medical help immediately if patient has hallucinations, falls into stupor or coma, shows signs of confusion, has a weak pulse, or is having trouble breathing.

STOPPING DRUG
Discontinue when you no longer need it.

OTHERS
Do not drive or operate machinery until you have determined how medication affects you.

drug or category:

METOCLOPRAMIDE

condition:

NAUSEA

warning

Tell your doctor if you have or have had:

- an allergic reaction to this medication, or to preservatives or food additives
- a history of stomach ulcers or gastrointestinal bleeding

drugs

GENERIC	BRAND	RX
metoclopramide	*Reglan*, others	Yes

form/usage

TABLETS, SYRUP, INJECTIONS: Tablets and syrup can be taken with food or liquid to prevent or lessen stomach irritation.

when

Half an hour before needed (before chemotherapy treatment, for example).

side effects and adverse reactions

Abnormal face movements, Parkinson-like trembling, breathing difficulties

Mild gastrointestinal problems, mild headache, inability to sleep, menstrual changes, swollen breasts, skin reactions, drowsiness

Dry mouth or throat

what to do

Stop taking. Get in touch with your doctor immediately.

Continue taking, but discuss with your physician.

Try sugarless candy or gum. If condition persists, discuss with your doctor or dentist.

special precautions

DRUG INTERACTIONS
1. Anticholinergics, medications with narcotics

because

1. Will counter effect of metoclopramide.

(continued)

DRUG INTERACTIONS

2. Central nervous system depressants, ethinamate fluoxetine, guanfacine, methyprylon, nabilone

3. Acetaminophen, aspirin, bromocriptine, digitalis, levodopa, lithium, nizatidine, pergolide

4. Antidiabetics, digoxin

5. Leucovorin

6. Phenothiazines, thiothixine

7. Elixirs

8. Tetracycline

2. Greater sedation and depressant effects. Possible toxicity.

3. Metoclopramide will increase their absorption and effects.

4. Metoclopramide will decrease their absorption and effectiveness.

5. Can cause changes in blood sugar levels. Discuss possible dose changes with doctor.

6. May cause shaking and trembling.

7. Contain alcohol, which may increase sedative effect.

8. Can cause trembling and muscle spasms.

DIET

Avoid coffee and other foods and beverages with caffeine.

Will counteract effect of drug.

ALCOHOL AND TOBACCO

Avoid both.

Alcohol will heighten drug's sedative effects. Tobacco will decrease impact of drug.

PREGNANCY

No negative interactions reported, but discuss with your doctor.

While no evidence of fetal harm has been found in animals. no sufficient, well-controlled studies have been done in humans.

BREAST-FEEDING

No problems reported, but discuss with your doctor.

Drug will migrate into breast milk.

AGE FACTOR

1. Give to children very cautiously.

2. People over 60 should use cautiously.

1. Children can develop muscle spasms.

2. Adverse and side effects may be worse in older people; may cause walking difficulties and trembling of hands if taken over long period of time.

MISSED DOSE
You can take a missed dose up to two hours after scheduled time. Otherwise, wait for next dose but do not double the amount taken.

OVERDOSE
Get emergency medical help immediately if patient falls into coma, has seizures, or muscle spasms, has a hard time staying awake, is confused, or is shaking.

STOPPING DRUG
You can stop taking when you feel better.

OTHERS
Do not drive or operate machinery until you have determined how medication affects you.

`drug or category:`

SCOPOLAMINE

`condition:`

NAUSEA; ALSO USED FOR DIGESTIVE SYSTEM SPASMS, RELIEF OF MENSTRUAL CRAMPS

---

warning

Tell your doctor if you have or have had:
- an allergic reaction to this medication, or to any preservatives or foods
- glaucoma, chronic constipation, or urinary retention

---

drugs

GENERIC	BRAND	RX
scopolamine	*Transderm Scōp* patch	Yes, for some dosages

---

form/usage

SKIN PATCHES: Follow directions on package. Change placement position on body every time you put on a new patch.

when

Half an hour before boarding plane, train, automobile, or boat.

---

side effects and adverse reactions

Severe allergic reaction (anaphylactic shock), severe skin reactions

Confusion, increased heartbeat, light-headedness, severe vision problems, delirium

Urination problems, constipation, inability to taste, headache

Dry mouth, nose, and throat

what to do

Get emergency medical help immediately.

Stop taking. Get in touch with doctor immediately.

Continue taking, but discuss with your physician.

Try sugarless candy or gum. If condition persists, discuss with your doctor or dentist.

special precautions	**because**

DRUG INTERACTIONS
1. Amantadine, other anticholinergics, tricyclic antidepressants, antihistamines, buclizine, fluoxetine, guanfacine, MAO inhibitors, meperidine, methylphenidate, methyprylon, molindone, nabilone, orphenadrine, phenothiazines, quinidine, sedatives, and sleeping agents

2. Digitalis

3. Encainide

4. Pilocarpine

5. Nitrates

1. Will increase effect of scopolamine, resulting in greater sedation, or have increased depressive action on central nervous system

2. Will decrease effect of scopolamine.

3. Risk of toxic effects on heart.

4. Antiglaucoma effect may be decreased.

5. May increase pressure inside the eye.

DIET
No restrictions.

ALCOHOL AND TOBACCO
Avoid alcohol.
No problems reported with tobacco.

Alcohol may increase the sedating effect of drug.

PREGNANCY
Discuss with your doctor.

No human or animal studies relating to pregnancy have been done.

BREAST-FEEDING
Discuss with your doctor.

Medication will migrate into breast milk, but there are no reports of problems with infants. Medication may affect milk flow.

AGE FACTOR
1. Do not give to children.

2. People over 60 should use cautiously.

1. Medication may make children excitable or nervous and more susceptible to heat.

2. Adverse and side effects may be worse in older people. Effects include confusion, memory problems, and increased nervousness or excitability.

(continued)

MISSED DOSE

Put on patch when you remember.

OVERDOSE

Get emergency medical help immediately if patient falls into a coma, or suffers breathing difficulties, hallucinations, dilated pupils, confusion, fever, excitability, or rapid pulse.

STOPPING DRUG

Remove patch as needed.

OTHERS

Do not drive or operate machinery until you have determined how medication affects you.

Drug may make you more sensitive to heat. Be careful exercising or exerting yourself in hot weather.

Getting up from a sitting or lying position may make you dizzy. Rise slowly from bed or chair. Check with your doctor if condition does not improve after a few days.

Medication may increase your sensitivity to light and may make one pupil larger than the other. Discuss with your doctor if condition persists.

TRIMETHOBENZAMIDE

condition:
NAUSEA

warning

Tell your doctor if you have or have had:
- an allergic reaction to this medication or local anesthetics such as benzocaine, or to preservatives or food additives

Tell your doctor if you:
- have been running a fever or have an intestinal infection
- are taking any medications that have an effect on the central nervous system

drugs

GENERIC	BRAND	RX
trimethobenzamide	*Tigan*, others	Yes

form/usage

CAPSULES, INJECTION, SUPPOSITORIES: Capsule may be opened and taken with beverage or food.

Unwrap suppository and insert in rectum, pointed end first. If suppository seems too soft, put in refrigerator for half an hour or place in cold, running water.

when

As needed; see package instructions for maximum per-day limits.

side effects and adverse reactions

Convulsions, seizures

Skin reactions, vision changes, sore throat, back pain, Parkinson-like symptoms, muscle spasms, tremors

Headaches, dizziness, mild gastrointestinal problems, fatigue

what to do

Get emergency medical help immediately.

Stop taking. Get in touch with doctor immediately.

Continue taking, but discuss with your physician.

(continued)

special precautions	because
DRUG INTERACTIONS 1. Antidepressants, barbiturates, belladonna, anticholinergics, fluoxetine, guanfacine, methyprylon, nabilone, sedatives or sleep medications, drugs containing narcotics, phenothiazines, tranquilizers	1. Increase sedative and depressant effects.
2. Leucovorin	2. Contains alcohol, which may increase sedative effects.
3. Clozapine, nabilone	3. Dangerous impact on central nervous system.
DIET No restrictions	
ALCOHOL AND TOBACCO Avoid alcohol. No problems reported with tobacco.	Alcohol may intensify effects of medication.
PREGNANCY No fetal impact reported, but discuss with your doctor.	May increase chance of miscarriage.
BREAST-FEEDING No problems reported.	
AGE FACTOR 1. Do not give to children unless specifically prescribed by physician.	1. Side effects may be more serious in children. Observe child carefully, if drug is given.
2. People over 60 should use cautiously.	2. Adverse and side effects may be worse in older people.

MISSED DOSE
Take when you remember, unless it is almost time for next dose. When you take next dose, do not double amount.

OVERDOSE
Get emergency medical help immediately if patient falls into coma, has convulsions, or is confused.

STOPPING DRUG

May be stopped when no longer needed.

OTHERS

Do not drive or operate machinery until you have determined how medication affects you.

May increase sensitivity to sun. If you go outdoors between 10 A.M. and 3 P.M., wear protective clothing and/or sunblock.

-22-

ANTIPSYCHOTIC MEDICATIONS, TRANQUILIZERS, AND SLEEP MEDICATIONS

IN RECENT DECADES, the development of highly effective psychoactive drugs has revolutionized the treatment of schizophrenia and other psychoses, as well as anxiety and milder forms of mental and emotional illness.

Hundreds of years ago, people with schizophrenia and other psychoses were either driven into the wilderness or burned at the stake. Until the late 1960s, on any given day half a million Americans with severe mental illness were confined to mental institutions. Dozens of drugs now help people with severe mental illness lead better lives. The drugs, some of which were first developed in French pharmaceutical laboratories, include:

- **Antipsychotics**. These drugs, also referred to as major tranquilizers, decrease paranoia, fear, hostility, and agitation. The mentally ill who receive them experience a decrease in delusions, hallucinations, restlessness, and hyperactivity. The **phenothiazines**, which include drugs like *Thorazine* and *Stelazine*, have also been found to be beneficial to children who

are hyperactive, combative, and manic-depressive. Medications like *Haldol, Halperon,* and *Peridol* are effective against schizophrenia, paranoia, and the manic swing in the manic-depressive cycle. From time to time haloperidols are successfully used to dampen the tics and the offensive language that are typical of Tourette's syndrome. Loxapine (*Loxitane*) is used with success in schizophrenics, and has also been used to treat patients with severe anxiety and depression. The major antipsychotics also include lithium (*Cibalith-S, Eskalith,* and others), a drug used to stabilize the manic phase of manic-depressive illness, and chlorprothixene (*Taractan*), used to treat psychosis, agitation, and anxiety.

- **Psychostimulants**. Methylphenidate (*Ritalin*) is sometimes prescribed for hyperactive children, as well as withdrawn older people or those with minimal brain damage. Dextroamphetamine (*Dexedrine*) is also used to control hyperactivity in children as well as narcolepsy, uncontrollable urges to sleep.

- **Minor tranquilizers and antianxiety medications**. These drugs, which include the **benzodiazepines**, (*Valium, Ativan, Xanax*, and many others) ease nervousness and anxiety by blocking the activity of the neurotransmitter dopamine in various parts of the brain.

Sleep Medications

The best way to cope with sleep problems is to find a nondrug way around them. Nevertheless, if you need a short-term sleeping medication to get through a trying period, there are prescription medications such as **temazepam** (*Restoril*), **flurazepam** (*Dalmane*), and **triazolam** (*Halcion*), which are related to the benzodiazepine class of tranquilizers. It should be stressed that these drugs are only for short-term use, generally only a few weeks. They carry a risk of possible overdose, especially if you are taking cold pills, antihistamines, or other medications with sedating ingredients. Potentially, they are psychologically and physiologically addictive. They also can lead to reactive, or "bounce-back," insomnia, meaning that your insomnia will return even worse than before when the drugs are stopped. (Also see Chapter 18 for information on drugs to treat depression.)

drug or category:

PHENOTHIAZINES (CHLORPROMAZINE, TRIFLUOPERAZINE)

condition:
PSYCHOTIC ILLNESS

warning

Tell your doctor if you have or have had:

- an allergic reaction to this medication, or to any preservatives or foods
- any blood disorders
- breast cancer
- urination or prostate problems
- cardiovascular or lung disease
- Parkinson's disease, seizures, or liver disease
- lupus erythematosus

If you are going to have surgery (including extensive oral procedures), tell the doctor that you are taking these medications.

drugs

GENERIC	BRAND	RX
chlorpromazine	*Thorazine*, others	Yes
trifluoperazine	*Stelazine*	

form/usage

CAPSULES (EXTENDED-RELEASE, REGULAR), ORAL CONCEN-TRATES, TABLETS, SYRUPS: May be taken with food, milk, or water. Do not open extended-release capsules.

when

Discuss with your doctor.

side effects and adverse reactions

Uncontrollable face, tongue, and mouth movements or spasms, inability to walk correctly

Vision problems, confusion, fainting, skin reactions, restlessness, uncontrolled lip and tongue movements

what to do

Get emergency medical help immediately.

Stop taking. Get in touch with doctor immediately.

ANTIPSYCHOTIC MEDICATIONS, TRANQUILIZERS, AND SLEEP MEDICATIONS

side effects and adverse reactions	what to do
Constipation, congestion in nose, urination difficulties	Continue taking, but discuss with your physician.
Dry mouth	Try sugarless candy or gum. If condition persists, discuss with your doctor or dentist.

special precautions	because
DRUG INTERACTIONS	
1. Anticholinergics, antihistamines, guanethidine, drugs containing narcotics, other tranquilizers	1. Phenothiazines will increase the effect of these drugs; they may interfere with phenothiazines' effectiveness. Do not take within one hour of taking this medication.
2. Tricyclic antidepressants, calcium supplements, dronabinol	2. Will increase effect of phenothiazines.
3. High blood pressure medications	3. Can cause dangerous drop in blood pressure.
4. Antithyroid medications	4. May cause blood disorders.
5. Diet pills	5. Their effect will be diminished.
6. Bupropion	6. Risk of seizures.
7. Clozapine, nabilone	7. Can have dangerous impact on central nervous system.
8. Isoniazid	8. Possible liver damage.
9. Lithium	9. Phenothiazines will diminish its effect.
10. Metyrosine	10. Toxic effects.
11. Quinidine	11. May interfere with heart activity.
12. Antacids, antidiarrheals	12. These drugs decrease effectiveness of phenothiazine; do not take them within one hour of taking this medication.

DIET
No restrictions.

(continued)

ALCOHOL and TOBACCO
Avoid alcohol.
No interaction reported with tobacco.

Alcohol increases sedative effect.

PREGNANCY
Avoid drug.

Drug has caused fetal abnormalities in animal experiments. There have been reports of jaundice and muscle disorders in human newborns.

BREAST-FEEDING
Avoid drug or avoid nursing.

Medication will migrate into breast milk and could affect child.

AGE FACTOR
1. Use caution in giving to children.

1. Children may be especially sensitive and develop muscle spasms and other uncontrollable body movements, especially if they are severely ill.

2. People over 60 should use cautiously.

2. Adverse and side effects may be worse in older people and may include dizziness; constipation; uncontrolled movements of mouth, tongue, and jaw; and trembling.

MISSED DOSE
You can take a missed dose up to two hours after scheduled time. Otherwise, wait for next dose but do not double the amount taken.

OVERDOSE
Get emergency medical help immediately if patient falls into coma, has convulsions, or is in a stupor.

STOPPING DRUG
Do not stop taking even if you feel better until you have talked with your doctor. You may have to come off drug slowly.

OTHERS
Do not drive or operate machinery until you have determined how medication affects you.

May increase sensitivity to sun. If you go outdoors between 10 A.M. and 3 P.M., wear protective clothing and/or sunblock. Wear sunglasses, even when it's cloudy.

May cause decreased sexual desire, inhibited ejaculation, painful and long-lasting erections of the penis, and impotence.

May cause enlargement of breasts and stop menstruation. Discuss these problems with your doctor.

Getting up from a sitting or lying position may make you dizzy. Rise slowly from bed or chair. Check with your doctor if condition does not improve after a few days.

Drug may make you more sensitive to heat because it decreases sweating and can cause an increase in body temperature. Be careful in hot environments.

Periodic laboratory tests might be necessary to check blood count and liver function. Periodic eye exams may also be required.

drug or category:

CHLORPROTHIXENE

condition:
PSYCHOTIC ILLNESS

warning

Tell your doctor if you have or have had:
- an allergic reaction to this medication, or to preservatives or food additives
- a history of drug abuse
- blood disease, glaucoma, cardiovascular disease
- severe asthma or liver disease
- Parkinson's disease
- ulcers, seizures

Tell your doctor if you are taking narcotic or anticholinergic drugs. If you are going to have surgery (including extensive oral procedures), tell the doctor that you are taking these medications.

drugs

GENERIC	BRAND	RX
chlorprothixene	*Taractan*	Yes

form/usage

TABLETS, CAPSULES (EXTENDED-RELEASE), SYRUP: May be taken with beverages.

Tablet may be crumbled and taken with liquid or food.

Do not open extended-release capsules.

when

Discuss schedule with your doctor.

side effects and adverse reactions

Body movements that cannot be controlled, fainting spells and palpitations

Uncontrolled movements of mouth, lips, and cheeks; heatstroke; unexplained bruising or bleeding; skin reactions; fainting; vision problems; increased heartbeat

what to do

Get emergency medical help immediately.

Stop taking. Get in touch with doctor immediately.

side effects and adverse reactions	what to do
Dizziness, gastrointestinal problems, weight gain, sensitivity to light, stuffy nose, swollen breasts, menstrual problems	Continue taking, but discuss with your physician.
Dry mouth	Try sugarless candy or gum. If condition persists, discuss with your doctor or dentist.

special precautions	because
DRUG INTERACTIONS	
1. Anticholinergics, dronabinol, antihypertensives	1. Chlorprothixene increases their effect.
2. Tricyclic antidepressants, antihistamines, barbiturates, medications containing narcotics, sedatives, sleep medications, tranquilizers	2. Increase effect of chlorprothixene.
3. Anticonvulsants	3. Can cause changes in seizures.
4. Bethanechol, guanethidine, levodopa, pergolide	4. Their effect is decreased.
5. Antacids, antidiarrheals	5. May interfere with chlorprothixene's effectiveness. Do not take within one hour of taking this medication.
DIET No restrictions	
ALCOHOL and TOBACCO Avoid alcohol. No problems reported with tobacco.	Alcohol will depress brain activity dangerously.
PREGNANCY Avoid drug if you want to become pregnant.	Drug may cause fertility problems.
BREAST-FEEDING Avoid drug or avoid nursing.	While no problems have been reported with this medication and doctors do not know if it enters breast milk, other tranquilizers and antipsychotics pass into breast milk and have caused problems for nursing infants, including drowsiness.

(continued)

AGE FACTOR

1. Use cautiously in children.

2. People over 60 should use cautiously.

1. Children are more likely to react with muscle spasms in upper body and head, as well as other muscular problems.

2. Adverse and side effects may be worse in older people, including constipation, dizziness, drowsiness, and involuntary movements of mouth, tongue, jaw, and limbs.

MISSED DOSE

You can take a missed dose up to two hours after scheduled time. Otherwise, wait for next dose but do not double the amount taken.

OVERDOSE

Get emergency medical help immediately if patient falls into coma or suffers breathing difficulties, a sharp drop in blood pressure, convulsions, tremors, confusion, or vision problems.

STOPPING DRUG

Do not stop taking even if you feel better until you have talked with your doctor. You may have to come off drug slowly.

OTHERS

Do not drive or operate machinery until you have determined how medication affects you.

Getting up from a sitting or lying position may make you dizzy. Rise slowly from bed or chair. Check with your doctor if condition does not improve after a few days.

May increase sensitivity to sun. If you go outdoors between 10 A.M. and 3 P.M., wear protective clothing and/or sunblock.

drug or category:

LOXAPINE

condition:

PSYCHOTIC ILLNESS

warning

Tell your doctor if you have or have had:
- an allergic reaction to this medication before, or if you are allergic to any preservatives or foods
- a history of alcohol abuse
- glaucoma, cardiovascular disease, liver disease, or breast cancer
- Parkinson's disease or seizures
- urination or prostate difficulties

If you are going to have surgery (including extensive oral procedures), tell the doctor that you are taking these medications.

drugs

GENERIC	BRAND	RX
loxapine	*Loxitane*	Yes

form/usage

CAPSULES, TABLETS, SOLUTION, INJECTION: Should be taken with food or beverage to avoid or lessen stomach irritation.

Solution should be taken with fruit juice to dispel taste.

when

Follow your doctor's instructions.

side effects and adverse reactions

Severe breathing difficulties, skin reactions, sweating, heart rhythm changes

Fast heartbeat, unexplained bleeding, sore throat, uncontrolled mouth movements, shaking hands, problems swallowing, stiff limbs, dizziness

Mild gastrointestinal problems, urination problems, vision problems, inability to sleep, eye sensitivity to light, mild headache, diminished sex drive

what to do

Get emergency medical help immediately.

Stop taking. Get in touch with doctor immediately.

Continue taking, but discuss with your physician.

(continued)

side effects and adverse reactions	what to do
Dry mouth	Try sugarless candy or gum. If condition persists, discuss with your doctor or dentist.

special precautions	because

DRUG INTERACTIONS

1. Anticonvulsants, guanadrel, guanethidine, pergolide

1. Medication decreases their effect.

2. Fluoxetine, methyprylon, nabilone

2. Increase depressant and sedative effects.

3. Clozapine, haloperidol, methyldopa, metoclopramide, metyrosine, molindone, pemoline, other antipsychotics, pimozide, rauwolfia

3. Increase toxicity.

4. Epinephrine

4. Causes dangerous increases in heart rate and drops in blood pressure.

5. Ethinamate

5. Sharply increases effects of ethinamate.

6. Antacids, antidiarrheal medications

6. May decrease antipsychotic's effectiveness. Do not take within one hour of taking this medication.

DIET
No interactions reported.

ALCOHOL and TOBACCO
Avoid both.

Alcohol may interfere with drug's effectiveness. Tobacco may make medication toxic.

PREGNANCY
Discuss with your doctor.

Drug has been reported to cause fetal problems in some animal experiments. There have been no reports of increased risk of fetal deformations in humans.

BREAST-FEEDING
Discuss with your doctor.

While there are no reports of problems, in humans, the drug is excreted in dog milk.

AGE FACTOR

1. Not recommended for children under 18.

2. People over 60 should use cautiously.

1. Safety and effectiveness have not been established.

2. Adverse and side effects may be worse in older people, including uncontrolled movements of tongue, mouth, and jaws as well as limbs.

MISSED DOSE

You can take a missed dose up to two hours after scheduled time. Otherwise, wait for next dose but do not double the amount taken.

OVERDOSE

Get emergency medical help immediately if patient falls into coma, or suffers muscle spasms, breathing difficulties, dizziness, or drowsiness.

STOPPING DRUG

Do not stop taking even if you feel better until you have talked with your doctor. You may have to come off drug slowly.

OTHERS

Do not drive or operate machinery until you have determined how medication affects you.

May increase sensitivity to sun. If you go outdoors between 10 A.M. and 3 P.M., wear protective clothing and/or sunblock.

Getting up from a sitting or lying position may make you dizzy. Rise slowly from bed or chair. Check with your doctor if condition does not improve after a few days.

Periodic laboratory tests might be necessary to check blood count and liver function. Periodic eye exam may also be necessary.

drug or category:

HALOPERIDOL

condition:

PSYCHOTIC ILLNESS

warning

Tell your doctor if you have or have had:
• an allergic reaction to this medication, or to any preservatives or foods
• Parkinson's disease, cardiovascular problems, or history of seizures or breast cancer
Tell your doctor if you are receiving anticoagulant medication.
If you are going to have surgery (including extensive oral procedures) tell the doctor that you are taking these medications.

drugs

GENERIC	BRAND	RX
haloperidol	*Haldol, Halperon*	Yes

form/usage

TABLETS, CAPSULES (INCLUDING EXTENDED-RELEASE CAP-SULES), SOLUTIONS, INJECTIONS: Tablets and capsules may be taken with food or liquid.

Tablets may be crushed. Do not open extended-release capsules.

Solutions should be taken as is, though they can be taken with liquid if necessary.

when

Discuss schedule with your doctor; then take at same time every day.

side effects and adverse reactions

Uncontrolled movements of muscles, including those in the face and mouth

Skin reactions, hallucinations, uncontrolled movements of the lips or tongue, pain in stomach, sore throat, vision and balance problems, spasms

what to do

Get emergency medical help immediately.

Stop taking. Get in touch with doctor immediately.

side effects and adverse reactions	what to do
Mild dizziness, mild gastrointestinal problems, stiffness, shaking	Continue taking, but discuss with your physician.
Dry mouth	Try sugarless candy or gum. If condition persists, discuss with your doctor or dentist.

special precautions	because

DRUG INTERACTIONS

1. Antidepressants, antihistamines, barbiturates, central nervous system medications, fluoxetine, guanfacine, nabilone, drugs containing narcotics, procarbazine, sedatives, tranquilizers	1. Increase sedation, depress central nervous system, increase other depressant effects.
2. Anticonvulsants, bupropion	2. Can cause seizures.
3. High blood pressure medications	3. Can cause dangerous drop in blood pressure.
4. Clozapine, loxapine, lithium	4. Increase toxicity.
5. Guanethidine, levodopa, pergolide, phenindione	5. Their effectiveness is decreased.
6. Leucovorin	6. Alcohol content may cause excessive sedation.

DIET
No interactions reported.

ALCOHOL and TOBACCO
Avoid alcohol.
No problems reported with tobacco.

Alcohol can increase sedation.

PREGNANCY
Avoid drug.

Drug has caused fetal abnormalities in animal experiments. Has not been studied in pregnant women.

BREAST-FEEDING
Avoid drug or avoid nursing.

Medication will migrate into breast milk and could affect child. Discuss with your doctor.

(continued)

AGE FACTOR

1. Drug is not recommended for children.

1. Children are more sensitive to the drug and more likely to develop side effects.

2. People over 60 should use cautiously.

2. Adverse and side effects may be worse in older people.

MISSED DOSE

You can take a missed dose up to two hours after scheduled time. Otherwise, wait for next dose but do not double the amount taken.

OVERDOSE

Get emergency medical help immediately if patient falls into coma; suffers breathing difficulties, convulsions, or a severe drop in blood pressure; has a weak pulse or tremors.

STOPPING DRUG

Do not stop taking even if you feel better until you have talked with your doctor. You may have to come off drug slowly.

OTHERS

Do not drive or operate machinery until you have determined how medication affects you.

May increase sensitivity to sun. If you go outdoors between 10 A.M. and 3 P.M., wear protective clothing and/or sunblock.

Drug may decrease sweating, thus increasing body temperature. Be careful in hot environments and ask your doctor for guidance.

Getting up from a sitting or lying position may make you dizzy. Rise slowly from bed or chair. Check with your doctor if condition does not improve after a few days.

Periodic laboratory tests might be necessary to check blood count and liver function. Periodic eye exams may also be necessary.

Long-term use of this drug may necessitate the use of an anticholinergic agent such as *Artane* or benztropine to control the side effects of haloperidol.

drug or category:

LITHIUM

condition:
PSYCHOTIC ILLNESS (MANIC-DEPRESSION)

warning

Tell your doctor if you have or have had:
- an allergic reaction to this medication, or to any preservatives or foods
- brain diseases, schizophrenia
- leukemia, Parkinson's disease, or seizures
- kidney, heart, or thyroid disease
- psoriasis, diabetes, or urinary problems

drugs

GENERIC	BRAND	RX
lithium	Cibalith-S, Eskalith, Lithonate, others	Yes

form/usage

CAPSULES, TABLETS (REGULAR AND EXTENDED-RELEASE), SYRUP: Should be taken after meal or snack.

Syrup should be diluted in fruit juice or flavored drink.

Extended-release tablets should not be crumbled or crushed. Ample quantities of water should be drunk during the day.

when

Discuss schedule with your physician.

side effects and adverse reactions

Vision problems or pain in eyes, skin reactions, abdominal pain, changes in heart rhythm, breathing difficulties, ringing or other noises in ears

Hair loss, uncontrolled movements of legs or arms, fatigue, thinking difficulty, muscle pain, menstrual irregularities, loss of sexual drive, severe loss of appetite, shaking

what to do

Stop taking. Get in touch with doctor immediately.

Continue taking, but discuss with your physician.

(continued)

side effects and adverse reactions	what to do
Dry mouth	Try sugarless candy or gum. If condition persists, discuss with your doctor or dentist.

special precautions	because

DRUG INTERACTIONS

1. Acetazolamide, nicardipine, nimodipine, phenothiazines, sodium bicarbonate, theophylline, verapamil	1. Decrease effectiveness of lithium.
2. Carbamazepine, diuretics, dronabinol, indomethacin, methyldopa, phenytoin, phenylbutazone, tetracyclines	2. Increase effect of lithium.
3. Antihistamines	3. May increase sedation.
4. Bupropion	4. May lead to seizures.
5. Desmopressin	5. Lithium will decrease its effect.
6. Diclofenac, muscle relaxants, potassium iodide	6. Effect of these drugs will be increased.
7. Molindone	7. May cause changes in brain.

DIET

Discuss your salt intake with your doctor. Do not go on a low-salt or salt-free diet without consulting your physician.	Eating too many salty foods could decrease effect of medication. Insufficient amount of salt could increase medication's impact.

ALCOHOL and TOBACCO

Avoid alcohol. No problems reported with tobacco.	Alcohol could enhance toxic effects of lithium.

PREGNANCY

Avoid drug.	Drug has caused fetal abnormalities in humans.

BREAST-FEEDING

Avoid drug or avoid nursing.	Medication will migrate into breast milk and could affect child. Discuss with your doctor.

ANTIPSYCHOTIC MEDICATIONS, TRANQUILIZERS, AND SLEEP MEDICATIONS

AGE FACTOR

1. Monitor children carefully.

2. People over 60 should use cautiously.

1. Lithium may cause bone weakness in children.

2. Adverse and side effects may be worse in older people. These may include diarrhea, muscle problems, gastrointestinal problems, and goiter.

MISSED DOSE

You can take a missed dose up to two hours after scheduled time. Otherwise, wait for next dose but do not double the amount taken.

OVERDOSE

Get emergency medical help immediately if patient falls into coma or stupor or has convulsions or severe gastrointestinal problems.

STOPPING DRUG

Do not stop taking even if you feel better until you have talked with your doctor. You may have to come off drug slowly.

OTHERS

Do not drive or operate machinery until you have determined how medication affects you.

Drug may make you more sensitive to heat. Be careful in hot environments and ask your doctor for guidance on taking hot showers or baths.

Periodic laboratory tests might be necessary to check blood lithium levels, blood count, and kidney function. Periodic evaluation of thyroid gland may also be needed.

drug or category:

BENZODIAZEPINES

condition:

SLEEP PROBLEMS, ANXIETY

warning

Tell your doctor if you have or have had:

- an allergic reaction to this medication, or to any preservatives or foods
- narrow-angle glaucoma
- alcohol or drug abuse problems
- serious mental problems
- respiratory ailments like asthma or emphysema

Tell your doctors and dentist that you are using these medications.

If you are having laboratory tests, tell the doctor that you are taking tranquilizers.

Tell your doctor if you are pregnant or planning to become pregnant while taking this drug.

drugs

GENERIC	BRAND	RX
alprazolam	*Xanax*	Yes
chlordiazepoxide	*Librium*, others	
diazepam	*Valium*, others	
flurazepam	*Dalmane*, others	
lorazepam	*Ativan*, others	
midazolam	*Versed*	
oxazepam	*Serax*	
temazepam	*Restoril*, others	
triazolam	*Halcion*	

form/usage

TABLETS, CAPSULES (REGULAR AND EXTENDED-RELEASE), SOLUTIONS, INJECTIONS: Can be taken with or without food or beverage.

Extended-release capsules should be taken whole.

when

Usually at bedtime, but discuss schedule with your doctor.

side effects and adverse reactions	what to do
Very slow heartbeat, breathing problems	Get emergency medical help immediately.
Sores in mouth or throat, hallucinations, depression, severe skin reactions, vision problems, fever or chills	Stop taking. Get in touch with your doctor immediately.
Sleepiness, mild gastrointestinal problems, urination problems, strange dreams, stomach pain, mild behavioral changes	Continue taking, but discuss with your physician.

special precautions	because
DRUG INTERACTIONS	
1. Antidepressants, antihistamines, oral contraceptives, disulfiram, dronabinol, erythromycin, ketoconazole, molindone, nabilone, drugs containing narcotics, nizatidine, probenecid, sedatives, sleep medications	1. Increase tranquilizer, sedative, or central nervous system depression effect.
2. Anticonvulsants	2. Change in seizure pattern.
3. High blood pressure medication	3. Blood pressure may drop too much.
4. Levodopa	4. Benzodiazepines will decrease its effects.
5. MAO inhibitors	5. Convulsions, severe temper outbursts.
6. Zidovudine	6. Benzodiazepines increase its toxicity.
DIET Avoid excessive use of beverages containing caffeine.	Can heighten anxiety.
ALCOHOL and TOBACCO Be cautious in use of alcohol and tobacco.	Alcohol can heighten depressive effect on brain. Tobacco/Smoking can counteract effect of tranquilizers.

(continued)

PREGNANCY
Avoid drug.

Some medications within this class of drugs have caused fetal abnormalities in animal experiments. There have been reports of increased fetal deformations in humans.

BREAST-FEEDING
Avoid drug or avoid nursing.

Medication will migrate into breast milk and could affect child.

AGE FACTOR
1. Use in children cautiously.

1. Side effects are more likely to affect children and, over long period of time, may affect physical and intellectual development.

2. People over 60 should use cautiously.

2. Adverse and side effects, including agitation, may be worse in older people.

MISSED DOSE
You can take a missed dose up to two hours after scheduled time. Otherwise, wait for next dose but do not double the amount taken.

OVERDOSE
Get emergency medical help immediately if patient falls into a coma or stupor, has severe shaking, or cannot stay awake.

STOPPING DRUG
Do not stop taking even if you feel better until you have talked with your doctor. You may have to come off drug slowly.

OTHERS
Do not drive or operate machinery until you have determined how medication affects you.

Although small doses of some benzodiazepines are given to help men deal with impotence and women with lack of orgasm, large doses of some of these medications can cause sexual dysfunction.

Drug may make you more sensitive to heat. Be careful in hot environments and ask your doctor for guidance on taking hot showers or baths.

drug or category:

BUSPIRONE

condition:
ANXIETY DISORDERS

warning

Tell your doctor if you have or have had:
- an allergic reaction to this medication, or to preservatives or food additives
- a history of drug or alcohol abuse
- kidney or liver disease

Tell your doctor if you are using anticoagulants.

drugs

GENERIC	BRAND	RX
buspirone	*BuSpar*	Yes

form/usage

TABLETS: May be taken with food or liquid.

when

As scheduled by your doctor; usually medication is taken three times a day.

side effects and adverse reactions

what to do

side effects and adverse reactions	what to do
Chest pains, fast and pounding heartbeat	Get emergency medical help immediately.
Depression; confusion; psychotic episodes; vision problems; sore throat; involuntary movements of lips, tongue, or limbs; headache; nausea; restlessness	Stop taking. Get in touch with your doctor immediately.
Drowsiness, nightmares, unexplained fatigue	Continue taking, but discuss with your physician.
Dry mouth	Try sugarless candy or gum. If condition persists, discuss with your doctor or dentist.

(continued)

special precautions

because

DRUG INTERACTIONS

1. Anthistamines, barbiturates, muscle relaxants, medications containing narcotics, sedatives, tranquilizers

1. May cause increased sedation.

2. MAO inhibitors

2. May cause higher blood pressure.

DIET

Avoid beverages with caffeine.

Will diminish effectiveness of medication.

ALCOHOL and TOBACCO

Avoid both.

Alcohol may increase sedation.
Tobacco may decrease effectiveness of drug.

PREGNANCY

No negative interactions reported.

BREAST-FEEDING

No problems reported.

Safety and effectiveness have not been established.

AGE FACTOR

1. Not recommended for children under 18.

1. Safety and effectiveness have not been established.

2. Adults over 60 have not had reactions different from those of younger adults.

MISSED DOSE

Take when you remember. If it is almost time for next dose, take the scheduled dose, but do not double the amount taken.

OVERDOSE

Get emergency medical help immediately if patient is extremely drowsy and cannot be roused, has small pupils, or is unconscious.

STOPPING DRUG
Discontinue only on advice of your physician.

OTHERS
Do not drive or operate machinery until you have determined how medication affects you.

DEXTROAMPHETAMINE

condition:

HYPERACTIVITY IN CHILDREN; ALSO USED FOR UNCONTROLLED SLEEPINESS (NARCOLEPSY)

warning

Tell your doctor if you have or have had:
- an allergic reaction to this medication, or to any preservatives or foods
- a history of mental illness or drug or alcohol abuse
- cardiovascular disease, hypertension, thyroid problems, Tourette's syndrome

If you are scheduled for surgery under general anesthesia, tell the surgeon you are taking this medication.

Tell your doctor if you are prone to anxiety or tension.

Do not use to lose weight.

drugs

GENERIC	BRAND	RX
dextroamphetamine	*Dexedrine*, others	

form/usage

TABLETS, CAPSULES (INCLUDING EXTENDED-RELEASE FORMULATIONS): Take with beverage.

Do not crush tablets. Extended-release formulations must also be taken whole.

when

Take at the same time every day.

Do not take short-acting forms less than six hours before you go to bed.

Extended-release formulations are best taken in the morning.

side effects and adverse reactions

Skin reactions, uncontrolled head movements, heart rhythm changes or fast and pounding heartbeat, visual problems, dizziness, unexplained sweating

Moodiness, breast enlargement, minor gastrointestinal problems, headaches, nervousness or irritability

what to do

Stop taking. Get in touch with doctor immediately.

Continue taking, but discuss with your physician.

side effects and adverse reactions	what to do
Dry mouth	Try sugarless candy or gum. If condition persists, discuss with your doctor or dentist.

special precautions	because
DRUG INTERACTIONS	
1. Tricyclic antidepressants, haloperidol, phenothiazines	1. Will decrease effect of amphetamines.
2. High blood pressure medications, doxazosin, prazosin	2. Their effect will be decreased.
3. Beta-blockers, furazolidone, MAO inhibitors	3. Will cause sudden and severe increases in blood pressure.
4. Thyroid medications	4. Will cause heartbeat problems.
5. Sympathomimetics	5. May cause seizures.
6. Nabilone	6. Could cause increased central nervous system depression.
DIET	
Avoid coffee and other drinks with caffeine.	Will add to stimulant effects.
ALCOHOL and TOBACCO	
Avoid alcohol.	Alcohol interferes with amphetamine's effect.
No problems reported with tobacco.	
PREGNANCY	
Avoid drug.	Drug has caused fetal abnormalities in animal experiments. No studies in humans.
BREAST-FEEDING	
Avoid drug or avoid nursing.	Medication will migrate into breast milk. Discuss with your doctor.

(continued)

AGE FACTOR

1. Give to children cautiously.

2. No specific reports on effects on older people, but people over 60 should use cautiously.

1. Prolonged use in children has been linked to physical and mental development problems.

2. Adults over 60 are more prone to side effects.

MISSED DOSAGE

If you are taking a short-lasting formulation, you can take a missed dose up to two hours after scheduled time. Otherwise, wait for next dose but do not double the amount taken.

If you are taking one dose a day, take the next one as soon as you remember. Wait 20 hours before taking yet another dose, then return to schedule. Do not double doses.

OVERDOSE

Get emergency medical help immediately if patient falls into coma or convulsions, if person expresses thoughts of committing suicide or killing someone else, or if there is high fever or excessive activity.

STOPPING DRUG

Do not stop taking even if you feel better until you have talked with your doctor. You may have to come off drug slowly.

OTHERS

Do not drive or operate machinery until you have determined how medication affects you.

Children taking this medication should have periodic examinations to determine effect on development.

drug or category:

METHYLPHENIDATE

condition:

HYPERACTIVITY IN CHILDREN; ALSO USED FOR UNCONTROLLED SLEEPINESS (NARCOLEPSY)

warning

Tell your doctor if you have or have had
- an allergic reaction to this medication, or to preservatives or food additives
- problems with alcohol or drugs
- seizure disorders, Tourette's syndrome or other tic disorders
- glaucoma or high blood pressure
- severe mental or emotional problems

drugs

GENERIC	BRAND	RX
methylphenidate	*Ritalin*	Yes

form/usage

TABLETS, INCLUDING EXTENDED-RELEASE FORM: Should be taken on an empty stomach, but may be taken with food or beverage to lessen risk of stomach irritation.

Regular tablets may be crushed.

when

Should be taken 30–45 minutes before meals. To avoid insomnia, avoid using after 6 P.M.

side effects and adverse reactions

Skin reactions, irregular or fast heart rhythm, pain in joints, psychotic incidents, vision problems

Fatigue, mood changes, inability to sleep, nervousness, mild headaches, stomach pain

what to do

Stop taking. Get in touch with doctor immediately.

Continue taking, but discuss with your physician.

(continued)

special precautions	because
DRUG INTERACTIONS	
I. Anticholinergics, anticoagulants, anticonvulsants, tricyclic antidepressants, oxyphenbutazone, phenylbutazone	I. Methylphenidate will increase their effect.
2. Acebutolol, high blood pressure medications, central nervous system depressants, guanadrel, guanethidine, minoxidil, nitrates, oxprenolol, terazosin	2. Their effect will be decreased.
3. MAO inhibitors	3. May cause sharp and dangerous rise in blood pressure.
DIET	
Avoid or be careful with foods that contain tyramine.	May cause increase in blood pressure.
ALCOHOL and TOBACCO	
No interactions reported for either.	
PREGNANCY	
Discuss with your doctor.	No studies done in animals or humans. Safety not established.
BREAST-FEEDING	
No problems reported.	
AGE FACTOR	
I. Use cautiously in children.	I. Children are especially likely to develop sleeping problems, stomach pain, and loss of weight. Prolonged use may also lead to physical development problems.
2. Adults over 60 years of age should use cautiously.	2. Increased likelihood of side effects.
MISSED DOSE	
You can take a missed dose up to two hours after scheduled time. Otherwise, wait for next dose but do not double the amount taken.	

OVERDOSE
Get emergency medical help immediately if patient falls into a coma or has severe gastrointestinal problems, hallucinations, fever, or fast heartbeat.

STOPPING DRUG
Do not stop taking even if you feel better until you have talked with your doctor. You may have to come off drug slowly.

OTHERS
Periodic laboratory tests might be necessary to check blood counts.

-23-

ASTHMA AND ALLERGY DRUGS

ASTHMA AND ALLERGIES are exceedingly common disorders that may occur together or independently. Allergies are the more common of the two, afflicting 35 to 50 million Americans. For unknown reasons, the incidence of asthma and the number of deaths from it have risen steadily in the last two decades. Although the precise number of Americans who have asthma is debated, the National Institute of Allergy and Infectious Diseases puts the figure at more than 15 million, an increase of 60 percent since 1980. An additional 40 million have inactive asthma, which can flare up given the right circumstances.

Asthma

Doctors once thought asthma was largely a psychosomatic disease triggered by anxiety or stress. In reality, asthma reflects hypersensitive lungs, and many attacks are set off by an allergic reaction to dust, pollens, foods, animals, and other allergens. Sensitivity to drugs like aspirin can bring on asthma attacks, as can exercise, cold air, infections, tobacco smoke, and stress. Whatever the trigger, the result is that the bronchial tubes tighten, narrowing the air passages.

During an asthma attack, the bronchial tubes also become inflamed, leading to increased production of mucus. The result is increasingly labored breathing. Left untreated—or treated too late—an asthma attack can be fatal. In fact, asthma claims more than 4,000 lives a year, and Americans now spend more than $6 billion a year for drugs to prevent or treat asthma attacks. The most commonly used asthma medications are:

- **Xanthine bronchodilators.** This class of drugs, which includes aminophylline, oxtriphylline, and theophylline (*Theo-Dur, Slo-Bid*), blocks production of an enzyme known as phosphodiesterase. When the enzyme is inhibited, tissues in the bronchial tube increase their production of adenosine monophosphate, or AMP. AMP helps relax the muscles of the bronchial tubes and blood vessels, increasing air flow in and out of the lungs. The xanthine bronchodilators can be taken as oral solutions, tablets, or enemas.

- **Adrenergic bronchodilators.** These drugs, which include albuterol (*Proventil, Ventolin*), metaproterenol (*Alupent*), also increase the production of adenosine monophosphate, relaxing the muscles controlling the bronchial tubes and alleviating lung congestion. These drugs are taken as aerosols or in capsules, syrups, and tablets. Ipratropium (*Atrovent*) is sometimes used to treat asthma, but is more commonly prescribed for bronchitis and emphysema.

• **Corticosteroids.** Steroids used to treat asthma include beclomethasone (*Beconase, Vancenase*), flunisolide (*Nasalide, Aerobid*), and triamcinolone (*Azmacort, Aristocort*). They counter inflammation and shrink swollen membranes. They are most often dispensed as aerosols, but some are also administered by injection or taken orally.

• **Cromolyn sodium** (*Intal*). This drug is a type of nonsteroidal anti-inflammatory medication that is used to prevent attacks by reducing inflammation in the bronchial tubes. It is taken as an inhalant or in capsule form.

None of these drugs cures asthma, but they go a long way toward mitigating the impact of the disease. The bronchodilators stop an asthma attack, and other medications, like cromolyn sodium, are used to prevent them. Still others, such as corticosteroids, are used both to treat attacks and to prevent frequently recurring flare-ups. Unfortunately, most have troublesome side effects, inducing facial flushing, nervousness, anxiety, insomnia, and palpitations. The inhaled corticosteroids have fewer side effects than their oral counterparts, but prolonged use of either can result in lowered resistance to infection, weight gain, mood swings, bleeding problems, bone thinning, and childhood growth problems.

Improper use of asthma medications has been identified as a factor contributing to the rising asthma death rate. According to some experts, up to half of the people who use inhalers do so incorrectly, thus allowing their asthma to worsen. If you or your child takes asthma medications, ask

your doctor to demonstrate how to use them step by step. This may include using a nebulizer, a tube that mists the drug and allows it to penetrate more deeply into the lungs.

If you have moderate to severe asthma, seek out medical care from an asthma specialist and follow your regimen faithfully, especially if it calls for an anti-inflammatory medication as a preventive medication.

Allergies

An allergic reaction comes about because the immune system inappropriately goes into action against a harmless substance such as pollen, animal dander, dust, certain foods, and drugs. To battle the perceived enemy, the immune system produces antibodies programmed to whenever the foreign substance enters the body. As part of this allergic reaction, certain tissues release histamines, which cause varied reactions throughout the body—nasal congestion, sneezing, runny eyes, itchiness, hives, even life-threatening anaphylaxis.

There are more than 35 generic variations and more than 200 brand name products to treat allergies. These medications fall into these general categories:

• **Antihistamines,** such as brompheniramine (*Bromfed*), chlorpheniramine (*Chlor-Trimeton*), dimenhydrinate (*Dramamine*), and diphenhydramine (*Benadryl*), among others, which counter the action of histamines. They work by blocking the histamine's access to their receptors on specific cells. Antihistamines, which are available both over the counter and as prescription drugs, can be taken as tablets, capsules, inhalants, syrups, elixirs, injections, and suppositories. Some are combined with decongestants such as phen-

ylephrine (*Codimal DH*), phenylpropanolamine (*Dimetane DH*), and pseudoephedrine (*Sudafed*).

- **Steroid nasal sprays.** These adrenocorticoid medications (*Beconase, Vancenase*) work directly and effectively on inflamed nasal tissues, but they are expensive and take several days to work.

- **Decongestants.** Medications such as oxymetazoline (*Afrin, Dristan,* and others) are widely used to ease the stuffiness of hay fever and colds.

Many antihistamines cause drowsiness and lethargy, although some of the newer prescription drugs have nondrowsy formulas. Others increase sensitivity to the sun, and some people who take them develop sore throats and other adverse effects. Nasal steroids have fewer serious side effects than oral medications, but they can irritate nasal tissues.

Desensitization with injections of small amounts of the offending allergens represents an alternative to drug therapy. The injections, which are usually given weekly for months or even years, gradually increase the body's resistance to the allergens. They must be given in an allergist's office, clinic, or other medical setting; thus, desensitization is a lengthy, costly process that doesn't always work.

drug or category:

ADRENOCORTICOIDS FOR ALLERGIES

condition:
NOSE DISCOMFORT AND STUFFINESS

warning

Tell your doctor if you have or have had:
• an allergic reaction to this medication, or to any preservatives or foods
• glaucoma
• herpes eye infection or other infections
• a recent nose injury or sores
• liver or thyroid disease, or tuberculosis
Tell your doctor if you have had surgery recently or are planning to have an operation.

drugs

GENERIC	BRAND	RX
beclomethasone	*Beconase, Vancenase*	Yes

form/usage

AEROSOL, SPRAY: Follow instructions with medicine carefully, or ask your doctor or pharmacist for directions.

when

As recommended by your physician.

side effects and adverse reactions

Pain in eyes, wheezing or other breathing difficulties

Nose problems including bleeding, sores, discharge, crusting; headache; nausea; white patches in throat or nose

Sneezing, dry nose

what to do

Get emergency medical help immediately.

Stop taking. Get in touch with doctor immediately.

Continue taking, but discuss with your physician.

special precautions

DRUG INTERACTIONS
No interactions reported.

because

(continued)

DIET
No interactions reported.

ALCOHOL and TOBACCO
No interactions reported.

PREGNANCY
Discuss with your doctor.

Drug has caused fetal abnormalities in animal experiments. While it may not cause defects in the human fetus, it may affect developing baby's growth and its adrenal gland development.

BREAST-FEEDING
Discuss with your doctor.

While there have been no reports of problems in infants, it is unknown whether drug is excreted in human milk.

AGE FACTOR
1. Nasally inhaled adrenocorticoids generally are considered safer for children and may allow cutback or ending of doses needed to control hay fever symptoms.

2. No special problems expected in people over 60 years of age.

MISSED DOSE
You can take a missed dose up to an hour after scheduled time. Otherwise, wait for next dose but do not double the amount taken.

OVERDOSE
No overdose problems expected.

STOPPING DRUG
You can discontinue when problem ends.

OTHERS

Do not drive or operate machinery until you have determined how medication affects you.

A brief gargle or mouth rinse with plain water after each inhaler administration may reduce the incidence of thrush infections in the mouth.

ADRENERGIC BRONCHODILATORS

ASTHMA, CHRONIC BRONCHITIS, EMPHYSEMA, AND OTHER LUNG DISEASES

warning

Tell your doctor if you have or have had:
- an allergic reaction to this medication or to any preservatives or foods
- brain damage, seizures, or Parkinson's disease
- diabetes, cardiovascular or thyroid disease
- high blood pressure or mental illness

Tell your doctor if you have:
- taken an MAO inhibitor or digitalis recently
- scheduled any kind of surgery

drugs

GENERIC	BRAND	RX
albuterol	*Proventil, Ventolin*	Yes
metaproterenol	*Alupent*	
terbutaline	*Brethine*	

form/usage

TABLETS (INCLUDING EXTENDED-RELEASE), SYRUP, ORAL SOLUTIONS, INJECTIONS, INHALERS, AEROSOLS: Extended-release tablets must be taken whole, without chewing or crushing.

Take other formulations according to instructions with medication.

when

When needed. Do not take more than four times a day.

side effects and adverse reactions

Cramps, chest pain or changes in heart rhythm, hallucinations

Minor gastrointestinal problems, urination difficulty, inability to sleep, excitability, rapid heartbeat, dilated pupils, coughing

what to do

Stop taking. Get in touch with doctor immediately.

Continue taking, but discuss with your physician.

special precautions	because
DRUG INTERACTIONS	
1. Tricyclic antidepressants, epinephrine, MAO inhibitors, pseudoephedrine, thyroid medications	1. Increase effect of albuterol.
2. Hypertension medications, beta-blockers, guanadrel, guanethidine, nitrates, rauwolfia, terazosin	2. Decrease effect of albuterol, other medicine, or both.
3. Digitalis	3. Causes heart rhythm changes.
4. Migraine medications, uterine contraction medications, furazolidone, methyldopa	4. Cause dangerous increase in blood pressure.
5. Phenothiazines	5. Increase toxic potential of albuterol.
6. Theophylline	6. Irritates stomach.
DIET No interactions reported.	
ALCOHOL and TOBACCO No interactions reported.	
PREGNANCY Avoid drug.	Drug has caused fetal abnormalities in animal experiments.
BREAST-FEEDING No problems reported, but it may be wise to discuss with your doctor.	
AGE FACTOR 1. No problems expected in children.	
2. Adults over 60 should use cautiously.	2. Older adults may be especially likely to have blood pressure and heart rhythm problems or to have angina.

MISSED DOSE
You can take a missed dose up to two hours after scheduled time. Otherwise, wait for next dose but do not double the amount taken.

(continued)

OVERDOSE

Get emergency medical help immediately if patient has irregular and fast pulse, is confused or delirious, or is showing extreme anxiety.

STOPPING DRUG

Discuss with your doctor.

OTHERS

Do not drive or operate machinery until you have determined how medication affects you.

Periodic tests might be necessary to check effect on your heart, internal eye pressures, and blood pressure.

ANTIHISTAMINES

ALLERGIES

warning

Do not take in the midst of an asthma attack.

Tell your doctor if you have or have had:

- an allergic reaction to this medication, or to any preservatives or foods
- glaucoma
- prostate or other urogenital problems

Tell your doctor if you are taking medications for stomach or muscle spasms (anticholinergics), any central nervous system depressants, or any MAO inhibitors.

drugs

GENERIC	BRAND	RX
astemizole	*Hismanal*	some
brompheniramine	*Bromfed*	
clemastine	*Tavist*	
chlorpheniramine	*Chlor-Trimeton,* others	
dimenhydrinate	*Dramamine*	
diphenhydramine	*Benadryl,* others	
terfenadine	*Seldane*	
others		

form/usage

ORAL SUSPENSIONS, TABLETS (EXTENDED-RELEASE AND REG-ULAR), SYRUPS, CAPSULES (EXTENDED-RELEASE AND REGU-LAR), PEDIATRIC ELIXIR: Most can be taken with food or beverage to avoid irritation to the stomach. However, astemizole should be taken on an empty stomach, an hour or two before eating.

Extended-release capsules or tablets must be taken whole.

when

As directed by your doctor or instructions with medication.

(continued)

side effects and adverse reactions

Severe agitation; sleeping problems, including nightmares; palpitations; fatigue; unexplained bleeding; vision changes; skin symptoms

Decreased appetite, contact lens irritation, urination problems, dry mouth, nausea

what to do

Stop taking. Get in touch with doctor immediately.

Continue taking, but discuss with your physician.

special precautions

DRUG INTERACTIONS
1. Anticholinergics, dronabinol
2. Oral anticoagulants, carteolol
3. MAO inhibitors, molindone, sotalol
4. Antidepressants, other antihistamines, sleep medications, medications containing narcotics, pro-carbazine, sedatives, tranquilizers
5. Dronabinol, nabilone

DIET
No interactions reported.

ALCOHOL and TOBACCO
Avoid alcohol.
No problems reported with tobacco.

PREGNANCY
Discuss with your doctor.

BREAST-FEEDING
Avoid drugs or avoid nursing.

because

1. Their effect is increased.
2. Decrease effect of antihistamines.
3. Increase effect of antihistamines.
4. Cause an increased sedative effect.

5. Possible central nervous system toxicity.

Alcohol cause increased drowsiness.

Some antihistamines have caused fetal abnormalities in animal experiments.

Medication will migrate into breast milk and could cause irritability and other problems in baby.

AGE FACTOR

1. Give to children cautiously.

2. People over 60 should use cautiously.

1. Children are more likely to have side effects, including seizures, irritability, and other behavioral problems.

2. Adverse and side effects may be worse in older people, including urinary retention, drowsiness, confusion, restlessness, and irritability.

MISSED DOSAGE

You can take a missed dose up to two hours after scheduled time. Otherwise, wait for next dose but do not double the amount taken.

OVERDOSE

Get emergency medical help immediately if patient falls into coma, or has hallucinations or convulsions.

STOPPING DRUG

Discontinue when problem stops.

OTHERS

Do not drive or operate machinery until you have determined how medication affects you.

drug or category:

CROMOLYN SODIUM

condition:

ASTHMA, INCLUDING EXERCISE-INDUCED ASTHMA—FOR PREVENTION

warning

Tell your doctor if you have or have had:
• an allergic reaction to this medication, or to any preservatives or foods, particularly milk or milk products (some formulations include lactose)
• kidney, liver, or heart disease

drugs

GENERIC	BRAND	RX
cromolyn	*Intal*	Yes

form/usage

INHALATION CAPSULES, AEROSOL, SOLUTION: Read instructions or follow your doctor's recommendations.

when

Every day as prescribed by your doctor.

Do not use to treat an asthma attack that has already started.

side effects and adverse reactions

Severe allergic reaction (anaphylactic shock), including skin reactions, fainting

Severe gastrointestinal problems, skin reactions, wheezing

Sedation, headache, inability to sleep, cough

what to do

Get emergency medical help immediately.

Stop taking. Get in touch with doctor immediately.

Continue taking, but discuss with your physician.

special precautions

DRUG INTERACTIONS
1. Cortisone drugs.

because

1. Cromolyn may increase the effects of cortisone, making it more difficult to reduce dosage or stop cortisone.

DRUG INTERACTIONS

2. Ipratropium

2. Increases effect of cromolyn.

DIET

No interactions reported.

ALCOHOL and TOBACCO

No reactions reported.

PREGNANCY

Avoid drug.

Drug has caused fetal problems in animal experiments.

BREAST-FEEDING

No problems reported.

AGE FACTOR

Both children and adults over 60 should use with caution.

Possible increased risk of side effects.

MISSED DOSE

Take when you remember, then space next dose according to recommended schedule. Do not double next dose.

OVERDOSE

No overdose problems are likely to occur.

STOPPING DRUG

Discuss with your doctor before discontinuing cromolyn or discontinuing other antiasthma drugs because cromolyn has been effective.

OTHERS

If you are on a bronchodilator, use it at least five minutes before the cromolyn. This will allow the dilator to relax the bronchial tubes and will make inhalation of the cromolyn more effective, because cromolyn will penetrate deeper into the respiratory system.

drug or category:

IPRATROPIUM

condition:
CHRONIC BRONCHITIS, EMPHYSEMA, ASTHMA

warning

Tell your doctor if you have or have had:
• an allergic reaction to this medication, other inhaled medications, or antinausea or antispasm medications, or to any preservatives or foods
• prostate or urination problems
• glaucoma

drugs

GENERIC	BRAND	RX
ipratropium	*Atrovent*	Yes

form/usage

INHALATION AEROSOL AND SOLUTION: Follow your doctor's or pharmacist's instructions.

Do not use drug by itself to alleviate asthma attack. Do not depend on this drug to prevent exercise-induced asthma.

when

According to your doctor's instructions.

side effects and adverse reactions

Pounding heart, skin reactions, sores in and around mouth

Vision problems, inability to sleep, coughing, dizziness, excitability, shaking

what to do

Stop taking. Get in touch with doctor immediately.

Continue taking, but discuss with your physician.

special precautions

DRUG INTERACTIONS
1. Cromolyn

because

1. Decreased effectiveness of cromolyn and ipratropium. Use five minutes apart.

DRUG INTERACTIONS

2. Other inhaled medications

2. Decreased effectiveness of both drugs. Use five minutes apart.

DIET

No interactions reported.

ALCOHOL and TOBACCO

No interactions reported with either.

PREGNANCY

Avoid drug.

Drug has caused fetal abnormalities in animal experiments. No human studies are available.

BREAST-FEEDING

No problems reported, but discuss with your doctor.

It is unknown whether drug is excreted in human breast milk.

AGE FACTOR

1. Use with caution in children.

1. Safety and effectiveness for children under 12 have not been established.

2. Adults over 60 should use with caution.

2. Side effects may be worse in all older adults; however, older men should be alert for signs of prostate problems as a result of taking this medication.

MISSED DOSE

You can take a missed dose up to two hours after scheduled time. Otherwise, wait for next dose but do not double the amount taken.

OVERDOSE

Overdose problems are unlikely.

STOPPING DRUG

No problems expected if you stop before your prescription runs out.

OTHERS

Do not drive or operate machinery until you have determined how medication affects you.

Periodic measurements of internal eye pressures may be necessary.

drug or category:

OXYMETAZOLINE

condition:

NASAL CONGESTION CAUSED BY HAY FEVER, COLDS, SINUS PROBLEMS

warning

Tell your doctor if you have or have had:
- an allergic reaction to this medication or any other nasal decongestant, or to preservatives or food additives
- diabetes, cardiovascular disease, thyroid problems

drugs

GENERIC	BRAND	RX
oxymetazoline	*Afrin, Dristan, Vicks, Sinex Long-Acting,* others	No

form/usage

DROPS: Follow label instructions.

when

As needed. Do not take more than four times a day.

side effects and adverse reactions

Headache, inability to sleep, runny or dry nose, increased sneezing, pounding heart

what to do

Continue taking, but discuss with your physician.

special precautions

DRUG INTERACTIONS

1. Tricyclic antidepressants, sympathomimetics

2. Phenothiazines

3. Beta-blockers, guanadrel, minoxidil, nitrates, rauwolfia, terazosin

4. MAO inhibitors, methyldopa

because

1. May increase oxymetazoline's effects.

2. May decrease effect of oxymetazoline or increase its toxic effects.

3. Decrease effects of either or both drugs.

4. Increase blood pressure.

DIET

Avoid caffeine drinks.

--   --

ALCOHOL and TOBACCO

No interactions reported.

--   --

PREGNANCY

No negative interactions reported.

--   --

BREAST-FEEDING

No problems reported.

--   --

AGE FACTOR

1. Should not be given to children without consulting doctor.

2. People over 60 should use cautiously.

1. Safety and effectiveness have not been established. Also, redness in eyes may be a sign of illness, not just irritation.

2. Adverse and side effects may be worse in older people.

--   --

MISSED DOSE

Take when you remember, then take next dose four hours later. Do not double dose.

OVERDOSE

Get emergency medical help immediately if you have headaches, unexplained sweating, extreme agitation and anxiety, or an irregular heartbeat.

STOPPING DRUG

No need to continue with prescription if symptoms disappear, but check with your doctor. Some inhalants may cause rebound symptoms.

PSEUDOEPHEDRINE

NASAL OR SINUS CONGESTION

warning

Tell your doctor if you have or have had:
- an allergic reaction to this medication, or to any preservatives or foods
- diabetes, a prostate or thyroid problem, cardiovascular disease, or high blood pressure

drugs

GENERIC	BRAND	RX
pseudoephedrine	*Sudafed*	Some

form/usage

CAPSULES AND TABLETS (INCLUDING EXTENDED-RELEASE), SOLUTION, SYRUPS: Extended-release capsule contents may be mixed into a food that can be swallowed without chewing (jelly, for example).

Extended-release tablets must be taken whole and should not be crushed or crumbled.

when

As directed on package or according to your doctor's instructions. Take last dose for the day at least five to six hours before retiring, as drug may interfere with ability to sleep.

side effects and adverse reactions

Gastrointestinal problems, changes in heart rhythm, pounding heart, sweating

Shaking, nervousness

what to do

Stop taking. Get in touch with doctor immediately.

Continue taking, but discuss with your physician.

special precautions

DRUG INTERACTIONS
1. High blood pressure medications, beta-blockers, guanadrel, guanethidine, nitrates, rauwolfia, terazosin

because

1. Effect of pseudoephedrine, other drug, or both will be decreased.

DRUG INTERACTIONS

2. Calcium supplements, MAO inhibitors, sympathomimetics

3. Epinephrine, migraine headache medications, methyldopa

4. Digitalis

2. Will increase effect of pseudoephedrine.

3. Will increase blood pressure, perhaps seriously. Some may also increase heart rate.

4. May cause heart rhythm disturbances.

DIET
Avoid caffeine.

Will increase nervousness, anxiety.

ALCOHOL and TOBACCO
No interactions reported.

PREGNANCY
Discuss with your doctor.

Drug has not caused fetal abnormalities in animal experiments, but has caused decreases in weight and size of offspring.

BREAST-FEEDING
Avoid drug or avoid nursing.

Medication will migrate into breast milk and could affect child. Discuss with your doctor.

AGE FACTOR
1. Infants and children should be given this drug in low doses, if at all.

2. People over 60 should use cautiously.

1. Increased risk of side effects.

2. Adverse and side effects may be worse in older people.

MISSED DOSE
You can take a missed dose up to two hours after scheduled time. Otherwise, wait for next dose but do not double the amount taken.

OVERDOSE
Get emergency medical help immediately if patient has convulsions or hallucinations, or is delirious or shaking, vomits, or has heartbeat changes.

(continued)

STOPPING DRUG

You can stop taking when symptoms disappear. Discuss with your doctor.

OTHERS

Do not drive or operate machinery until you have determined how medication affects you.

drug or category:

STEROID INHALERS (ADRENOCORTICOIDS OR CORTICOSTEROIDS)

condition:
ASTHMA

warning

Tell your doctor if you have or have had:

- an allergic reaction to this medication, or to any preservatives or foods
- any respiratory illnesses (including lung problems) other than asthma
- mouth, lung, or throat infections

If your doctor prescribes *Azmacort*, tell him or her if you have or have had:

- bone disease, diabetes, high blood pressure, or cardiovascular illness
- ulcers or herpes or fungus infections
- kidney or liver disease
- thryoid problems
- tuberculosis
- myasthenia gravis, cholesterol problems, or glaucoma

Any doctor or dentist you consult should be told that you are taking this medication. You should give this information for up to two years after you stop taking this drug.

drugs

GENERIC	BRAND	RX
beclomethasone	*Beclovent, Vanceril*, others	Yes
flunisolide	*Nasalide*	
triamcinolone	*Azmacort*	

form/usage

AEROSOL, CAPSULES: Ask your doctor or pharmacist to demonstrate how to use inhalers.

when

Use as directed by your physician.

(continued)

side effects and adverse reactions

Increase in asthma symptoms, lung inflammation

Skin problems, mouth and throat discomfort

what to do

Stop taking. Get in touch with doctor immediately.

Continue taking, but discuss with your physician.

special precautions

because

DRUG INTERACTIONS
Other bronchodilators, including albuterol, amino-phylline, bitolterol, ephedrine, epinephrine, isoethar-ine, isoproterenol, pirbuterol, terbutaline, and theophylline

Will increase effects of triamcinolone, flunisolide, and beclomethasone.

DIET
No interactions reported.

ALCOHOL and TOBACCO
Avoid both.

Alcohol may increase risk of ulcers.

Tobacco may increase effect of triamcinolone and may increase danger of drug poisoning.

PREGNANCY
Avoid drug.

Adrenocorticoids taken by mouth or injection have caused fetal abnormalities in animal experiments. While they may not cause defects in a human fetus, they may affect developing baby's growth and its adrenal gland development.

BREAST-FEEDING
No problems reported, but discuss with your doctor.

It is not known whether drug(s) will migrate into breast milk.

AGE FACTOR

1. Inhaled adrenocorticoids generally are considered safer for children and may allow cutback or ending of medication needed to control hay fever symptoms.

2. In adults over 60 effects are not likely to differ from those experienced by younger adults.

MISSED DOSAGE

Triamcinolone

If you are taking several doses a day, you can take a missed dose up to two hours after scheduled time. Otherwise, wait for next dose but do not double the amount taken.

If you are taking medication once a day, wait for next dose and *double the dose taken.*

Flunisolide

If you missed a dose, take it up to two hours later. Otherwise, wait for next scheduled dose, but do not double dose.

Beclomethasone

You can take a missed dose up to two hours after scheduled time. Otherwise, wait for next dose but do not double the amount taken.

OVERDOSE

Overdose is unlikely.

STOPPING DRUG

Do not stop taking even if you feel better until you have talked with your doctor.

OTHERS

If you are taking beclomethasone you may have to have periodic checks to guard against mouth fungal infections. A brief gargle or mouth rinse with plain water may reduce the incidence of fungal infections in the mouth. You should have periodic X-ray exams if you have had tuberculosis.

drug or category:

THEOPHYLLINE

condition:
ASTHMA

warning

Tell your doctor if you have or have had:
• an allergic reaction to this or similar medication, aminophylline, dyphylline or oxtriphylline, or to any preservatives or foods
• a seizure disorder or ulcers
• high blood pressure, heart disease, or heart rhythm problems
Tell your doctor if you are scheduled for surgery.

drugs

GENERIC	BRAND	RX
theophylline	*Theo-Dur, Slo-Bid,* others	Yes

form/usage

CAPSULES AND TABLETS (INCLUDING EXTENDED-RELEASE), ELIXIR, ORAL SOLUTION, AND SUSPENSION: Should be taken on an empty stomach, but may be taken with food to prevent or reduce stomach irritation.

Regular capsules may be opened and regular tablets may be crushed or crumbled, but extended-release formulations should be taken whole.

Oral suspension should be shaken well.

Liquid formulations should not be refrigerated.

when

Dosage and schedule must be set by your physician according to your individual needs.

side effects and adverse reactions

Gastrointestinal bleeding, fall in blood pressure, heart rhythm changes, behavioral changes

Minor gastrointestinal problems, appetite loss, fatigue, shaking, inability to sleep

what to do

Get emergency medical help immediately.

Continue taking, but discuss with your physician.

special precautions

because

DRUG INTERACTIONS
1. Lithium

2. General anesthetics

3. Phenytoin

4. Allopurinol, cimetidine, ciprofloxacin, disulfiram, erythromycin, mexiletine, norfloxacin, oral contraceptives, ranitidine, ticlopidine, troleandomycin

5. Barbiturates, beta-blockers, carbamazepine, primidone, rifampin

1. Effectiveness of lithium will be decreased.

2. May cause heart rhythm disturbances.

3. Decreases effectiveness of both drugs.

4. Will increase effect of theophylline.

5. Will decrease effect of theophylline.

DIET
Avoid caffeine drinks.

Will cause insomnia and nervousness.

ALCOHOL and TOBACCO
Avoid both.

Alcohol may cause stomach irritation.

Tobacco may interfere with effectiveness of drug.

PREGNANCY
Avoid drug, particularly in first three months.

Drug has caused fetal abnormalities in animal experiments, though there have been no reports of fetal problems in the very limited number of cases of pregnant women who have taken this medication.

BREAST-FEEDING
Avoid drug or avoid nursing.

Medication will migrate into breast milk and could affect child. Discuss with your doctor.

AGE FACTOR
1. Monitor children carefully. Children on this medication should have periodic laboratory tests.

2. People over 60 should use cautiously.

1. Excessive amounts can cause seizures and heart rhythm disturbances. You should also monitor child for irritation, agitation, and other behavioral problems that may be caused by the drug.

2. Adverse and side effects, including gastrointestinal problems, may be worse in older people.

(continued)

MISSED DOSE

You can take a missed dose up to two hours after scheduled time. Otherwise, wait for next dose but do not double the amount taken.

OVERDOSE

Get emergency medical help immediately if patient is in coma or has seizures, heart rhythm abnormalities, muscle twitching, or bloody stool.

STOPPING DRUG

Discuss with your doctor. Phase out use over several days.

OTHERS

Do not drive or operate machinery until you have determined how medication affects you.

Periodic laboratory tests might be necessary to check effect on some body functions, including sugar levels.

Blood pressure and heart rate may need to be checked regularly.

chapter

-24-

BLOOD MODIFIERS

Cholesterol-Lowering Drugs

Over the last quarter of a century or so, the American people have participated in what may well be one of the largest, most extensive public health experiments of all time. Heeding the warnings of heart disease specialists, nutritionists, and others that a diet high in cholesterol and fats could increase the risk of heart disease, heart attacks, strokes, and other cardiovascular disasters, millions of Americans have cut back on meat, choosing low-fat or nonfat dairy products, reducing consumption of fried foods, and increasing fiber intake. As a result, between 1976 and 1991, the number of adults who had serum cholesterol levels of 240 milligrams or more—levels considered to increase the risk of heart attacks—dropped by almost 25 percent. And the number of adults whose cholesterol levels dropped below 200—the point at which the risk of heart attack drops precipitously—grew by almost 10 percent.

Some heart researchers still question whether there is a direct correlation between blood cholesterol levels and heart disease. Nevertheless, most public health specialists maintain that reducing blood cholesterol levels—along with regular exercise, control of high blood pressure, and cessation of cigarette smoking—has had a significant impact on heart disease in the United States. And there is statistical evidence that this is true; between 1972 and 1990, the heart attack mortality fell by 50 percent while the death rate from strokes fell by nearly 57 percent.

Cholesterol, of course, is essential to carry out a vast array of vital functions, including maintaining cell walls and manufacturing hormones. There are also different types of cholesterol, depending on the weight of the protein that carries it through the bloodstream. Thus, low-density lipoproteins, or LDL cholesterol, are considered detrimental because they tend to collect in the arteries, leading to the buildup of fatty plaque, or atherosclerosis. Conversely, high-density lipoproteins, or HDL cholesterol, are beneficial because they gravitate away from the artery walls. So, while total cholesterol readings are important, the ratio of LDL to HDL cholesterol is perhaps even more indicative of risk. In other words, high levels of LDL cholesterol increase the risk of heart disease, whereas high HDL cholesterol levels lower it. Increased physical activity raises the HDL cholesterol level, and a low-fat, low-calorie diet can lower total cholesterol.

Unfortunately, for an estimated 13 million Americans, these measures are inadequate; for them, drugs that lower cholesterol (and triglycerides—another fatty substance linked to heart disease), along with life-style changes, are the answer. Categories of these drugs include:

- **Drugs that reduce the body's manufacture of cholesterol.** These agents include the HMG-CoA reductase inhibitors, which block an enzyme in the liver that the body needs to make cholesterol. The drugs—lovastatin (*Mevacor*), pravastatin (*Pravachol*), and simvastatin (*Zocor*)—are taken orally in tablet form. High doses of niacin (*Endur-Acin, Niac, Nicobid*), also known as nicotinic acid or vitamin B_3, also inhibit the production of cholesterol and lipoproteins. Although high-dose niacin is available without prescription, its use should be monitored by a doctor because it can alter liver function and also raise blood glucose levels.

    Other drugs such as clofibrate (*Atromid-S*), gemfibrozil (*Lopid*), and probucol (*Lorelco*), work in the liver to inhibit the production of cholesterol.

- **Drugs that increase the body's elimination of cholesterol.** Some of these drugs—cholestyramine (*Questran*) and colestipol (*Colestid*)—act on bile salts, which contain large amounts of cholesterol that finds its way back into the bloodstream. These drugs lower cholesterol by attaching to bile salts and carrying them out of the body. Because of the increased secretion of bile, the liver uses up cholesterol to make more bile acids and salts, further lowering the amount of cholesterol in the bloodstream. Because the drugs are not absorbed into the bloodstream from the in-

testinal tract, they have few side effects, although they can cause constipation and nausea and also interfere with absorption of fat-soluble vitamins.

Anticoagulants

Though anticoagulants are often referred to as blood thinners, they do not dilute the blood; instead, they alter its chemistry to reduce its propensity to form clots. Blood clots, although essential to stop bleeding from a cut, are a major hazard when they travel through the bloodstream. A clot lodged in a coronary artery—coronary thrombosis—can cause a heart attack. In the brain, a clot (cerebral thrombosis) can result in a stroke; in the lung, it is a life-threatening pulmonary embolism. And a clot blocking a vein—usually in the leg—can lead to thrombophlebitis.

Although anticoagulants do not dissolve existing clots, they can prevent new clots from forming. One group of anticoagulants—dicumarol, heparin, and warfarin (*Panwarfin, Sofarin, Coumadin*)—interferes with the metabolism of vitamin K, which is instrumental in making clotting factors. Antiplatelet drugs—such as aspirin (see Chapter 14), dipyridamole (*Dipridacot, Persantine*), and sulfinpyrazone (*Anturane*) (see Chapter 16)—block enzymes that prompt blood platelets to form clots.

Thrombolytic agents, streptokinase (*Kabikinase, Streptase*), and tissue plasminogen activator, or TPA (*Activase*), work by breaking up, or dissolving, clots. These drugs are now used to short-circuit heart attacks and strokes.

---

drug or category:

CHOLESTYRAMINE

condition:
EXCESS BILE ACIDS

---

warning

Tell your doctor if you have or have had:
- an allergic reaction to this medication or to preservatives or food additives
- bleeding disorders, constipation, hemorrhoids, or gallstones
- cardiovascular disease
- ulcers
- thyroid problems, kidney disease, or phenylketonuria

Tell your doctor if you are using anticoagulants, digitalis, diuretics, penicillin, phenylbutazone, propranolol, tetracyclines, or thyroid medications.

---

drugs

GENERIC	BRAND	RX
cholestyramine	*Questran*, others	Yes

---

form/usage

CHEWABLE BAR, POWDER: Powder should never be taken dry. Add to 2 ounces of liquid and mix. Add another 2 to 4 ounces of liquid, mix and drink. When finished, add more liquid to the glass and drink. Any beverage, including milk and fruit juices, can be used for dissolving powder.

Bar should be chewed thoroughly before swallowing.

when

Three to four times a day, one hour before or two hours after meals.

Other medicines should be taken at least one hour before or four to six hours after cholestyramine.

---

side effects and adverse reactions

Skin reactions, gastrointestinal problems, weight gain, blood in urine or stool

Mild gastrointestinal problems, sore tongue

what to do

Stop taking. Get in touch with doctor immediately.

Continue taking, but discuss with your physician.

(continued)

special precautions	because
DRUG INTERACTIONS	
1. Anticoagulants	1. Increases anticoagulant effect.
2. Dextrothyroxine, digitalis, indapamide, thyroid drugs, ursodiol	2. May decrease their absorption into the body and/or effect.
3. Thiazides, trimethoprim	3. Decrease absorption of cholestyramine.
4. Vancomycin	4. May cause hearing loss, kidney damage, decreased effect of vancomycin.

DIET
Ask your doctor about taking vitamin supplements.

Medication may interfere with vitamin absorption.

ALCOHOL and TOBACCO
No interactions reported.

PREGNANCY
No negative interactions reported.

BREAST-FEEDING
No problems reported.

AGE FACTOR

1. Not recommended for children.

1. Safety and effectiveness have not been established.

2. People over 60 should use cautiously.

2. Adverse and side effects may be worse in older people.

MISSED DOSE
You can take a missed dose up to two hours after scheduled time. Otherwise, wait for next dose but do not double the amount taken.

OVERDOSE
Get in touch with poison control center, emergency room, or doctor if you have blood in stool or severe stomach pain.

STOPPING DRUG
Do not stop taking until you have talked with your doctor.

OTHERS
Periodic laboratory tests for blood cholesterol, bleeding times, and red blood cell counts might be necessary to guard against development of anemia.

drug or category:

DIPYRIDAMOLE

condition:
BLOOD CLOT FORMATION

warning

Tell your doctor if you have or have had:
- an allergic reaction to this medication, or to preservatives or food additives
- hypotension

Tell your doctor if you are taking vasodilators.

drugs

GENERIC	BRAND	RX
dipyridamole	*Persantine, Dipridacot,* others	Yes

form/usage

TABLETS: Take with 8 ounces of water (full glass). May be taken with food to lessen stomach irritation.

when

One or two hours after eating.

side effects and adverse reactions

Angina, headache, fainting spells, severe gastrointestinal effects, skin symptoms

Dizziness

what to do

Stop taking. Get in touch with doctor immediately.

Continue taking, but discuss with your physician.

special precautions

DRUG INTERACTIONS
Anticoagulants, aspirin, and medications containing aspirin

because

May increase anticoagulant effect of medication.

DIET
No interactions reported.

ALCOHOL and TOBACCO
Avoid both.

Alcohol may lead to an excessive blood pressure drop.

Tobacco may decrease the effectiveness of the drug.

PREGNANCY
No negative interactions reported.

BREAST-FEEDING
No problems reported.

AGE FACTOR
1. Discuss with your doctor.

2. People over 60 years of age should begin treatment with small doses and gradually build up.

1. No information on effect in children.

2. Increased risk of side effects in older people.

MISSED DOSE
You can take a missed dose up to two hours after scheduled time. Otherwise, wait for next dose but do not double the amount taken.

OVERDOSE
Get emergency medical help immediately if patient is unconscious or has a severe drop in blood pressure and a weak and fast pulse.

STOPPING DRUG
Do not stop taking even if you feel better until you have finished prescription.

OTHERS
Do not drive or operate machinery until you have determined how medication affects you.

Periodic laboratory tests might be necessary to check blood functions.

drug or category:

GEMFIBROZIL

condition:

HIGH BLOOD CHOLESTEROL AND TRIGLYCERIDE LEVELS

warning

Tell your doctor if you have or have had:
- an allergic reaction to this medication, or to preservatives or food additives
- Severe liver or kidney problems or gallbladder disease

Tell your doctor if you are taking anticoagulant medications.

drugs

GENERIC	BRAND	RX
gemfibrozil	*Lopid*	Yes

form/usage

CAPSULES, TABLETS: May be taken with food or liquid to lessen risk of stomach irritation.

when

Usually taken twice a day, half an hour before breakfast and before dinner.

side effects and adverse reactions

Severe skin symptoms, swollen legs, painful or bloody urination, severe gastrointestinal effects

Headache, indigestion, dry skin, backache, muscle cramps, extreme fatigue

what to do

Stop taking. Get in touch with doctor immediately.

Continue taking, but discuss with your physician.

special precautions

DRUG INTERACTIONS

1. Oral anticoagulants

2. Oral contraceptives, other estrogen drugs

because

1. Increase anticoagulant effect.

2. Decrease effect of gemfibrozil.

DRUG INTERACTIONS

3. Oral antidiabetics

4. Mevacor

3. Increase effect of antidiabetic medications.

4. May cause kidney and muscle damage.

DIET
Avoid foods high in fats.

Will interfere with medication.

ALCOHOL and TOBACCO
No interaction with alcohol. Avoid tobacco.

Tobacco may decrease effectiveness of drug.

PREGNANCY
Discuss with your doctor.

Animal studies show increased rate of fetal death.

BREAST-FEEDING
Avoid drug or discuss with your doctor.

Animal studies have linked medication with some kinds of tumors.

AGE FACTOR
1. Not used in children.

2. People over 60 should use cautiously.

1. Safety and efficacy have not been established.

2. Adverse and side effects may be worse in older people.

MISSED DOSE
You can take a missed dose up to two hours after scheduled time. Otherwise, wait for next dose but do not double the amount taken.

OVERDOSE
Get in touch with poison control center, emergency room, or doctor if you have diarrhea, headaches, and pain in muscles.

STOPPING DRUG
Do not stop taking even if you feel better until you have talked with your doctor.

OTHERS
Do not drive or operate machinery until you have determined how medication affects you.

Periodic laboratory tests might be necessary to check liver function, blood lipids, and blood counts.

drug or category:

HMG-COA REDUCTASE INHIBITORS

condition:

HIGH CHOLESTEROL AND SATURATED FAT BLOOD LEVELS

warning

Tell your doctor if you have or have had:
- an allergic reaction to this medication, or to any preservatives or foods
- liver disease
- convulsions, infections, severe injuries, or low blood pressure
- immunosuppressant therapy

Tell your doctor if you:
- have abused alcohol
- are taking cyclosporine, erythromycin, gemfibrozil, or niacin (nicotinic acid)

drugs

GENERIC	BRAND	RX
lovastatin	Mevacor	Yes
simvastatin	Zocor	

form/usage

TABLETS: Best taken with food.

when

At evening meal.

side effects and adverse reactions

Muscle pain, vision problems, fever

Lovastatin
Impotence, inability to sleep

Lovastatin, simvastatin
Mild gastrointestinal problems, rash, headaches

what to do

Stop taking. Get in touch with doctor immediately.

Continue taking, but discuss with your physician.

special precautions

DRUG INTERACTIONS
Cyclosporine, erythromycin, gemfibrozil, niacin

because

May cause kidney and heart damage.

DIET
No restrictions.

--   --

ALCOHOL and TOBACCO
No interactions reported.

--   --

PREGNANCY
Avoid drug.

Fetus needs cholesterol to develop. Drug has caused congenital defects in animals.

--   --

BREAST-FEEDING
Avoid drug or avoid nursing.

Medication will migrate into breast milk and could affect child.

--   --

AGE FACTOR
1. Not recommended for children.

2. People over 60 should use cautiously.

1. Safety and efficacy have not been established. Also, cholesterol plays a role in child development.

2. Adverse and side effects may be worse in older people.

--   --

MISSED DOSE
You can take a missed dose up to two hours after scheduled time. Otherwise, wait for next dose but do not double the amount taken.

OVERDOSE
No overdose problems likely.

STOPPING DRUG
Do not stop taking even if you feel better until you have talked with your doctor. You may have to come off drug slowly.

OTHERS
Periodic laboratory tests might be necessary to check effect on liver, eyes, and blood fat levels.

NIACIN (NICOTINIC ACID, VITAMIN B$_3$)

condition:

HIGH CHOLESTEROL LEVELS

warning

Tell your doctor if you have or have had:

- an allergic reaction to this medication, or to preservatives or food additives
- diabetes or bleeding disorders
- glaucoma
- gout
- liver disease, low blood pressure, or ulcers

drugs

GENERIC	BRAND	RX
niacin	*Endur-Acin, Niac, Nicobid,* others	some

form/usage

TABLETS, CAPSULES (INCLUDING EXTENDED-RELEASE FORMU-LATIONS), SOLUTIONS, INJECTIONS: May be taken with milk or food.

Extended-release capsules should not be chewed or crushed. May be opened and contents mixed into a food you can swallow without chewing (i.e., jelly or jam).

Scored tablets (with a line down the middle) may be broken before swallowing. Do not crumble or crush.

when

Discuss with your doctor. Then take at the same time every day.

side effects and adverse reactions

Severe skin reactions, vision problems, difficulty getting up from bed or chair, pain in stomach, diarrhea

Dry skin, feeling of flushing or heat, headache, dizziness, tingling in extremities

what to do

Stop taking. Get in touch with doctor immediately.

Continue taking, but discuss with your physician.

special precautions	**because**
DRUG INTERACTIONS	
1. Antidiabetics, probenecid, sulfinpyrazone	1. Effect of these drugs will be decreased.
2. Guanethidine	2. Its effect will be increased.
3. Beta-blockers, mecamylamine, methyldopa, pargyline	3. Blood pressure may be lowered beyond safe levels.
4. Isoniazid	4. Will decrease effect of niacin.
DIET	
No interactions reported.	
ALCOHOL and TOBACCO	
Avoid both.	Alcohol will lower blood pressure to dangerous levels.
	Tobacco will interfere with niacin.
PREGNANCY	
No negative interactions reported.	
BREAST-FEEDING	
No problems reported.	
AGE FACTOR	
1. Children should not be given doses higher than recommended daily amounts unless specifically suggested by your physician.	1. No data on safety and effectiveness of high doses.
2. People over 60 should discuss with their doctors.	2. May cause low blood pressure and heart rhythm disturbances.
MISSED DOSE	
Take when you remember. Wait four hours before next dose. No need to double dose. Return to regular schedule.	

(continued)

OVERDOSE
Get in touch with poison control center, emergency room, or doctor if you have severe gastrointestinal problems, feel weak, have fainted, or have unexplained sweating.

STOPPING DRUG
No problems if discontinued without finishing prescription. Discuss with your doctor.

OTHERS
Do not drive or operate machinery until you have determined how medication in high doses affects you.

Getting up from a sitting or lying position may make you dizzy. Rise slowly from bed or chair. Check with your doctor if condition does not improve after a few days.

Periodic laboratory tests might be necessary to check effect on liver and blood.

Generalized skin flushing may occur frequently in the first few weeks of therapy; however, typically this diminishes after longer use of the drug.

drug or category:

WARFARIN

condition:
EXCESSIVE BLOOD CLOT FORMATION

warning

Tell your doctor if you have or have had:
- an allergic reaction to this medication, or to any preservatives or foods
- inflammatory bowel disease, any bleeding disorder, ulcers, high blood pressure, or kidney or liver disease
- heavy menstrual periods
- spinal anesthesia
- injuries to your head or body
- radiation therapy

Tell your doctor if you:
- are scheduled to have surgery within two months
- have recently had a baby or had an intrauterine device inserted

Take special care using cutting utensils, flossing, and shaving.

Report any injuries or accidents to your doctor immediately.

Any doctor or dentist you consult should know that you are taking this drug. Carry an information card or wear a bracelet stating you are taking an anticoagulant.

drugs

GENERIC	BRAND	RX
warfarin	*Coumadin, Panwarfin, Sofarin*	Yes

form/usage

TABLETS: Take with liquids. Tablets may be crumbled or crushed and taken with food.

when

Follow your doctor's directions. Take at the same time every day.

side effects and adverse reactions

Unusual or heavy bleeding; blood in stool, urine, or sputum, or bruising under the skin

Vision problems, skin reactions, chills, fever, fatigue, headaches, lessened output during urination, bleeding gums

Minor gastrointestinal problems, swelling in extremities, hair loss

what to do

Get emergency medical help immediately.

Stop taking. Get in touch with doctor immediately.

Continue taking, but discuss with your physician.

(continued)

special precautions	**because**
DRUG INTERACTIONS	
1. Acetaminophen, allopurinol, amiodarone, androgens, antibiotics, aspirin, bismuth subsalicylate, oral antidiabetics, cefixime, clofibrate, dextrothyroxine, diclofenac, fluconazole, nicardipine, nizatidine, nonsteroidal anti-inflammatory drugs, omeprazole, suprofen, testolactone, vitamin E	1. Increase effect of anticoagulant; increase risk of bleeding.
2. Aminoglutethimide, antacids in large quantities, barbiturates, oral contraceptives, calcium supplements, griseofulvin, phenytoin, rifampin, vitamin K	2. Decrease anticoagulant effect.
3. Antihistamines, benzodiazepines	3. May increase *or* decrease anticoagulant effect. Unpredictable.
4. Fluoxetine	4. Confusion, convulsions, high blood pressure.
5. Phenytoin	5. Phenytoin levels may drop.
6. Sulfadoxine, pyrimethamine	6. May be toxic.
DIET	
Ask your doctor how much of the following you should include in your diet: fish, liver, spinach, cabbage, cauliflower, brussels sprouts.	These foods are high in vitamin K and may interfere with the anticoagulant effect of the medication.
ALCOHOL and TOBACCO	
Avoid alcohol or use cautiously.	Alcohol may interfere with anticoagulant effect.
No problems reported with tobacco.	
PREGNANCY	
Avoid drug.	May cause fetal defects.
BREAST-FEEDING	
Discuss with your doctor.	Medication will migrate into breast milk and could affect child.

AGE FACTOR
Use with caution in children and older adults.   Both age groups are highly sensitive to side effects.

MISSED DOSE
You can take a missed dose up to 12 hours after scheduled time. Otherwise, wait for next dose but do not double the amount taken. Call your doctor if you miss a dose.

OVERDOSE
Get emergency medical help immediately if patient vomits or coughs up blood or passes blood in stool or urine.

STOPPING DRUG
Do not stop taking even if you feel better until you have talked with your doctor. You may have to come off drug slowly.

OTHERS
Do not drive or operate machinery until you have determined how medication affects you.

Caution is required when exercising or performing any kind of contact play to avoid the risks of internal bleeding.

-25-

DRUGS TO TREAT CARDIOVASCULAR DISORDERS

DESPITE TREMENDOUS GAINS in recent decades, heart disease remains our number one cause of death and disability. One in every five Americans—more than 56 million people—suffer some form of cardiovascular disease, which kills more than 923,000 people each year. Coronary artery disease—clogging of the blood vessels that nourish the heart muscle—is responsible for most of the 1.5 million heart attacks in the United States each year.

Coronary Artery Disease

According to the American Heart Association, more than 3 million Americans experience periodic bouts of angina—chest pains that develop when the heart muscle does not get enough oxygen. There are numerous approaches to treating coronary artery disease, and most heart patients undertake one or more of the following:

• Life-style changes—adopting a low-fat, low-cholesterol diet, losing excess weight, stopping smoking, increasing exercise, and

managing stress—are central to a prudent, heart-healthy approach.

• Surgical procedures, such as coronary bypass operations and balloon angioplasty to increase coronary blood flow. Angioplasty is the more conservative of the two procedures; it involves inserting a balloon-tipped catheter into the diseased arteries and then inflating the balloon to flatten the fatty deposits and widen the channel. Unfortunately, not all arteries can be reached by angioplasty, and in many cases, the arteries become blocked again in a few months or years. Coronary bypass surgery, in which healthy blood vessels from elsewhere in the body are grafted onto the heart to bypass severely clogged coronary arteries, produces longer-lasting results than angioplasty, but the operation is much more expensive and also carries its own risk of death and disability.

For most heart patients, a combination of life-style changes and medication can keep angina under control. The major classes of cardiovascular drugs are:

- **Nitrates, in the form of nitroglycerin.** These drugs are prescribed to both treat and prevent angina. During an attack, nitroglycerin tablets (*Nitrong, Nitrostat*) are placed under the tongue or in the cheek, or the drug is taken as an aerosol (*Nitrolingual*). In these forms, most of the drug is absorbed directly into the bloodstream and works by opening or dilating the coronary arteries, allowing more blood to reach the heart muscle. Slower-acting forms, such as medicated skin patches (*Nitro-Dur, Minitran*) or ointments (*Nitrol, Nitro-Bid*), are used to prevent attacks. With time, however, the heart develops a tolerance for nitrates and higher doses are required to attain a positive effect.

- **Beta-adrenergic blocking drugs.** These drugs, also called beta-blockers, which are also prescribed to treat high blood pressure and cardiac arrhythmias, have been used since the 1960s to alleviate angina. They work through the sympathetic nervous system to block the effects of norepinephrine, a chemical produced by the adrenal glands and other tissues, resulting in a slower, less forceful heartbeat. This category includes atenolol (*Tenormin*), nadolol (*Corgard*), and propranolol (*Inderal*). (See Chapter 20.)

- **Calcium channel blockers.** Like the beta-blockers, calcium blockers are used to treat both angina and high blood pressure. They reduce angina by relaxing the muscles in blood vessels, allowing them to open wider and allow increased blood flow. Calcium blockers are especially effective in treating variant angina—the kind that develops even during rest and is caused by spasms of a coronary artery. Diltiazem (*Cardizem*), nifedipine (*Procardia*), and verapamil (*Calan*) are a few

examples of this category. (See Chapter 20 for more specific information on these drugs.)

In addition to medications to treat or prevent angina, **low-dose aspirin** also may be prescribed to help prevent heart attack and stroke. A single aspirin taken daily or even every other day reduces the clotting action of blood platelets, thereby lowering the risk of a heart attack caused by a clot blocking an already narrowed coronary artery. However, consult your doctor before taking aspirin on a regular basis. It can cause stomach irritation and bleeding. (See the table on aspirin in Chapter 14; also see Chapter 24 for information on anticoagulants.)

Heart Failure

Heart failure refers to the inability of the heart to pump enough blood to meet the body's needs for oxygen, resulting in shortness of breath, fatigue, and swelling (edema) caused by a buildup of fluids in the legs. In congestive heart failure, the lungs may become waterlogged, interfering with the movement of oxygen into the blood supply.

Some 2 million Americans suffer from heart failure, which can result from coronary artery disease, a heart attack, heart valve disorders, and diseases of the heart itself. Treatment varies depending on the underlying cause, and may include use of the following drugs:

- **Diuretics.** These drugs, which are often used to treat high blood pressure, are also a mainstay in treating congestive heart failure. By reducing the body's volume of fluids, they ease the burden on the heart. Thiazide diuretics such as *Diuril* and loop diuretics such as *Lasix* are two types of this drug. (See Chapter 20.)

- **Angiotensin-converting enzyme (ACE) inhibitors.** This class of drugs, which is also used to treat hypertension, works against congestive heart failure by dilating blood vessels, thus reducing the heart's workload. Some studies indicate that these drugs may also prevent heart enlargement after a heart attack—a common contributor to heart failure. ACE inhibitors include captopril (*Capoten*) and enalapril (*Vasotec*). (See Chapter 20.) Other vasodilator drugs that may be prescribed to treat heart failure include nitrates such as isosorbide dinitrate (*Isordil, Sorbitrate*).

- **Digitalis.** This drug, which is derived from the leaves of the foxglove plant, has been used to treat edema (dropsy) for centuries, and digoxin (*Lanoxin*) and digitoxin (*Crystodigin*)—two modern forms—are still prescribed to treat congestive heart failure. Use of these drugs is limited by their toxicity, so they are used mostly for patients who have not responded well to diuretics or vasodilators.

Cardiac Arrhythmias

From time to time, everyone experiences sudden, unexplained palpitations in which the heartbeat speeds up. In most instances, these changes in heart rhythm are of no significance, but for many men and women aberrant heart rhythms—or cardiac arrhythmias—are a serious issue, causing problems ranging from dizziness and fainting to sudden death. To help the heart maintain its normal beating pattern, doctors may prescribe beta-blockers, calcium channel blockers, or digoxin (see the preceding sections of this chapter). Other specific antiarrhythmia drugs include:

- **Quinidine, procainamide, and similar medications.** The various drugs made of quinidine (*Cardioquin, Quinaglute, Quinidex*) and procainamide (*Procan SR, Promine, Pronestyl*) can be administered in shots, capsules, or tablets. These drugs act on the heart's pacemaker cells, which control the heart's electrical system. The medications are used most often to prevent very rapid heartbeats, such as atrial or ventricular tachycardia.

- **Disopyramide** (*Norpace, Rhythmodan*). This drug, which acts very much like quinidine, comes in capsules. Its targets are premature heartbeats that originate in both the upper chambers (atria) and lower chambers (ventricles) of the heart.

- **Anesthetic drugs, like lidocaine.** Lidocaine usually is given by injection or IV following a heart attack or during heart surgery. Mexiletine (*Mexitil*), which is chemically related to lidocaine, is also used to combat arrhythmias.

Cardiac arrhythmias that are not adequately controlled by drugs may be treated by implantation of an artificial pacemaker.

drug or category:

NITRATES

condition:
ANGINA, CONGESTIVE HEART FAILURE

warning

Tell your doctor if you have or have had:
- an allergic reaction to this medication, or to preservatives or food additives
- severe anemia
- glaucoma

drugs

GENERIC	BRAND	RX
nitroglycerin	*Nitro-Dur, Nitrostat*, others	Yes
isosorbide dinitrate	*Isordil*	

form/usage

TABLETS, CAPSULES (SOME EXTENDED-RELEASE FORMULA-TIONS), SPRAY, OINTMENT, PATCHES: Tablets and capsules should be taken whole with liquid, but preferably on an empty stomach.

Do not crush tablets.

You may open capsules, but don't crush or chew them.

Nitrates that come in chewable form should be held in the mouth for up to two minutes.

Allow buccal tablets to dissolve at the side of mouth.

Sublingual tablets are to be placed directly under the tongue, and sprays are to be directed to the underside of tongue.

Ointment and patch formulations have precise, step-by-step, illustrated instructions in package.

when

Tablets and capsules should be taken one hour before meals or two hours after, at the same time every day.

Sublingual tablets and sprays and buccal tablets are taken when angina begins.

Your physician will tell you when to use patches and ointments.

(continued)

side effects and adverse reactions	what to do
Rashes, skin irritations, blurry vision, dry mouth	Stop taking. Get in touch with doctor immediately.
Headaches, palpitations, stomach problems	Continue taking, but discuss with your physician.

special precautions	because
DRUGS	
I. Hypertension medications, beta-blockers, calcium channel blockers, carteolol, lisinopril, narcotic-based medications, phenothiazines, sotalol; tricyclic antidepressants	I. Could cause blood pressure to drop too much.
2. Aspirin	2. In doses exceeding 500 mg, will heighten the effect of nitrates.
3. Any medication with ephedrine	3. Decreases the effectiveness of nitrates.
DIET No restrictions.	
ALCOHOL AND TOBACCO Avoid both.	Alcohol could lead to an excessive blood pressure drop. Tobacco can reduce the impact of nitrates.
PREGNANCY Discuss with your physician.	Though studies have not uncovered any impact on the fetus, pregnancy should be avoided while taking nitrates.
BREAST-FEEDING Discuss with your doctor.	It is unknown whether nitrates migrate into breast milk. There are not likely to be any problems, but you should keep a close eye on the baby.

AGE FACTOR

1. Nitrates are not recommended for infants and children.

2. People over 60 should use cautiously.

1. Not of much use in children, and little is known of long-term effects.

2. Adverse and side effects may be worse in older people.

MISSED DOSE

If you have forgotten a dose and remember within two hours, take your pill. If you remember after two hours, wait until your next regularly scheduled dose.

OVERDOSE

Get emergency medical help immediately in case of fever, accelerated heartbeat, convulsions, pressure in head, fainting, or breathing problems.

STOPPING DRUG

Never stop taking the drug without consulting your doctor.

OTHERS

Don't drive or operate machinery until you have determined how drug affects you.

Since nitrates increase the ability of the heart to work, be especially careful when exercising.

Be careful in hot environments like saunas and steam rooms. Heat can cause an excessive drop in blood pressure.

Periodic laboratory tests might be necessary to check blood counts.

drug or category:

DISOPYRAMIDE

condition:
ARRHYTHMIA

warning

Tell your doctor if you have or have had:
- an allergic reaction to this medication, or to preservatives or food additives
- other disorders of the heart's electrical system
- kidney or liver disease
- glaucoma
- myasthenia gravis
- prostate difficulties or urinary disorders

Tell your doctor if you are taking digitalis or any diuretic.

drugs

GENERIC	BRAND	RX
disopyramide	*Norpace, Rhythmodan*	Yes

form/usage

CAPSULES (REGULAR AND EXTENDED-RELEASE): Should be taken on an empty stomach, but if medication irritates stomach, may be taken with food.

Regular capsules can be opened. Do not open extended-released capsules.

when

Follow your doctor's recommendations. Take one hour before eating or two hours after.

side effects and adverse reactions

Cold sweats, extreme hunger, nervousness, and other signs of hypoglycemia; dizziness; confusion; emotional or behavioral abnormalities; changes in heartbeat; shortness of breath

Loss of sex drive, pain in eyes, swollen feet, constipation, problems urinating, blurry vision

what to do

Stop taking. Get in touch with doctor immediately.

Continue taking, but discuss with your physician.

special precautions	because
DRUG INTERACTIONS I. Phenytoin, other antiarrhythmia drugs, lidocaine, propranolol, anticholinergic drugs, anticoagulants, antihypertensives, phenobarbital, rifampin	I. Effects of disopyramide or other medications could be heightened, diminished, or altered in some other fashion.
2. Flecainide, nicardipine, nimodipine	2. Adverse impact on heart rhythm.
DIET No restrictions.	
ALCOHOL AND TOBACCO Use alcohol cautiously until you have established your reaction to the drug.	Drug lowers blood pressure, and alcohol can magnify this effect.
Avoid tobacco.	Tobacco diminishes effect because nicotine adds to irritability of heart.
PREGNANCY Discuss with your doctor.	Effects of drug on pregnancy or fetus have not been established.
BREAST-FEEDING Avoid drug or avoid nursing.	Drug enters breast milk.
AGE FACTOR I. Children's dosages are determined according to weight.	
2. Dosages for elderly must be individualized.	2. Administration is based on individual weight and health history to avoid urinary problems, constipation, and other side effects.
MISSED DOSE You can take a missed dose up to two hours after scheduled time. If more time has elapsed, wait until next dose is due, but do not double dose.	
OVERDOSE **Get emergency medical help immediately** in case of apnea (breathing interruptions during sleep), unconsciousness, or irregular heartbeat.	

(continued)

STOPPING DRUG
Do not stop abruptly. Discuss how to stop medicine with your doctor.

OTHERS
May cause breast enlargement in men and, in a few instances, impotence if taken in doses exceeding 300 mg a day.

drug or category:

PROCAINAMIDE

condition:

ARRHYTHMIA

warning

Tell your doctor if you have or have had:
- an allergic reaction to this drug or local anesthetics like procaine
- complete heart block
- lupus erythematosus
- kidney or liver disease
- myasthenia gravis
- enlarged prostate

Tell your doctor if you are taking another heart drug.

drugs

GENERIC	BRAND	RX
procainamide	*Procan SR, Promine, Pronestyl,* others	Yes

form/usage

TABLETS (REGULAR AND EXTENDED-RELEASE), CAPSULES, INJECTIONS: Drug should be taken on an empty stomach, but if it irritates stomach, it may be taken with food or milk.

Regular tablets may be crushed and capsules may be opened.

Extended-release tablets must be taken whole.

when

One hour before eating or two hours afterward.

side effects and adverse reactions

Difficult breathing, pain in joints, depression and other mood or behavioral changes, bleeding, fever, sore throat

Tiredness, diarrhea, lack of appetite, other gastrointestinal disturbances

what to do

Stop taking. Get in touch with doctor immediately.

Continue taking, but discuss with your physician.

(continued)

special precautions	**because**
DRUG INTERACTIONS	
1. High blood pressure drugs	1. Procainamide can increase their effect and cause excessive blood pressure drop.
2. Anticholinergics, guanfacine, nicardipine, propafenone, other antiarrhythmia drugs	2. Procainamide increases the effects of these medications.
3. Amiodarone, acetazolamide, cimetidine, nizatidine	3. Increase procainamide's impact.
4. Anti-myasthenia drugs	4. Their effect will be decreased.
5. Dapsone	5. Amplifies potential adverse impact on blood cells.
DIET	
Avoid beverages with caffeine.	Caffeine affects heart rhythm.
ALCOHOL AND TOBACCO	
Use alcohol carefully until interaction with drug is determined.	Alcohol can magnify blood-pressure-lowering capacity of medication.
Avoid tobacco.	Nicotine irritates the heart and diminishes the effect of this medication.
PREGNANCY	
Discuss with your doctor.	Effects on pregnancy or fetus have not been determined.
BREAST-FEEDING	
Avoid drug or avoid nursing.	Medication passes into breast milk.
AGE FACTOR	
1. This drug is not recommended for children, but if given, it should be done only under close medical supervision, and blood counts should be done regularly.	1. Safety and effectiveness have not been established. Medication could adversely affect white blood cells.

AGE FACTOR

2. Adults over 60 may require lower doses.

2. Reduced kidney function could allow drug to have greater impact and cause dizziness, putting patient at risk of falling.

MISSED DOSE

Missed dose can be taken up to two hours after scheduled time. After two hours, wait for next dose, but do not double the amount taken.

OVERDOSE

Get emergency medical help immediately if heart starts beating fast or beat is irregular, if there is a drop in blood pressure, or if patient has fainted or gone into cardiac arrest.

STOPPING DRUG

Do not discontinue abruptly. Discuss with your doctor how to stop taking medicine.

OTHERS

Don't drive or operate machinery until you have determined how drug affects you.

Your doctor may order regular laboratory tests to check on changes in the amount of the drug in your body.

Electrocardiogram tests also may be routinely ordered when you are taking this drug.

drug or category:

DIGOXIN

condition:
CONGESTIVE HEART FAILURE

warning

Do not take any other medications, whether prescribed or over-the counter, unless you have checked with your physician first.

Tell your doctor if you have or have had:

- an allergic reaction to this medication, or to preservatives or dyes
- kidney, liver, or lung disease or thyroid problems
- rheumatic fever

Tell your doctor if you:

- are taking beta-blocker or calcium channel blocker drugs
- have had any kind of surgery—including oral surgery—within the last two months

drugs

GENERIC	BRAND	RX
digoxin	*Lanoxin*, others	Yes

form/usage

TABLETS, CAPSULES, ELIXIR, AND INJECTIONS: Tablets and cap-sules should be taken with a liquid.

Liquid forms of medications should be diluted in a beverage.

Pills may be broken or crushed and capsules can be opened. Take with food or liquid.

when

At the same time every day.

side effects and adverse reactions

Severe headaches, hallucinations, changes in heart rhythm, fainting spells, disorientation

Loss of appetite, diarrhea, pain in lower stomach; changes in vision, in-cluding yellow or green halos around objects; depression; a feeling of weakness or a sense of being tired; sensitivity or soreness in breast tissues in men

what to do

Stop taking. Get in touch with doctor immediately.

Continue taking, but discuss with your physician.

special precautions	**because**
DRUG INTERACTIONS	
1. Antacids, calcium supplements, carteolol, cholestyramine, colestipol, dextrothyroxine	1. Decrease the effect of digoxin.
2. Amiodarone, anticonvulsants, anticholinergics, beta-blockers, calcium channel blockers, diuretics, amphetamines	2. May amplify the impact of digoxin.
3. Cortisone, diuretics, hydroxychloroquine	3. May cause digoxin toxicity.
4. Ephedrine, epinephrine, beta-blockers	4. May cause heartbeat irregularities.
DIET	
1. Don't overload your meals with fiber.	1. Fiber foods can interfere with the absorption of digoxin in the stomach, thus decreasing the drug's effect.
2. Avoid milk products for two hours before and after taking digoxin.	2. Milk could impact effectiveness of drug.
3. Don't indulge excessively in drinks containing caffeine (coffee, colas, etc.).	3. Caffeine contributes to heart rhythm irregularities.
ALCOHOL AND TOBACCO	
No reported interactions with alcohol.	
Abstinence from tobacco is advised.	Nicotine contributes to heartbeat irregularities.
PREGNANCY	
No problems linked to drug in animals or humans have been reported. Discuss with your doctor.	Reproduction studies have not been done in either animals or humans.
BREAST-FEEDING	
Avoid nursing or avoid drug.	Medication enters breast milk. If you cannot avoid drug, observe baby closely for reactions.

(continued)

AGE FACTOR

1. Do not give to infants or children unless prescribed, and be sure to follow instructions very precisely.

2. People over 60 should use very carefully.

1. Could induce slow heartbeat and heart rhythm problems.

2. Adverse reactions and side effects may be worse in older people.

MISSED DOSE

Take missed dose as soon as possible, even if you remember it 10 to 12 hours later. If more than 12 hours go by, just take your next dose—but do not double the amount.

OVERDOSE

Get emergency medical help immediately in case of nausea, vision problems, hallucinations, or convulsions.

STOPPING DRUG

Do not stop taking this medicine until your doctor tells you to do so.

OTHERS

Don't drive or operate machinery until you have determined how drug affects you.

If something other than the medicine causes you to vomit or have a spell of diarrhea right after you have taken digoxin, seek your doctor's advice because you may have flushed some of the drug out of your body.

Your doctor may prescribe potassium supplements or encourage you to follow a potassium-rich diet when you are taking digoxin for long periods of time.

Periodic laboratory tests might be necessary to check levels of calcium, potassium, and magnesium in your blood.

ISOXSUPRINE

condition:
POOR CIRCULATION

warning

Tell your doctor if you have or have had:
- an allergic reaction to this drug or any other blood vessel dilator
- any bleeding disorder

drugs

GENERIC	BRAND	RX
isoxsuprine	*Vasodilan, Vasoprine*	Yes

form/usage

TABLETS: May be taken with food or milk.

Tablets may be crumbled into liquid or food.

when

At the same time every day.

side effects and adverse reactions

Fast or slow heartbeat, chest pain, breathing difficulties, loss of appetite, other gastrointestinal disturbances

Lethargy, feeling of weakness

what to do

Stop taking. Get in touch with doctor immediately.

Continue taking, but discuss with your physician.

special precautions

DRUG INTERACTIONS
No interactions reported.

DIET
No interactions reported.

because

(continued)

ALCOHOL AND TOBACCO

No interaction with alcohol reported.

Avoid tobacco.

Tobacco decreases impact of drug and narrows blood vessels.

PREGNANCY

Discuss with your doctor.

While drug has not been shown to cause birth defects in humans, it may cause fast heartbeat and other problems in the baby if given shortly before delivery.

BREAST-FEEDING

No problems reported. Discuss with your doctor.

While no problems have been reported in nursing babies, drug may migrate into breast milk.

AGE FACTOR

1. Not recommended for children.

2. People over 60 should use cautiously.

1. Safety and efficacy have not been established. No specific information on drug's effect on children is available.

2. Adverse and side effects may be worse in older people.

MISSED DOSE

May be taken up to two hours after scheduled time. If longer than two hours, wait until next dose is due, but do not double dose.

OVERDOSE

Get emergency medical help immediately in case of coma, headache, sweating, or breathing difficulties.

STOPPING DRUG

Always finish prescription and do not discontinue unless you have discussed it with your doctor.

OTHERS

May cause dizziness or bring on fainting. Do not drive or use machinery until you have established how drug affects you.

-26-

CONTRACEPTIVES

Oral Contraceptives

Birth control pills, or oral contraceptives, offer numerous advantages, especially for women. They are 99 percent effective, giving women virtually total control over their fertility; they are relatively safe; and they remove the need to interrupt sexual activity to use a barrier device. Most of today's oral contraceptives combine two hormones, estrogen and progestin, which halt ovulation; this is similar to what happens during pregnancy. As secondary lines of defense, the hormones thicken the cervical mucus to block the passage of sperm and also alter the lining of the uterus to prevent implantation of a fertilized egg. Brands include *Loestrin* Fe, *Ovcon,* and *Ortho-Novum.*

Current combination pills have lower doses of hormones than earlier pills, and—consequently—fewer side effects. Even so, they may be contraindicated for women with heart disease, clotting disorders, certain cancers, or migraine headaches, as well as for women over 35 who smoke, because of an increased risk of heart attacks and stroke.

Oral contraceptives containing only progestin (*Ovrette, Micronor, Nor Q D*)—the so-called minipill—halt implantation of any fertilized eggs. The minipill has a somewhat higher failure rate than combination pills, and "breakthrough" bleeding or irregular periods may be a problem.

Before starting any oral contraceptive, a woman should have a gynecological examination and Pap smear. Thereafter, checkups every six to nine months are advisable.

Implantable Contraceptives

In 1990, the Food and Drug Administration approved *Norplant,* an implantable birth control device that prevents pregnancy for five years. The device consists of five small tubes—each roughly the size of a match—that are placed just under the skin of the arm. The tubes then release small amounts of levonorgestrel, a synthetic form of progestin.

During its first year in place, *Norplant* is 99.9 percent effective—protection that is matched only by sterilization. Efficiency ebbs slightly each year, but even by the fifth year it is as effective as conventional birth control pills. Serious side effects are uncommon, but they may include formation of blood clots, mood changes, and intestinal problems.

Morning-After Pill

Some oral contraceptives can be used as morning-after, or postcoital, pills to prevent pregnancy after unprotected sex. This strategy calls for taking double doses of a combination pill, such as *Norinyl* or *Ortho-Novum*, that has a high level of estrogen.

Alternatively, a high dosage of estrogen or DES will also prevent pregnancy. Taken in this manner, the drugs postpone or prevent ovulation and also prevent implantation.

Barrier Contraceptives

These include condoms, diaphragms, cervical caps, spermicides, foams, and sponges that provide a barrier to keep sperm from entering a woman's cervix. In addition, **spermicides**—which come in foams, gels, jellies, and suppositories—destroy sperm on contact. They also offer some protection against sexually transmitted diseases. To achieve maximum protection against both pregnancy and diseases, however, spermicides should be used with a condom and diaphragm. Spermicide products include *Because, Conceptrol Gel, Gynol II, Semicid,* and *Kormex Cream.*

The vaginal sponge *Today,* a 2-inch device that contains a spermicide, is a nonprescription alternative to a diaphragm. Its greatest advantage is that it can be used for 24 hours and does away with the need for inserting fresh spermicide for every sex act. However, it offers less protection to a woman who has had a child and whose cervix may be larger than the sponge. Some women also have encountered difficulty in removing the sponge.

drug or category:

ESTROGEN AND PROGESTIN

condition or use:

TO PREVENT CONCEPTION, REGULATE MENSTRUAL CYCLES

warning

Smoking increases the risk of cardiovascular disease in women taking oral contraceptives. Risk is highest among women older than 35. Tell your doctor if you have or have had:

- a previous allergic reaction to the pill
- clotting problems or liver disease
- breast cancer or other cancers, or a family history of breast or ovarian cancer
- unexplained vaginal bleeding or sickle-cell disease

Discuss all other serious illnesses you have or have had with your doctor before starting.

Oral contraceptives may increase cholesterol levels.

Be sure you are not pregnant before starting contraceptives.

drugs

GENERIC	BRAND	RX
estrogen and progestin	*Loestrin* Fe, *Ovcon, Tri-Levlen, Ortho-Novum, Lo-Ovral,* others	Yes

form/usage

TABLETS: To decrease potential stomach irritation, may be taken with or after food. May be taken with milk.

when

Every 24 hours, at same time every day. Pills are taken on 21- or 28-day cycles.

side effects and adverse reactions

Nausea, drowsiness, vomiting, vaginal bleeding

Jaundice, fever, inability to wear your contact lenses, headache, pain in joints or abdomen, enlarged clitoris, leg swelling, depression

Insomnia, hair loss, gastrointestinal problems, acne, breakthrough bleeding, depression, behavioral changes

what to do

Contact doctor or get emergency advice from a poison control center.

Stop taking. Get in touch with doctor immediately.

Continue taking, but discuss with your doctor.

(continued)

special precautions	because
DRUG INTERACTIONS Oral contraceptives interact with more than two dozen drugs, including antibiotics, anticoagulants, antidepressants, barbiturates, anticonvulsives, tranquilizers, steroid drugs, bronchial dilators, and vitamins A and C. Discuss with your doctor all drugs you are taking, whether they are prescription or over the counter.	Use of these drugs with contraceptives may increase, decrease, or change the impact or effectiveness of the drugs or the contraceptives.
DIET Avoid excessively salty foods.	
ALCOHOL and TOBACCO No problems with alcohol reported. Avoid or cut down on tobacco.	Research shows that heavy smoking and use of oral contraceptives can increase greatly the risk of heart attack.
PREGNANCY Have pregnancy test done before starting drug. Avoid pregnancy for three to six months after stopping pill.	Oral contraceptives are not recommended for use during pregnancy and could cause birth defects.
BREAST-FEEDING Do not start taking oral contraceptives immediately after delivery.	Contraceptives, if started too soon after birth, may interfere with milk supply. The drug enters breast milk in very small amounts but is not considered harmful to the baby.
AGE FACTOR Use with caution if you are over 35 and are a smoker.	Heightened risk of cardiovascular problems.
MISSED DOSE Take additional precautions against pregnancy.	

OVERDOSE
Get medical help immediately if you have symptoms indicating a stroke or heart attack.

STOPPING DRUG
Do not discontinue because of bleeding problems. Discuss with your physician; the estrogen content of the pill may be too low.

Skipping a dose may result in pregnancy.

OTHERS
May cause decrease in sexual desire, change in menstruation, or breast enlargement and fluid retention.

Regular breast and pelvic exams are recommended.

May increase sensitivity to sun.

drug or category:

LEVONORGESTREL

condition or use:
TO PREVENT PREGNANCY

warning

Tell your doctor if you have or have had:
- an allergic reaction to progestin, or to preservatives or dyes
- breast cancer, blood clot problems, or unexplained vaginal bleeding

Tell your doctor if you retain fluids.

Be sure you are not pregnant before starting.

drugs

GENERIC	BRAND	RX
levonorgestrel	*Norplant*	Yes

form/usage

IMPLANT: Capsules containing progestin are inserted by your doctor in upper arm, under skin.

when

Implants are left in place for five years.

side effects and adverse reactions

Bleeding or pus, swelling, tenderness at site of implant; tenderness in breast; abdominal pain; nausea; vaginal infection; changes in menstruation; headache; hair loss; dizziness; acne

what to do

For bleeding, pus, or infection, get in touch with your physician immediately; for others, call when you have time.

special precautions

DRUG INTERACTIONS
Phenytoin, carbamazepine, barbiturates, phenylbutazone, isoniazid, rifampin

DIET
No restrictions.

because

Decrease the implant's effectiveness.

ALCOHOL and TOBACCO
No reaction to alcohol reported.

No reaction to tobacco noted, but discuss with your doctor.

It is not known whether levonorgestrel carries a risk of serious cardiovascular side effects similar to that of combination oral contraceptives.

PREGNANCY
Have pregnancy test done before having implant.

BREAST-FEEDING
Avoid nursing or discuss with your doctor.

Progestin passes into breast milk.

AGE FACTOR
None.

MISSED DOSE
Not possible.

OVERDOSE
No overdose problems reported.

STOPPING DRUG
Can only be done by removing implant.

OTHERS
Implants lose effectiveness after five years. Replace, if prolonged contraception is desired.

drug or category:

VAGINAL SPERMICIDES

condition or use:
TO PREVENT PREGNANCY

warning

Tell your doctor if you have or have had an allergic reaction to a spermicide or to octoxynol-9, nonoxynol-9, or benzalkonium chloride.

Do not use without additional contraceptives such as condoms, a diaphragm, or additional preparations, because failure rate can be high. However, spermicide contraceptives can provide some protection against sexually transmitted diseases.

drugs

GENERIC	BRAND	RX
nonoxynol-9	*Today Sponge, Encare, Because, Conceptrol Gel, Semicid,* others	No (for most)

form/usage

FOAMS, GELS, JELLIES, SPONGES: Insert foams, gels, and creams into the vagina, in combination with diaphragm or other mechanical contraceptive devices.

For sponges, follow package instructions.

when

Foams and gels should be used before every act of sexual intercourse. Sponges do not need to be replaced before every sex act, but should not be left in vagina for more than 30 hours.

side effects and adverse reactions

Toxic shock syndrome, including chills, fever, confusion; redness in vagina, eyes, mouth, and throat; muscle aches

Vaginal discharge, rash, urination difficulties, bloody or cloudy urine

what to do

Get emergency medical help immediately.

Stop using. Get in touch with doctor immediately.

special precautions

because

DRUG INTERACTIONS
1. Soaps, disinfectants, peroxides, aspirin compounds

2. Douches

1. Decrease the effectiveness of spermicide.

2. May interfere with spermicide. Avoid for eight hours after sexual intercourse.

DIET
No interactions.

ALCOHOL and TOBACCO
No interactions.

PREGNANCY
No problems reported.

BREAST-FEEDING
No problems reported. Discuss with your doctor.

It is unknown if vaginal spermicides pass into human breast milk.

AGE FACTOR
None.

MISSED DOSE
If you forget to use, contact your doctor to determine what other options are open to you.

OVERDOSE
No problems anticipated.

STOPPING DRUG
May be stopped when no longer needed.

-27-

COUGH AND COLD MEDICATIONS

THE COMMON COLD is indeed common. On average, adult Americans catch at least one cold each winter, and some 60 million suffer three to six bouts. Schoolchildren are particularly vulnerable, averaging six to 12 colds a year.

Two hundred or more different viruses produce colds, but the most prevalent are the more than 100 strains of rhinoviruses. So if you develop antibodies against one strain, there are many more waiting their turn.

Flu, or influenza, produces symptoms similar to the common cold, but they are likely to be more severe and last longer. There are only three strains of flu viruses, but they keep mutating, so immunity against one does not necessarily protect against the next generation.

Experts agree that the best approach to treating colds and flu is to rest, drink plenty of fluids (including broth and chicken soup), and take aspirin or acetaminophen every few hours to alleviate aches and pains. (Older people and those with chronic diseases, however, should protect themselves with an annual shot that provides immunity against that season's prevalent strain of influenza virus). There are also hundreds of nonprescription cold, flu, and cough remedies that provide varying degrees of relief from cold and flu symptoms. Remember, though, aspirin should not be given to anyone under the age of 18 who has flu, a cold, or other viral illness because of the increased risk of Reye's syndrome, a rare but potentially fatal liver and brain disease.

Cold Medications

There are more than 125 different drug combinations and hundreds of different formulations of cold and flu medication. (See the tables in this chapter for a few examples.) Not one of them will cure the cold or flu, but they can relieve symptoms such as sneezing, nasal congestion, runny nose and teary eyes, headache, fever, and general achiness. Many cold medications combine decongestants, antihistamines, pain-killers, and other ingredients. The safest approach is to select a product with the fewest possible ingredients, ones that are targeted for your particular symptoms. For example, if fever, aches, and congestion head your list of symptoms, pick a drug that contains aspirin or acetaminophen for the fever and achiness and a decongestant. Also, read the label and list of ingredients carefully. If you have high blood pressure, diabetes, heart disease, glaucoma, or some other chronic condition, check with your doctor or pharmacist before taking any cold medication.

Cough Medications

There are two broad categories of cough medications: expectorants such as guaifenesin (*Robitussin*), which thin and loosen phlegm, making it easier to bring up, and cough suppressants such as dextromethorphan (*Pertussin Cough Suppressant, Robitussin Pediatric, Vicks Formula 44*, and others), which works through the brain's cough center to halt the reflexes that set off coughing spells.

In general, doctors discourage using cough suppressants, especially to stop "wet" coughs that produce sputum and help clear the airways. Exceptions might be dry, hacking coughs that keep you awake at night. Paradoxically, overuse of cough suppressants can keep you awake.

There are other factors to consider before taking a cough medication. Some contain ingredients that interact with prescription drugs, so it's a good idea to check with your pharmacist or doctor. Also, many cough medications are as much as 25 percent alcohol, which means you should be especially careful not to give them to children. Nor should you take them yourself if you have hypertension because just two doses a day could raise your blood pressure significantly.

Certainly, you don't want to take any kind of cough medication for too long. A lingering cough may be a sign of serious illness such as tuberculosis, lung cancer, bronchitis, or asthma. So if a cough lasts more than a week or ten days, it's a good idea to see a doctor. Go sooner if the cough is accompanied by a high fever or if you are coughing up blood or thick, malodorous phlegm.

drug or category:

GUAIFENESIN

condition:
COUGHS

warning

Tell your doctor if you have or have had an allergic reaction to this medication, or to preservatives or food additives.

drugs

GENERIC	BRAND	RX
guaifenesin	*Robitussin*	No

form/usage

CAPSULES AND TABLETS (INCLUDING EXTENDED-RELEASE FORMULATIONS), SYRUP, SOLUTIONS: Can be taken with food or liquid.

Drink 8 ounces of water (full glass) after taking medication.

All tablets may be crumbled and all capsules may be opened.

when

When you need it, but no more often than every three to four hours.

side effects and adverse reactions

Gastrointestinal problems, skin reactions

Drowsiness

what to do

Stop taking. Get in touch with doctor immediately.

Continue taking, but discuss with your physician.

special precautions

DRUG INTERACTIONS
Anticoagulants

because

Increase risk of bleeding.

DIET
No interactions reported.

Drink ample amounts of fluids while taking medication.

Fluids help to loosen mucus or phlegm and to facilitate drug's work.

ALCOHOL AND TOBACCO
No interactions reported.

PREGNANCY
No negative interactions reported.

BREAST-FEEDING
No problems reported.

AGE FACTOR
1. May be given to children and infants.

2. People over 60 should use cautiously. Older people should drink ample fluids throughout day while taking medication.

2. Adverse and side effects may be worse in older people.

MISSED DOSE
Take when you remember, but do not take next dose for another three hours. Do not double dose.

OVERDOSE
Get in touch with poison control center, emergency room, or doctor in case of gastrointestinal problems, drowsiness, or weakness.

STOPPING DRUG
Medication need not be finished if symptoms stop. However, if cough lasts longer than one week, consult your doctor.

OTHERS
Do not drive or operate machinery until you have determined how medication affects you.

drug or category:

COMBINATION DRUGS

condition:
COUGHS AND COLDS

warning

Tell your doctor if you have or have had:
- an allergic reaction to this medication, or to preservatives or food additives
- cardiac arrhythmias
- high blood pressure, thyroid problems, or urination difficulties
- asthma, glaucoma or prostate problems; liver disease

Do not use any of these products if you are taking an MAO inhibitor antidepressant drug such as *Nardil* or *Parnate*.

Double-check all labels to determine active and inactive ingredients; make sure that you or patient taking them is not allergic and has had no previous reactions to them.

Avoid giving any medications that include aspirin to children.

If you are having surgery involving general or spinal anesthesia within two months, discuss with your doctor before taking any drug containing phenylpropanolamine.

Tell your doctor if you are going to take a medication containing doxylamine.

Consult with your doctor before taking any medication containing dextromethorphan.

For warnings relating to codeine, see Chapter 15.

For warnings relating to acetaminophen, see Chapter 14.

For warnings relating to pseudoephedrine, see Chapter 23.

For warnings relating to guaifenesin, see table on medication in this chapter.

drugs

GENERIC	BRAND	RX
phenylephrine, phenylpropano-lamine, guaifenesin	*Entex*	Some
chlorpheniramine, dextromethor-phan, acetaminophen	*Comtrex*	
doxylamine, pseudoephedrine, dextromethorphan, acetamino-phen	*NyQuil*	
phenylpropanolamine, codeine, guaifenesin	*Naldecon-CX Adult*	
phenylpropanolamine	*Naldecon-DX* (Adult and Children)	

drugs

GENERIC	BRAND	RX
phenylpropanolamine, guaifenesin	*Naldecon EX*	
guaifenesin, dextromethorphan	*Naldecon Senior Dx*	
brompheniramine, phenylpropan-olamine, dextromethorphan	*Dimetapp DM*	

form/usage

CAPSULES, TABLETS (INCLUDING EXTENDED-RELEASE FORMU-LATIONS), SYRUPS, ORAL SOLUTIONS: Medications should be followed with full glass of water (8 ounces).

Extended-release tablets should be taken whole, without crushing or crumbling.

Extended-release capsules may be mixed into food that can be swallowed without chewing (applesauce, jellies, etc.).

when

Follow directions in medication package.

side effects and adverse reactions

For warnings relating to codeine, see Chapter 15.

For warnings relating to acetaminophen, see Chapter 14.

For warnings relating to pseudoephedrine, see Chapter 23.

For warnings relating to brompheniramine see Chapter 23.

For warnings relating to guaifenesin, see table on this medication in this chapter.

Phenylephrine
Dizziness, shaking, sweating, heart rhythm changes

Phenylpropanolamine
Heart rhythm changes, tight feeling in chest

Dextromethorphan
Confusion, extreme nervousness, dizziness, gastrointestinal problems

what to do

Stop taking. Get in touch with doctor immediately.

(continued)

side effects and adverse reactions	**what to do**
Phenylephrine Headache, watery or burning eyes	Continue taking, but discuss with your physician.
Phenylpropanolamine Minor gastrointestinal problems, nightmares or inability to sleep, urination problems	

special precautions	**because**
DRUG INTERACTIONS **Phenylephrine**	
1. Amphetamines, asthma medications, sympathomimetics	1. May cause nervousness.
2. Antidepressants	2. Possible increased effects of phenylephrine and these drugs.
3. Hypertension medications, beta-blockers, digitalis, guanadrel, nicotine, nitrates, oxprenolol, phenothiazines, rauwolfia, sedatives, tranquilizers	3. Possible decreased effectiveness of phenylephrine and these drugs as well.
4. Furazolidone, MAO inhibitors, methyldopa	4. May cause increase in blood pressure, perhaps to dangerous levels.
Phenylpropanolamine	
1. Anesthetics, high blood pressure medications, tricyclic antidepressants, MAO inhibitors, sympathomimetics	1. Increased effect of phenylpropanolamine.
2. Beta-blockers, guanethidine, guanadrel, nitrates, rauwolfia, terazosin	2. Decreased effect of phenylpropanolamine and these drugs.
3. MAO inhibitors, methyldopa, ergotamine	3. Increased blood pressure, perhaps to dangerous levels.
4. Digitalis	4. Disturbances in heart rhythm.
Dextromethorphan	
1. MAO inhibitors	1. Fall in blood pressure, possible fainting, disorientation, or fever.
2. Any medication containing sedative ingredients	2. Increased sedation.

DRUG INTERACTIONS

For drug interaction warnings relating to codeine, see Chapter 15.

For drug interaction warnings relating to acetaminophen, see Chapter 14.

For drug interaction warnings relating to pseudoephedrine, See Chapter 23.

For drug interaction warnings relating to brompheniramine, see Chapter 23.

For drug interaction warnings relating to guaifenesin, see table on this medication in this chapter.

DIET

No restrictions.

ALCOHOL and TOBACCO

Avoid alcohol with drugs containing codeine, pseudoephedrine, phenylpropanolamine, or doxylamine.

No interactions with tobacco.

Alcohol will cause increased drowsiness and sedation.

PREGNANCY

Discuss with your doctor.

Some components of these medications have caused fetal defects in animals; others have not. Some, while not causing defects in humans, do have a negative impact on baby.

BREAST-FEEDING

Discuss with your doctor, though generally you may want to avoid drug or nursing.

Many of the ingredients in these combination medications enter breast milk and can affect baby.

AGE FACTOR

1. Give to children and infants only after checking with your doctor. Children under 12 should not be given medications containing doxylamine.

2. People over 60 should use cautiously.

1. Some may be too strong for children. Some also contain large percentages of alcohol and should be avoided by children.

2. Adverse and side effects may be worse in older people.

(continued)

MISSED DOSE
Follow directions on package. For most medications, you can take when you remember, then take next dose three to four hours later without doubling dose.

OVERDOSE
For likely overdose problems relating to codeine, see Chapter 15.

For likely overdose problems relating to acetaminophen, see Chapter 14.

For likely overdose problems relating to pseudoephedrine, see Chapter 23.

For likely overdose problems relating to brompheniramine, see Chapter 23.

For likely overdose problems relating to guaifenesin, see table on this medication in this chapter.

Phenylephrine
No overdose reactions expected.

Phenylpropanolamine
Get emergency medical help immediately in case of confusion, tremors, irregular pulse, or high degree of anxiety.

Dextromethorphan
Get emergency medical help immediately in case of hallucinations, breathing difficulties, coordination problems, hyperactivity, or visual problems.

STOPPING DRUG
Discontinue when symptoms have eased.

OTHERS
Do not drive or operate machinery until you have determined how medications affect you.

Contact your doctor if symptoms and illness persist for more than a week.

-28-

INSULIN AND ORAL HYPOGLYCEMICS

FOR MOST OF US, digestion and metabolism are straightforward processes that require only periodic intake of food. But for some 10 to 14 million Americans who have diabetes, the metabolic process has broken down. Some 10 to 15 percent of people with diabetes—those who have the juvenile, or type 1, form of the disease—have ceased to produce insulin, a hormone that is essential to metabolize glucose, a simple sugar that is the body's principal fuel. The remaining 85 to 90 percent of diabetic patients develop the disease later in life, usually between the ages of 45 and 60. This is known as type II, adult-onset, or insulin-resistant diabetes. In some cases, the body does not make enough insulin; more commonly, there is adequate insulin, but the body does not utilize it. Obesity is a common factor in type II diabetes, and researchers believe that excess fatty tissue somehow increases insulin resistance.

Both types of diabetes are characterized by a buildup of glucose in the bloodstream. As a result, the body starts to break down protein and fats for fuel and becomes overburdened trying to rid the body of excess sugar and the by-products of fat and protein metabolism. Urine production increases and the person feels extraordinarily thirsty and hungry. Body chemistry becomes upset, and, without treatment, the person eventually slips into

a diabetic coma and dies. This scenario can be prevented by prompt diagnosis and treatment to control the diabetes.

Although diabetes cannot be cured, appropriate medications can keep it under control and prevent or delay serious consequences, including heart disease, kidney failure, blindness, and gangrene.

By and large, type I diabetes is treated with injections of insulin (*Lente, Regular Iletin, Ultralente Iletin I, Novolin N, Velosulin Human,* and others), diet, and exercise. Patients are taught to monitor their own blood glucose and adjust their insulin doses to match food intake and exercise in order to maintain normal glucose levels.

Type II diabetes calls for a somewhat different approach. About 70 to 80 percent of patients can control their diabetes by losing weight. Unfortunately, this has proven very difficult for most patients, so medications called oral hypoglycemics such as glyburide (*Diaβeta, Micronase*) and glipizide (*Glucotrol*), are used. These drugs prompt the pancreas to make more insulin or reduce insulin resistance. About 30 percent of type II patients, however, ultimately have to take insulin shots. (Insulin must be administered directly into the bloodstream by injection because an oral form is destroyed in the digestive process.) People with type II diabetes are also encouraged to monitor their blood glucose levels to help prevent complications of the disease.

Many factors affect insulin needs—pregnancy, infection, physical activity, growth, menstruation, and stress, among others—and patients must be very attentive to their bodies and to symptoms pointing to high glucose levels as well as excessive insulin.

For more information:
American Diabetes Association, National Center
1660 Duke Street
Alexandria, VA 22314
(703) 549-1500
(800) ADA-DISC

Juvenile Diabetes Foundation International
432 Park Avenue South, 16th Floor
New York, NY 10016
(800) 223-1138
(212) 889-7575
Fax: (212) 725-7259

| drug or category: |

INSULIN

condition:
DIABETES

warning

Tell your doctor if you have or have had:
- an allergic reaction to this medication, or to any preservatives or foods
- liver, kidney, or thyroid disease

Be sure that you or someone close to you is intimately familiar with emergency procedures should you go into hypoglycemic shock.

drugs

GENERIC	BRAND	RX
Insulin	*Novolin, Velosulin Human, Lente Ilentin I, Semilente Iletin I,* others	No

form/usage

INJECTIONS: Follow your physician's instructions.

when

Same time each day.

side effects and adverse reactions

Anaphylactic shock

Skin reactions, including redness and swelling at site of injection

what to do

Get emergency medical help immediately.

Continue taking, but discuss with your physician.

special precautions

DRUG INTERACTIONS
1. Anticonvulsants, oral contraceptives, cortisone, diuretics, furosemide, thyroid medications

because

1. Decrease effect of insulin.

(continued)

DRUG INTERACTIONS

2. Oral antidiabetics, bismuth subsalicylate, MAO inhibitors, antismoking preparations containing nicotine, oxyphenbutazone, phenylbutazone, drugs containing aspirin, sulfa drugs, tetracyclines

2. Increase insulin's impact.

3. Beta-blockers

3. May cause problems with regulation of blood sugar and may also mask the warning signs of hypoglycemic shock.

4. Carteolol, sotalol

4. May extend insulin's time of impact.

DIET

No interactions reported.

ALCOHOL AND TOBACCO

Avoid alcohol or use very carefully.
No problems expected with tobacco.

Alcohol can cause hypoglycemia, brain damage.

PREGNANCY

Discuss with your doctor.

Doctor should know of your plans to become pregnant in order to help you change drug regimen, if necessary.

BREAST-FEEDING

No interactions reported.

AGE FACTOR

1. Children should use under adult supervision only.

1. To assure proper use of injections, children will need adult assistance.

2. Adults over 60 should use with caution.

2. Repeated episodes of hypoglycemia could affect behavior and mental processes permanently.

MISSED DOSE

Take injection as soon as you remember, then wait four hours until next dose. Resume schedule.

OVERDOSE

Overdose is characterized by chills, cold sweats, paleness, excessive hunger, shaking. Eat a sandwich, crackers, or sugar cubes, or drink juice. If patient loses consciousness, administer glucagon injection or call for emergency medical help.

STOPPING DRUG

Do not discontinue unless you have discussed with your doctor.

OTHERS

Do not drive or operate machinery until you have determined how medication affects you.

Periodic laboratory tests might be necessary to check effect on sugar levels.

Insulin requirements may change with alterations in diet and exercise habits.

ORAL ANTIDIABETICS

condition:
DIABETES

warning

Tell your doctor if you have or have had:
- an allergic reaction to this medication, or to any preservatives or foods
- liver or kidney problems
- thyroid disease, cardiovascular disease, or severe infection

Tell doctors and dentists you consult about other medical problems that you are taking this medication.

drugs

GENERIC	BRAND	RX
glyburide	Diaβeta, Micronase	Yes
glipizide	Glucotrol	

form/usage

TABLETS: As directed by your doctor.

when

Follow your doctor's recommendations.

side effects and adverse reactions

Low blood sugar symptoms, including cold sweats, intense hunger, and fast pulse

Skin symptoms, fever, unexplained bleeding, confusion, headaches, dizziness

Minor gastrointestinal problems

what to do

Get emergency medical help immediately.

Stop taking. Get in touch with your doctor immediately.

Continue taking, but discuss with your physician.

special precautions	because
DRUG INTERACTIONS	
1. Beta-blockers, NSAIDs, aspirin, sulfonamides, *Coumadin,* others	1. May increase the effects of the antidiabetic drug and lower blood sugar to potentially dangerous levels.
2. Thiazide diuretics, phenothiazines, phenytoin, calcium channel blockers, others	2. May reduce the glucose control effects of antidiabetic and raise blood glucose levels.
DIET	
No interactions reported.	
ALCOHOL AND TOBACCO	
Avoid alcohol. No interactions with tobacco reported.	Consuming alcohol with oral antidiabetics will cause severe reactions, including severe headaches and gastrointestinal problems, chest pains, and breathing difficulties.
PREGNANCY	
Discuss with your doctor.	You may have to switch to insulin for more effective control of blood sugar. Sugar fluctuations could cause fetal defects or fetal death.
BREAST-FEEDING	
Avoid drug or avoid nursing.	Medication will migrate into breast milk and could affect child. Discuss with your doctor.
AGE FACTOR	
1. Children rarely develop diabetes treatable by oral hypoglycemics; therefore not much is known about the impact of these drugs on them.	
2. Adults over 60 should use these drugs with caution.	2. Older adults may suffer more severe side effects. They may also retain water.

MISSED DOSE
You can take a missed dose up to two hours after scheduled time. Otherwise, wait for next dose but do not double the amount taken.

(continued)

OVERDOSE
Get emergency medical help immediately in case of coma or if patient is unconscious, has greatly increased heartbeat, feels weak, suffers cold sweats, or has severe gastrointestinal problems.

STOPPING DRUG
Do not stop taking even if you feel better until you have talked with your doctor. You may have to come off drug slowly.

OTHERS
May increase sensitivity to sun. If you go outdoors between 10 A.M. and 3 P.M., wear protective clothing and/ or sunblock.

Periodic laboratory tests might be necessary to check sugar levels as well as status of other blood components.

-29-

DIARRHEA MEDICATIONS

DIARRHEA IS AN extremely common condition marked by passage of loose watery stools. In many cases, it is a symptom of an underlying infection or disease, but it can also result from food sensitivities, allergies, or poisoning. Stress can also bring on an attack of diarrhea.

In most cases, simple diarrhea can be alleviated by over-the-counter drugs such as loperamide (*Imodium*), kaolin and pectin (*Kao-tin, Kapectolin*), attapulgite (*Kaopectate*), and bismuth subsalicylate (*Pepto-Bismol*). Some compounds work by slowing the intestinal contractions (peristalsis) that move food and fluids through the gastrointestinal tract. Other medications work by removing excess water from the stools or by countering the bacterial poisons that cause diarrhea.

In cases of prolonged diarrhea, especially if it is accompanied by fever or vomiting, it may be necessary to replenish salts and fluids to prevent dehydration. There are special electrolyte solutions for this (see Diarrhea in Children).

In some instances, doctors advise that it is best to let nature take its course. For example, diarrhea associated with uncomplicated *Salmonella* poisoning, which affects some 2 million Americans every year, is usually self-limiting and will disappear in a few days. Similarly, diarrhea due to staphylococcal bacteria, another form of food poisoning, is usually gone within 18 hours, with complete recovery in two to three days. In such cases, diarrhea is actually beneficial because it helps rid the body of the offending organism. Rest and a bland diet with plenty of fluids, extra salt, and sugar is usually all that is needed. Of course, in case of prolonged diarrhea, blood in the stools, and the presence of other symptoms a doctor should be consulted. In some cases—for example, if you have irritable bowel syndrome—your doctor may choose to recommend a prescription drug such as diphenoxylate and atropine (*Lomotil*).

Diarrhea in Children

Many doctors recommend that infants with diarrhea be put on a clear liquid diet for 24 to 48 hours and then be given the so-called BRAT diet—*b*ananas, *r*ice, *a*pplesauce, and *t*oast. The American Academy of Pediatrics has somewhat different recommendations; namely, that simple diarrhea in very young babies be handled by giving them clear liquids for 4 to 6 hours and then half-strength formula and full-strength formula or solid foods that were previously tolerated by the child within 24 hours.

Remember, however, that diarrhea in children

under age two always poses a risk of dehydration. In fact, diarrhea is a major cause of infant mortality in Third World countries. Thus, the American Academy of Pediatrics recommends that babies also be given a dextrose–electrolyte solution, such as *Pedialyte*. Such electrolyte solutions are designed specifically to replace the sodium, potassium, and sugar lost during a bout of diarrhea. (Water alone is not adequate.) The electrolyte solution should be given in small frequent doses—an ounce or two every half hour, for example. However, since the demands of the body for these solutions vary from person to person, exact amounts should be determined by instructions from doctors and those packaged with the electrolyte formulas. For older children, diluted broth, flat ginger ale or 7UP, and decaffeinated sodas may be sufficient.

DIPHENOXYLATE AND ATROPINE

condition:

DIARRHEA, INTESTINAL CRAMPS

warning

May be habit-forming.

May aggravate heart disease.

May cause severe eye pain in people with glaucoma or serious breathing problems in people with emphysema and bronchitis.

Do not take if you have jaundice or diarrhea that was caused by a germ or set off by another medication.

If you are consulting a doctor about diarrhea, tell the physician if you have or have had:

- an allergic reaction to this medication, or to preservatives or food additives
- colitis or liver disease

Tell your doctor if you are thinking about becoming pregnant or are taking any other medication.

Use of antidiarrhea drugs should be accompanied by a regimen to replace fluids and vital salts and potassium.

drugs

GENERIC	BRAND	RX
diphenoxylate and atropine	*Lomotil,* others	Yes

form/usage

TABLETS, DROPS, LIQUIDS: Tablets should be taken with liquid or food to prevent stomach irritation.

Drops and liquids should be used according to instructions with medication. Use measuring device to dispense correct dose.

when

Follow directions on label.

side effects and adverse reactions

Dry mouth, swollen gums, rapid heartbeat, restlessness, headache, vomiting, constipation, bloating, numb hands or feet

what to do

Stop taking. Get in touch with doctor immediately.

(continued)

special precautions

DRUG INTERACTIONS

1. Barbiturates, fluoxetine, guanfacine, sedatives, tranquilizers

2. Clozapine

3. Ethinamate, methyprylon, narcotics

4. Leucovorin

5. MAO inhibitors

6. Naltrexone

DIET
No interaction.

ALCOHOL AND TOBACCO
Avoid alcohol.
No nicotine interaction.

PREGNANCY
Avoid drug, if possible.

BREAST-FEEDING
Avoid drug or avoid nursing.

AGE FACTOR

1. Do not give to children under 2, and discuss with your doctor if you want to give it to a child with Down syndrome.

2. People over 60 should use cautiously.

because

1. Effects of antidiarrheal and these other drugs will be increased.

2. May be toxic to nervous system.

3. Effects are increased by antidiarrheals.

4. Has high alcohol content and may cause adverse effects.

5. Could increase blood pressure.

6. May cause drug withdrawal symptoms.

Effects of alcohol are increased. May result in excessive depression of brain activity..

In animal studies drug seemed to induce weight loss in pregnant rats and to interfere with conception when given in very high doses.

Medication enters breast milk.

1. Children, particularly those with Down syndrome, are highly sensitive to diphenoxylate and atropine, which may increase the chance of more pronounced side effects.

2. Side and adverse effects, especially shortness of breath, may be greater than younger adults. Elderly people should not take without consulting a physician and should follow a regimen that will replace fluids lost by diarrhea.

MISSED DOSE
You can take a missed dose up to two hours later. Otherwise, wait until the next dose is scheduled to be taken, but do not double the amount.

OVERDOSE
Get emergency medical help immediately in case of excitement, constriction of pupils, labored breathing, or coma.

STOPPING DRUG
May be discontinued if diarrhea abates, but check with your doctor. Call the doctor if you vomit or experience muscle or stomach cramps or sweating after you stop medication.

OTHERS
Consult with your doctor if diarrhea persists for longer than two to four days or if you develop fever.

If medication is taken for two to four days without any real improvement, contact your doctor, who may order further laboratory studies. If medication is taken for more than four days, you may need laboratory tests.

Rebound constipation may occur after two or more days of treatment of diarrhea with this drug. Some people may find that it may take several days after discontinuing the drug before bowel habits return to normal.

drug or category:

KAOLIN, PECTIN, AND ATTAPULGITE

condition:
DIARRHEA

warning

If you are consulting a doctor about diarrhea, tell the physician if you have or have had:
- an allergic reaction to this medication, or to preservatives or food additives
- dysentery, ulcers, heart disease, or asthma

Call a physician if diarrhea does not stop in a day or two or if you develop a fever. Use of antidiarrhea drugs should be accompanied by a regimen to replace fluids and vital salts and potassium.

drugs

GENERIC	BRAND	RX
kaolin and pectin	*Kao-tin, Kapectolin PG*	No
attapulgite	*Kaopectate*	

form/usage

SUSPENSION: Follow directions on package.

when

Follow recommendation with medication, usually after each loose bowel movement.

side effects and adverse reactions

Constipation

what to do

Continue taking, but discuss with your physician.

special precautions

DRUG INTERACTIONS
Most medications.

DIET
No interactions reported.

because

Antidiarrheal may interfere with their absorption.

ALCOHOL AND TOBACCO
Avoid both.

Alcohol can aggravate diarrhea and interfere with medication.

Tobacco can aggravate diarrhea.

PREGNANCY
No negative interactions reported.

BREAST-FEEDING
No problems reported.

AGE FACTOR
1. Give to children with great caution; for children under six, administer only under doctor's supervision.

2. For older adults, use only under doctor's supervision.

1. Children may have more serious side effects and loss of fluids must be closely monitored and treated.

2. Older adults are more likely to suffer side effects. Loss of fluids due to diarrhea also calls for close supervision and treatment.

MISSED DOSE
Take when you remember unless it's almost time for next dose. If it is almost time for next dose, simply return to schedule. Do not double dose.

OVERDOSE
Get in touch with a poison control center, emergency room, or doctor if there is fecal impaction—feces that have hardened and cannot be moved.

STOPPING DRUG
You can stop medication when diarrhea ends.

drug or category:

LOPERAMIDE

condition:
DIARRHEA

warning

If you are consulting a doctor about diarrhea, tell the physician if you have or have had:
- an allergic reaction to loperamide, or to preservatives or dyes
- liver or kidney disease

In high doses, medication may be habit-forming.

Use of antidiarrhea drugs should be accompanied by a regimen to replace fluids and vital salts and potassium.

drugs

GENERIC	BRAND	RX
loperamide	*Imodium*	No, for liquid and tablet forms Yes, for capsules only

form/usage

CAPSULES, TABLETS, ORAL SOLUTIONS: May be taken on an empty stomach. If irritation occurs, take with food or liquids.

Capsules may be opened.

when

Follow directions on label.

side effects and adverse reactions

Distended, immobile colon if taken for diarrhea of ulcerative colitis, rash, fever, nausea, vomiting

Drowsiness, dizziness, dry mouth, reduced appetite

what to do

Stop taking. Get in touch with doctor immediately.

Continue taking, but discuss with your physician.

special precautions	**because**

DRUG INTERACTIONS

1. Antibiotics

2. Narcotic-based drugs

1. Some antibiotics cause diarrhea. Problem is best managed by stopping antibiotic and allowing bowel function to return to normal without using an anti-diarrheal drug such as loperamide. Contact your physician if you suspect you have an antibiotic-induced diarrhea.

2. May cause severe constipation if taken with anti-diarrheal drug.

DIET
No interactions.

ALCOHOL AND TOBACCO
Use alcohol conservatively until you have chance to see if the combination affects your thinking and behavior. No problems reported with tobacco.

Drug may increase alcohol's impact on brain.

PREGNANCY
Discuss with your doctor.

No studies on humans. No problems seen in animal experiments.

BREAST-FEEDING
Avoid drug or avoid nursing.

Not known if drug passes into breast milk. No reported problems in babies.

AGE FACTOR
1. Do not give to children under two years old. In older children, follow physician's dosage instructions precisely.

2. People over 60 should start with small doses.

1. Children are very sensitive to loperamide. Watch child for drowsiness, irritability, or unusual behavior.

2. Older people are more sensitive to side effects, including constipation and sedation.

MISSED DOSE
You can take a missed dose up to two hours after it was to have been taken. Otherwise, wait until next dose is due, but do not double up.

(continued)

OVERDOSE
Get in touch with a poison control center, emergency room, or doctor if patient is lethargic, unconscious, unable to stay awake, or constipated.

STOPPING DRUG
No need to continue taking medication once diarrhea stops. However, check with your doctor, especially if you have severe gastrointestinal problems after stopping.

OTHERS
Drug has to be used for two days to determine effectiveness in controlling a single attack of diarrhea and may have to be taken for ten days to see if it controls chronic diarrhea. Consult doctor if diarrhea continues.

drug or category:

BISMUTH SUBSALICYLATE

condition:

DIARRHEA; ALSO USED FOR NAUSEA, INDIGESTION

warning

If you are consulting a physician about diarrhea, tell the doctor if you are allergic to bismuth subsalicylate, salicylates (aspirin), oil of wintergreen, or nonsteroidal anti-inflammatory drugs (ibuprofen, *Naprosyn, Indocin,* etc.).

Use of antidiarrhea drugs should be accompanied by a regimen to replace fluids and vital salts and potassium.

drugs

GENERIC	BRAND	RX
bismuth subsalicylate	*Pepto-Bismol*	No

form/usage

ORAL SUSPENSION, CHEWABLE TABLETS: Be sure to chew tablets thoroughly.

Take suspension as directed on label.

when

Follow instructions on label or those given by your doctor.

side effects and adverse reactions

Hearing loss, mild headaches, hearing and vision disturbances, rapid breathing, abdominal pains, sweating, trembling, uncontrolled movements of hands

Constipation

Black stool or darkened tongue

what to do

Stop taking. Get in touch with doctor immediately.

Continue taking, but discuss with your physician.

Do nothing. The symptoms have no medical meaning.

(continued)

special precautions	because
DRUG INTERACTIONS	
1. Anticoagulants and other "blood thinners," insulin medications	1. Increases their impact.
2. Probenecid, tetracyclines, sulfinpyrazone	2. Decreases their effectiveness.
DIET	
No restrictions.	
ALCOHOL AND TOBACCO	
No interactions.	
PREGNANCY	
Avoid drug.	Other similar drugs, including aspirin, have been shown to cause birth defects in animals and may cause bleeding problems in the human fetus during the last two weeks of pregnancy or during delivery. Excessive use of salicylates during the last trimester has been linked to extended pregnancies and labor, and may cause other problems during delivery.
BREAST-FEEDING	
Avoid drug or avoid nursing.	Medication passes into breast milk and large amounts of salicylates may cause problems in baby.
AGE FACTOR	
1. Do not give to children.	1. Children react more sensitively to salicylates, and the use of these drugs in connection with viral diseases has been associated with Reye's syndrome.
2. Adults over 60 should take with care.	2. Older persons are also more sensitive to salicylates.
MISSED DOSE	

Take when you remember it, but don't double up on dose. However, if it is almost time for your next dose, skip the missed dose and return to your regular schedule. Do not double dose.

OVERDOSE
Get in touch with a poison control center, emergency room, or doctor if patient is anxious, confused, or depressed; is trembling or having muscle spasms; or is having trouble talking.

STOPPING DRUG
Okay to stop when diarrhea stops.

OTHERS
Salicylates may increase bleeding problems in people predisposed to them and may worsen stomach ulcers.

May interfere with urine tests for sugar.

d r u g   o r   c a t e g o r y :

FLUID AND ELECTROLYTE SOLUTIONS

c o n d i t i o n :
DEHYDRATION AFTER DIARRHEA

warning

Do not use if kidneys are not functioning.
All doctors attending to the patient should be told that he or she is taking an electrolyte solution.
Should not be used with any other medicine or drug without consulting your physician.

drugs

GENERIC	BRAND	RX
dextrose and electrolytes	*Pedialyte, Rehydralyte*	Some
rice syrup solids and electrolytes	*Ricelyte*	

form/usage

FLUIDS: Usage will vary according to patient. Follow your doctor's instructions and instructions on label.

when

Follow your doctor's or label's instructions.

side effects and adverse reactions

Excessive fluid buildup

Vomiting

what to do

Stop taking. Get in touch with doctor immediately.

If vomiting is severe, discontinue. Otherwise, continue taking, but discuss with your physician.

special precautions

DRUG INTERACTIONS
None.

DIET
Discuss with your doctor.

because

Some foods will promote diarrhea and in turn continued dehydration. Doctor may have dietary suggestions.

ALCOHOL AND TOBACCO
Avoid both.

Alcohol dehydrates body further.

Tobacco is an intestinal stimulant and could increase severity of diarrhea.

PREGNANCY
No side effects reported.

BREAST-FEEDING
No side effects reported.

AGE FACTOR
1. If patient is under six months of age, discuss with doctor before administering.

2. No problem reported in patients over 60.

1. Safety and efficacy not established.

MISSED DOSE
Can be taken up to two hours after scheduled dose. If more than two hours have elapsed, wait until next regularly scheduled dose, but do not double amount taken.

OVERDOSE
Get emergency medical help immediately in case of seizures or convulsions.

STOPPING DRUG
Check with doctor.

OTHERS
Periodic blood pressure monitoring, blood component tests, and check on weight may be advisable.

-30-

- - - - - - - - - - - - - - - -

FERTILITY DRUGS

INFERTILITY IS A growing problem in the United States, affecting an estimated one out of every five to seven couples. In general, infertility is defined as failure to conceive after a year of regular intercourse without birth control. There are many reasons for the decline, including the growing trend to delay parenthood, thereby bypassing a woman's most fertile years—ages 18 to 25. The increased incidence of pelvic inflammatory disease and sexually transmitted diseases contributes to infertility, as can endometriosis, uterine malformations or tumors, adhesions that have formed after surgery, hormonal problems, and obesity. Smoking and alcohol abuse reduce both male and female fertility. Causes of male infertility range from varicose veins in the scrotum (varicocele) to low sperm counts and hormonal imbalances. Even wearing tight-fitting clothing or regular use of a hot tub can damage sperm, which are very sensitive to heat.

The rise in infertility has been paralleled by an increase in fertility clinics and specialists offering a wide range of treatments—microsurgery to repair damaged fallopian tubes, test tube fertilization, artificial insemination, and a host of other procedures. There are also numerous fertility drugs that help many thousands of patients conceive.

If tests show that the man, woman, or both have a deficit or imbalance in reproductive hormones, the treatment of choice involves the administration of hormone drugs. The key ones are:

- **Clomiphene** (*Clomid, Serophene*), which stimulates the hypothalamus to prod the pituitary gland to increase hormone production, thereby stimulating the gonads.

- **Menotropins** (*Pergonal*), which directly affect the pituitary gland to increase stimulation of the ovaries.

Extreme care is needed when using these drugs to avoid overstimulation, which can result in multiple births and even ovarian rupture. Side effects include mood swings, physical discomfort, and rapid weight gain. *Pergonal* and *Clomid* may also slightly increase the risk of ovarian cancer.

---

drug or category:

CLOMIPHENE

condition:
FEMALE/MALE INFERTILITY

---

warning

Can lead to multiple births.
Drug could spur increases in size of existing ovarian cysts or fibroid tumors, or worsen endometriosis.
Tell your doctor if you have or have had:
• an allergic reaction to this drug, or to dyes or preservatives
• inflammations of the veins
• liver disease
• depression or unusual vaginal bleeding
Inform your doctor and pharmacist of all medications you are taking, whether prescription or over-the-counter.

---

drugs

GENERIC	BRAND	RX
clomiphene	Clomid, Serophene	Yes

---

form/usage

TABLETS: Follow your doctor's instructions on dosage and frequency. May be taken with water.

when

Men should take at same time every day; women should follow doctor's instructions.

---

side effects and adverse reactions

Abdominal pain, vomiting, bloating, vision problems, jaundice

Breast tenderness, dizziness, headache, heavy menstrual flow, depression, nausea and other gastrointestinal problems, insomnia, restlessness, fatigue, hot flashes

what to do

Stop taking. Get in touch with doctor immediately.

Continue taking, but discuss with your physician.

---

special precautions

DRUG INTERACTIONS
Thyroid preparations

because

Could increase their effect.

(continued)

DIET
No restrictions.

ALCOHOL AND TOBACCO
No restrictions.

PREGNANCY
Stop taking immediately if you believe you are pregnant. Call your doctor.

May cause severe fetal defects.

BREAST-FEEDING
Drug is discontinued long before breast-feeding starts.

AGE FACTOR
Not a factor.

MISSED DOSE
Take as soon as possible. If you forget until next dose is due, take a double dose, then return to schedule. You should check with your doctor if you forget to take more than one dose.

OVERDOSE
Get emergency medical help immediately if person taking drug is suddenly short of breath.

STOPPING DRUG
Discontinue immediately if pregnant. Discuss with your physician.

OTHERS
Schedule regular checkups to determine if drug is working and to monitor for side effects.

Determine your reaction to medication before driving or operating machinery.

May make eyes more sensitive to light.

drug or category:

MENOTROPINS

condition:

MALE/FEMALE INFERTILITY

warning

May cause multiple births.

Tell your doctor if you have had:

- an allergic reaction to menotropins
- asthma
- epilepsy or heart or kidney disease
- migraines
- ovarian cysts, fibroid tumors in uterus, or unusual vaginal bleeding
- any pituitary gland problems

Tell your doctor or pharmacist if you are taking other prescription or over-the-counter medications, particularly diuretics.

drugs

GENERIC	BRAND	RX
menotropins	*Pergonal*	Yes

form/usage

INJECTIONS: May be self-administered. Discuss with your physician.

when

Discuss with your physician.

side effects and adverse reactions

1. Women: Bloating, stomach pain, reaction at injection site, fever and chills, rapid weight gain

2. Men: Dizziness, fainting, headache, change in heartbeat, loss of appetite, shortness of breath

what to do

1. Get in touch with your doctor immediately.

---

1. Women: Abdominal or stomach pain, bloating, decreased urine output, gastrointestinal problems, pelvic pain, rapid weight gain

2. Men: Enlargement of breasts

1. Call your physician.

2. Continue taking drug, but discuss with your physician.

(continued)

special precautions	because
DRUG INTERACTIONS May interact with other hormone products. Check with your doctor.	While no clinically significant interactions have been reported, some combinations may produce adverse side effects. Physician may have to adjust your dosage.
DIET No restrictions.	
ALCOHOL AND TOBACCO Discuss with your doctor.	While no problems have been reported, alcohol and tobacco may decrease fertility.
PREGNANCY Discontinue as soon as you know you are pregnant.	May cause severe fetal defects.
BREAST-FEEDING Avoid drug or avoid nursing.	Safety has not been established and drug may pass into breast milk.
MISSED DOSE Discuss with your doctor.	
OVERDOSE **Call your doctor or poison control center** if you have abdominal pain (in women, this may point to ovarian enlargement) or if you feel you have taken too much.	
STOPPING DRUG Discuss with your doctor.	
OTHERS Schedule regular checkups to determine efficacy of medicine and to monitor its effect on your body. It is important that women take their temperature every day as directed by doctor so that intercourse can take place at correct time to increase chances of pregnancy.	

-31-

GASTROINTESTINAL PREPARATIONS

HEARTBURN, INDIGESTION, AND other stomach upsets are exceedingly common complaints, as evidenced by the fact that there are more than a hundred different over-the-counter antacids—products such as *Mylanta, Maalox, Rolaids, Tums,* and milk of magnesia. These products also may alleviate the symptoms of peptic ulcers, although they do not provide a cure or long-term relief.

The passage of intestinal gas, or flatulence, is a common problem that is more embarrassing than a threat to health. Products made of simethicone (*Mylicon, Gas Relief,* and others) are promoted to counter flatulence, but gastroenterologists tend to downplay their effectiveness and stress dietary modification instead. Beans, onions, brussels sprouts, and certain sugars and starches are common offenders, as is lactose, the sugar in milk. People who are lactose-intolerant, meaning they lack lactase, the enzyme needed to digest lactose, are especially prone to develop intestinal bloating, cramps, and flatulence. Lactase pills are available to improve lactose digestion; there also are numerous lactose-free dairy products on the market.

For detailed tabular information on *Pepto-Bismol* (bismuth subsalicylate), see Chapter 29.

Peptic Ulcers

Recent studies indicate that these ulcers are actually caused by a bacterium, and treatment involves prescribing antibiotics as well as ulcer medications. The offending organism, *Helicobacter pylori,* normally resides in the human intestinal tract but causes ulcers in only 5 to 10 percent of the people who harbor it. Why only some people are affected by the bacterium is unknown, but a genetic predisposition is suspected. Use of cigarettes, alcohol, caffeine, and aspirin and other anti-inflammatory drugs, as well as stress, may play a role in susceptible people. Trauma, especially severe burns and surgery, can also provoke ulcers.

There is little or no evidence to support earlier recommendations to follow a bland diet. However, it is important to abstain from caffeine, smoking, and alcohol, all of which exacerbate peptic ulcers.

In addition to antibiotics (see Chapter 19), drugs that are prescribed for ulcers include:

• **Coating agents.** Drugs such as sucralfate (*Carafate, Sulcrate*) promote ulcer healing by forming a protective coating over the ulcer that keeps acid away from it. It may also block pepsin, a digestive enzyme that contributes to the formation of ulcers.

- **H₂ receptor blockers.** As their name implies, these drugs—which include cimetidine (*Tagamet*), ranitidine (*Zantac*), famotidine (*Pepcid*)—work by blocking the histamines that contribute to the production of hydrochloric acid.

Inflammatory Bowel Disease

Inflammatory bowel disease, or IBD, afflicts an estimated 2 million Americans; although there are medications and strategies that help control IBD, a cure is not expected in the foreseeable future.

There are two major forms of IBD—**ulcerative colitis**, marked by inflammation and ulceration of the entire colon, and **Crohn's disease**, which affects sporadic portions of both the colon and small intestine. Both forms produce severe diarrhea, rectal bleeding, weight loss, and abdominal pain. Both illnesses also show a predilection for the young. They usually are diagnosed in people less than 30 years old—including 200,000 children under the age of 16.

At one time, stress and diet were thought to be causative factors in inflammatory bowel disorders, but neither appears to play a role. Researchers now think that an autoimmune system response, in which the immune system attacks healthy tissue, is responsible. What triggers the response is unknown—viruses, stress, a genetic predisposition, and other factors may play a role.

Typically, inflammatory bowel diseases come and go, and each flare-up requires intensive treatment. Drugs commonly used include:

- **Sulfasalazines.** These drugs—including *Azalin, PMS Sulfasalazine, SAS-Enteric*, and others—probably work by interfering with the production of prostaglandins and other compounds that lead to inflammation and the destruction of intestinal tissues. The medications can be taken as oral solutions, tablets, capsules, or enemas.

- **Corticosteroids.** Medicines like prednisone and hydrocortisone (*Cortenema*) work by countering the inflammatory process. Although mainstays in the treatment of colitis, their long-term use produces numerous adverse effects, including lowered resistance to infections, weight gain, bone thinning, and bleeding problems.

- **Mesalamine.** Drugs like *Rowasa*, which are administered as rectal suspensions, suppositories, and sustained-release tablets, are thought to work by blocking the prostaglandins that produce inflammation.

Gallstones

Gallstones, a common problem especially in overweight middle-aged women, can cause attacks of severe abdominal pain, especially if a stone becomes lodged in the common bile duct. Surgical removal of the gallstones is the usual treatment, but in some cases, drugs such as ursodiol (*Actigall*) may be prescribed to dissolve the stones, which are composed mostly of cholesterol crystals.

drug or category:

OVER-THE-COUNTER ANTACIDS

condition:

ACID STOMACH, PEPTIC ULCER, GASTRITIS, HIATAL HERNIA

warning

Tell your doctor if you have or have had:
- an allergic reaction to this medication
- high calcium levels, kidney problems, continuing and severe gastrointestinal problems
- an irregular heartbeat or congestive heart failure

drugs

GENERIC	BRAND	RX
Many generic ingredients	*Mylanta, Maalox, Gaviscon, Rolaids, Tums,* and many others	No

form/usage

TABLETS, SUSPENSIONS: According to instructions on package.

when

One to three hours after meals. If you are using in combination with other antiulcer drugs, discuss schedule with your doctor.

side and adverse effects

Irregular heartbeat (especially in heart patients), constipation, distended stomach, frequent urination, muscle pain, weight gain, mood and behavior changes

Feelings of lethargy, mild diarrhea, bad taste in mouth, stomach pain

what to do

Stop taking. Get in touch with doctor immediately.

Continue taking, but discuss with your physician.

(continued)

special precautions	because
DRUG INTERACTIONS	
1. No medications should be taken simultaneously with antacids. Wait a minimum of two hours.	1. Antacids will slow absorption of all other medications.
2. Chlorpromazine, digitalis, isoniazid, ketoconazole, methenamine, nalidixic acid, nicardipine, nizatidine, ofloxacin, oxyphenbutazone, *para*-aminosalicylic acid, penicillin, tetracycline, iron supplements	2. Antacids diminish their effect.
3. Aspirin, levodopa, meperidine, pseudoephedrine	3. Their effect is increased.
4. Ciprofloxacin	4. May cause kidney problems.
DIET	
Take antacids one hour after eating.	Food will diminish their effect.
ALCOHOL AND TOBACCO	
Avoid both.	Both diminish the effect of antacids.
PREGNANCY	
Avoid drug.	While no studies have been done in either humans or animals, drug may cause fetal problems or side effects in babies following long-term use, particularly in high doses during pregnancy .
BREAST-FEEDING	
Avoid antacids or avoid nursing.	Antacids pass into breast milk and could affect child.
AGE FACTOR	
1. Give to children only under doctor's supervision.	1. Side effects of antacids may be more severe in children. Also, symptoms may be caused by other problems.
2. If over 60, use carefully.	2. Side effects of antacids may be more pronounced in older people.
MISSED DOSE	
Take when you remember it unless it is almost time for your next dose; in this case, skip your missed dose and return to regular schedule. Do not double dose.	

OVERDOSE

Get in touch with poison control center, emergency room, or doctor in case of dry mouth, pain in bones, fatigue, breathing difficulties, or diarrhea.

STOPPING DRUG

Stop taking when you no longer have discomfort.

OTHERS

Do not take continuously or for more than two weeks without consulting a physician. You may have a peptic ulcer and require more precise medication. Also, continuing use of antacids could lead to kidney problems or kidney stones and excessive buildup of calcium.

Avoid antacids containing aluminum if you have chronic constipation or chronic kidney failure. Avoid antacids containing only magnesium if you have chronic diarrhea.

drug or category:

SUCRALFATE

condition:
ULCERS

warning

Tell your doctor if you have or have had:
- have or have had an allergic reaction to this medication
- have or have had kidney failure
- have constipation regularly
- are taking any other medication
- have surgery scheduled within eight weeks

drugs

GENERIC	BRAND	RX
sucralfate	*Carafate, Sulcrate*	Yes

form/usage

TABLETS: Take with water on an empty stomach.

Take tablet whole. Do not chew or crumble.

If you need to take an antacid for pain, take it half an hour or more before or after you take sucralfate.

when

One hour before or two hours after meals and at bedtime.

side effects and adverse reactions

Diarrhea

Constipation, dizziness, rash or itch, nausea, dry mouth, back pain

what to do

Stop taking. Get in touch with doctor immediately.

Continue taking, but discuss with your physician.

special precautions	because
DRUG INTERACTIONS 1. Antacids containing aluminum	1. May increase risk of aluminum poisoning in patients with kidney failure.
2. Cimetidine, digoxin, phenytoin, tetracycline, warfarin	2. Sucralfate decreases their effectiveness.
DIET Avoid foods that increase stomach acidity, such as protein-rich foods and beverages with caffeine.	
ALCOHOL AND TOBACCO Avoid both.	Alcohol irritates the stomach. Nicotine delays effectiveness of this drug.
PREGNANCY Discuss with your doctor.	Impact of drug on fetus has not been established.
BREAST-FEEDING Avoid drug or avoid nursing.	Drug enters breast milk and could affect child.
AGE FACTOR 1. Administer to children with caution only under doctor's supervision.	1. Safety and efficacy have not been determined.
2. People older than 60 should take this drug carefully.	2. Adverse effects in elderly can be more severe.
MISSED DOSE May be taken up to two hours after scheduled time; if it is later, wait for next scheduled dose, but do not double amount.	
OVERDOSE **Get in touch with a poison control center, emergency room, or doctor** if you think you have taken too much. However, there has been no previous experience with overdose in humans; taking excessive amounts of this medication has not been reported to threaten life.	

(continued)

STOPPING DRUG

Do not stop taking even if you feel better until you have talked with your doctor. You may have to come off drug slowly.

OTHERS

Long-term use may cause deficiencies of vitamins A, D, E, and K. Discuss with your doctor.

Do not drive or operate machinery until you have determined how medication affects you.

drug or category:

CIMETIDINE

condition:
ULCERS

warning

Tell your doctor if you have or have had:
- a previous allergic reaction to this medication
- liver or kidney disease
- a low sperm count

Tell your doctor if you are taking aspirin or anticoagulants, propranolol, quinidine, theophylline, or cyclosporine.

drugs

GENERIC	BRAND	RX
cimetidine	*Tagamet*	Yes

form/usage

TABLETS, SOLUTION, INJECTIONS: Tablets may be crushed and may be taken with liquids.

Take solution with liquid.

when

For existing ulcer, four times a day at meals and at bedtime. For prevention, at bedtime only.

For condition in which acid washes back into esophagus, twice a day.

side effects and adverse reactions

Rash, sore throat, irregular heartbeat, muscle pain, fever

Constipation or diarrhea, decline in libido, headache, hair loss, breast enlargement in men

what to do

Stop taking. Get in touch with doctor immediately.

Continue taking, but discuss with your physician.

(continued)

special precautions	because
DRUG INTERACTIONS	
1. Antacid, metoclopramide	1. Decrease absorption of cimetidine.
2. Anticoagulants, carbamazepine, chlordiazepoxide, diazepam, digitalis, flurazepam, glipizide, labetalol, methadone, metoprolol, metronidazole, morphine, nicardipine, nimodipine, phenytoin, procainamide, propafenone, propranolol, quinidine, triazolam, verapamil, theophylline, cyclosporine	2. Cimetidine increases their effect. May lead to toxicity in some cases.
3. Ketoconazole, tamoxifen	3. Its effect is decreased.
4. Anticholinergics, encainide, moricizine	4. Increase the effect of cimetidine.
DIET	
Avoid foods that increase stomach acidity, including beverages with caffeine and protein-rich foods.	
ALCOHOL and TOBACCO	
Avoid alcohol or use sparingly.	Alcohol does not interact with drug, but it does stimulate acid production.
Avoid tobacco.	Nicotine interferes with drug.
PREGNANCY	
Discuss with your doctor, though there are no reports of harm to child.	There has been no fetal harm reported in animals, but no studies have been done in humans.
BREAST-FEEDING	
No adverse effects on baby have been reported.	
AGE FACTOR	
1. Do not give to children under 16. If absolutely necessary, monitor child closely.	1. Safety and effectiveness in children have not been determined.
2. People over 60 and especially those who have difficulty chewing should use very carefully.	2. Drug can lead to aggregation of masses of undigested vegetables in stomach. Can also cause mood and behavior changes.

MISSED DOSE

Can be taken up to two hours later; otherwise, wait until next scheduled dose, but do not double amount taken.

OVERDOSE

Get emergency medical help immediately in case of speech and breathing difficulties, confusion, or delirium.

STOPPING DRUG

Do not discontinue abruptly, and consult with your doctor about stopping use. Tell your physician immediately if ulcer symptoms return after you have stopped.

OTHERS

Patients on dialysis should take medication after treatment because dialysis can remove up to 14 percent of drug.

Do not drive or operate machinery until you have determined if drug makes you drowsy or affects your reflexes in any way.

Periodic laboratory tests might be necessary to check blood count, liver and kidney function, sperm count, and blood clotting times.

drug or category:

HYDROCORTISONE

condition:

INFLAMMATORY BOWEL DISEASE

warning

Tell your doctor if you have or have had:
- an allergic reaction to this or other steroid medications
- ulcers or diabetes
- viral or fungus infections
- thyroid, heart, kidney, or liver problems

If you are scheduled for allergy tests or surgery, or if you get an infection up to two years after using this drug, tell the physician with whom you are consulting.

Prolonged use may cause glaucoma, high blood pressure, and water retention.

drugs

GENERIC	BRAND	RX
hydrocortisone	*Cortenema*	Yes

form/usage

ENEMA: Follow doctor's or package label's instructions.

when

At night. Try to retain all night.

side effects and adverse reactions

Vision problems, frequent urination; rectal problems, including bleeding

Roundness in face, weakness, nausea, bloody stool, skin problems, stomach pain, increased appetite, unusual hair growth

what to do

Stop taking. Get in touch with doctor immediately.

Continue taking, but discuss with your physician.

special precautions

DRUG INTERACTIONS
1. Amphotericin B, digitalis

because

1. Decrease potassium in blood and cause heart problems.

DRUG INTERACTIONS

2. Antidiabetics

2. Increase in blood sugar levels.

3. Diuretics, medicines with potassium

3. May decrease effectiveness of diuretics and may disturb blood levels of potassium.

4. Avoid vaccination while taking drug or until your doctor approves. Avoid people who have had recent vaccinations.

4. Drug suppresses immune response and could increase your susceptibility to organisms used to make vaccines.

DIET

Your doctor may want you to follow a diet:
   low in salt
   high in potassium and calcium
   rich in proteins

Hydrocortisone will cause an increase in salt retention, a loss of potassium, and an increased use of protein by the body. It also leads to an increase in calcium excretion.

ALCOHOL and TOBACCO

Discuss alcohol use with your doctor.

Though no interactions have been reported, alcohol may produce adverse effects including gastro-intestinal problems.

Avoid tobacco.

Tobacco may increase the drug's effect and cause poisoning.

PREGNANCY

Discuss with your doctor.

Effect on pregnancy or fetus has not been established.

BREAST-FEEDING

Avoid drug or avoid nursing.

Drug passes into breast milk.

AGE FACTOR

1. Administer to children carefully and follow doctor's instructions precisely.

1. May inhibit growth in children and teenagers.

2. People over 60 years of age should use cautiously.

2. Increases risk of high blood pressure and bone disease.

MISSED DOSE

Take it as soon as you remember it. However, if it is almost time for your next dose, skip the missed dose and just return to your regular dosage schedule. Do not take double doses.

(continued)

OVERDOSE
No overdose problems with use of this drug are anticipated.

STOPPING DRUG
Enemas are usually taken for three weeks, though difficult cases may require two to three months. Discuss with your doctor how to discontinue drug, though usual procedure is to discontinue slowly, usually by switching to an every-other-night schedule for three weeks.

drug or category:

DICYCLOMINE

condition:

INFLAMMATORY BOWEL DISEASE

warning

Tell your doctor if you have or have had:
- an allergic reaction to this medication or similar medication
- myasthenia gravis
- open-angle glaucoma
- liver, kidney, or thyroid disorders
- heart disease or respiratory difficulties

Tell your doctor if you are going to have surgery.

drugs

GENERIC	BRAND	RX
dicyclomine	*Bentyl, Antispas, Di-Spaz,* others	Yes

form/usage

CAPSULES, TABLETS, SYRUP: Take with food or beverage to prevent stomach irritation.

when

Usually half an hour before meals, but consult your doctor.

side effects and adverse reactions

Rash, hives, light-headedness, confusion, change in heart rhythm, vision changes, eye pain

Vomiting, nausea, constipation, headache, urination problems, nasal congestion

Dry mouth

what to do

Stop taking. Get in touch with doctor immediately.

Continue taking, but discuss with your doctor.

Chew gum or melt ice in your mouth. Consult with your dentist if dryness persists for more than two weeks.

(continued)

special precautions	because

DRUG INTERACTIONS

1. Amantadine, anticholinergics, tricyclic antidepressants, antihistamines, buclizine, MAO inhibitors, meperidine, methylphenidate, orphenadrine, phenothiazines, quinidine, sedatives

2. Antacids, antidiarrheal medications, large doses of vitamin C

3. Digitalis

4. Haloperidol

5. Ketoconazole, pilocarpine

6. Potassium supplements

1. Increase effect of dicyclomine.

2. Decrease effect of dicyclomine.

3. May decrease digitalis's effectiveness.

4. Increases pressures within eyes.

5. Decreases effectiveness of these two drugs.

6. Could lead to ulcers.

DIET

No interactions, though a low-fiber diet may help relieve symptoms.

ALCOHOL and TOBACCO

No interactions. However, both should be avoided since they both exacerbate symptoms of IBD.

PREGNANCY

Avoid drug unless absolutely necessary. Discuss with your doctor.

Medication has increased birth defects in animals.

BREAST-FEEDING

Avoid drug or avoid nursing.

Drug passes into breast milk.

AGE FACTOR

1. Administer very carefully to children, and follow doctor's instructions precisely.

2. Adults over 60 should use very carefully.

1. May cause behavioral changes, skin problems.

2. Can cause confusion, behavior and mood problems. May worsen or cause glaucoma.

MISSED DOSE

May be taken up to two hours after scheduled time. If more than two hours have passed, wait until next dose but do not double amount taken.

OVERDOSE

Get emergency medical help immediately in case of hallucinations, coma, convulsions, dizziness, dilated pupils, slurred speech, or rapid pulse and breathing.

STOPPING DRUG

Discuss with your doctor. You may not have to finish entire prescription, but may have to discontinue gradually.

OTHERS

Do not drive or operate machinery until you have determined how medication affects you, especially if you are taking other drugs that cause drowsiness or dizziness or if you use alcoholic beverages.

May cause your body temperature to rise. Exercise cautiously. Use caution in hot weather.

Wear sunglasses because drug could make your eyes more sensitive to light.

BELLADONA ALKALOIDS AND BARBITURATES

condition:
INFLAMMATORY BOWEL DISEASE

warning

Tell your doctor if you have or have had:
- an allergic reaction to this medication, its components, or similar medications
- myasthenia gravis
- liver, kidney, or thyroid disorders
- heart disease, glaucoma, urinary retention, or respiratory difficulties

Tell your doctor if you are:
- following a low-sodium or low-sugar diet
- pregnant
- taking any other drugs that cause drowsiness
- going to have surgery

Can cause a decrease in effectiveness of oral contraceptives.

drugs

GENERIC	BRAND	RX
phenobarbital, atropine, scopolamine, hyoscyamine	*Donnatal*	Yes

form/usage

CAPSULES (REGULAR AND EXTENDED-RELEASE), ELIXIR, TABLETS (REGULAR, CHEWABLE, AND EXTENDED-RELEASE): Take tablets, capsules, and liquid with food or beverage to prevent stomach irritation.

Regular tablets can be crushed and regular capsules can be opened, but extended-release tablets and capsules should be swallowed whole.

when

Usually half an hour before bedtime, but consult your doctor.

side effects and adverse reactions

Rash, hives, light-headedness, confusion, change in heart rhythm, vision changes

Vomiting, nausea, constipation, headache, urination problems

Dry mouth

what to do

Stop taking. Get in touch with doctor immediately.

Continue taking, but discuss with your doctor.

Chew gum or melt ice in your mouth. Consult with your dentist if dryness persists for more than two weeks.

special precautions

DRUG INTERACTIONS
1. Do not take within one hour of antacids or anti-diarrheals.

2. Any drug with sedative effect (antihistamines, antianxiety medications, etc.)

3. Anticoagulants, beta-blockers, cortisone, doxycy-cline, griseofulvin, oral contraceptives, quinidine, the-ophylline

4. Valproic acid

DIET
No interactions, but a low-fiber diet may relieve IBS symptoms.

ALCOHOL AND TOBACCO
Avoid both.

PREGNANCY
Avoid drug.

BREAST-FEEDING
Avoid drug or avoid nursing.

because

1. Will make *Donnatal* less effective.

2. Will increase their effect.

3. Will decrease their effect.

4. Will increase effects of *Donnatal*.

Will increase the sedative effect of the drug.

Some ingredients in medication increase risk of birth defects and may cause bleeding in newborns.

Drug passes into breast milk.

(continued)

AGE FACTOR

I. Administer very carefully to children, follow doctor's instructions precisely.

2. Adults over 60 should use very carefully.

I. May cause behavioral changes, skin problems.

2. Can cause confusion, behavior and mood problems. May worsen or cause glaucoma.

MISSED DOSE

Take as soon as you remember. However, if you remember when it is almost time for next dose, wait. Do not double the next dose.

OVERDOSE

Get emergency medical help immediately in case of hallucinations, coma, convulsions, dizziness, dilated pupils, slurred speech, or rapid pulse and breathing.

STOPPING DRUG

Discuss with your doctor. In most cases the drug should not be discontinued suddenly.

OTHERS

Do not drive or operate machinery until you have determined how medication affects you, especially if you are taking other drugs that cause drowsiness or dizziness.

May cause your body temperature to rise. Exercise cautiously. Use caution in hot weather.

Wear sunglasses because drug could make your eyes more sensitive to light.

May cause decrease in sexual desire.

Can lead to psychological and physiological dependence.

drug or category:

FAMOTIDINE

condition:
ULCERS

warning

Tell your doctor if you have or have had:
• an allergic reaction to *Pepcid* or other antiulcer drugs, including *Tagamet* or *Zantac*
Use carefully if you have kidney disease.

drugs

GENERIC	BRAND	RX
famotidine	*Pepcid*	Yes

form/usage

SUSPENSION, TABLETS, INJECTION: May be used concurrently with antacids to help relieve ulcer pain.

Tablet may be crushed.

Oral suspension requires reconstitution with water prior to use.

when

Best to take with a meal. Consult instructions provided by your doctor or label on medication.

side effects and adverse reactions

Pain in abdomen, constipation, bleeding problems, skin problems

Gastrointestinal problems, decreased sex drive, mood changes, loss of hair, bad taste in mouth

what to do

Stop taking. Get in touch with doctor immediately.

Continue taking, but discuss with your physician.

special precautions

DRUG INTERACTIONS
Ketoconazole, tamoxifen

because

May decrease their effectiveness.

(continued)

DIET

1. Follow a diet recommended by your doctor; generally it is wise to avoid protein-rich foods.

2. Avoid drinks with caffeine.

1. Foods high in protein spur stomach to increase production of acid.

2. Decreases drug's effectiveness.

ALCOHOL and TOBACCO

Avoid alcohol or use sparingly.

Alcohol does not interfere with drug per se but is thought to increase stomach acidity and reduce ability of drug to work.

Avoid tobacco.

Tobacco decreases effectiveness of drug and its ability to reduce acid secretion.

PREGNANCY

Discuss with your doctor.

Effects of *Pepcid* on pregnancy and fetus have not been determined.

BREAST-FEEDING

Avoid drug or avoid nursing.

Medication is passed into breast milk.

AGE FACTOR

1. Do not give to children.

2. People over 60 should use cautiously and should watch for signs of gastrointestinal distress after taking medicine.

1. Effectiveness and safety have not been established.

2. Masses of undigested vegetables may form in stomach of people who are unable to chew foods well or have had stomach surgery.

MISSED DOSE

You may take a missed dose up to two hours after scheduled time. If more than two hours have elapsed, wait for next scheduled dose, but do not double amount taken.

OVERDOSE

Get emergency medical help immediately in case of seizures, coma, or rapid increase in heartbeat.

STOPPING DRUG

Drug should not be taken at high dosages for longer than six to eight weeks. If drug gives you relief, the amount you take will be cut back. Do not discontinue without discussing with your doctor. If you do discontinue and ulcer symptoms return, let your doctor know immediately.

OTHERS

Be sure to ask your physician if you should be checked for stomach malignancy even if symptoms disappear with medication.

Avoid driving or operating machinery until you determine whether drug makes you dizzy.

May interfere with allergy tests.

Periodic laboratory tests might be necessary to check blood counts.

drug or category:

SIMETHICONE

condition:
FLATULENCE (INTESTINAL GAS)

warning

Tell your doctor if you have or have had a previous allergic reaction to this medication or food additives, including sulfites.

drugs

GENERIC	BRAND	RX
simethicone	*Mylicon, Gas Relief,* others	No

form/usage

CAPSULES, TABLETS (REGULAR AND CHEWABLE), SUSPENSIONS: Chewable tablets must be chewed thoroughly. Take suspension by mixing recommended amount in liquid.

when

After meals and at bedtime.

side effects and adverse reactions

None expected.

what to do

special precautions

DRUG INTERACTIONS
None reported.

DIET
No interactions, but avoid foods that contribute to gas formation (see Miscellaneous Intestinal Problems at the beginning of this chapter).

ALCOHOL AND TOBACCO
No interactions reported.

because

PREGNANCY

No problems reported.

---   ---

BREAST-FEEDING

No problems reported.

---   ---

AGE FACTOR

1. Acts the same in children as in adults.

2. Older adults should use cautiously.   2. No studies have been performed to determine effect on people over 60.

---   ---

MISSED DOSE

If you are on a schedule, take missed dose as soon as you remember. If you remember an hour or so before next dose, wait until that one, but do not double amount taken.

OVERDOSE

No life-threatening impact.

STOPPING DRUG

When problem is resolved.

drug or category:

MESALAMINE

condition:
INFLAMMATORY BOWEL DISEASE

warning

Tell your doctor if you have or have had:
- a previous allergic reaction to this medication or to aspirin, olsalazine, or sulfasalazine
- kidney disease
- allergies, including hay fever and asthma

drugs

GENERIC	BRAND	RX
mesalamine	*Rowasa, Asacol, Salofalk*	Yes

form/usage

RECTAL SUSPENSION, SUPPOSITORIES, SUSTAINED-RELEASE TABLETS: Suspension is used as an enema. It is most effective in an empty bowel and should therefore be administered after a bowel movement.

Take tablet on an empty stomach with water. Do not crush or crumble.

when

Enema: At bedtime. Should be retained all night.

Tablet: One hour before or two hours after meals. However, may be taken with food if drug irritates the stomach.

side effects and adverse reactions

Gastrointestinal problems like diarrhea or vomiting; fever; rash

Hair loss, nausea, headache

what to do

Stop taking. Get in touch with doctor immediately.

Continue taking, but discuss with your doctor.

special precautions

DRUG INTERACTIONS
Sulfasalazine

because

May cause kidney damage.

DIET
No interactions.

--   --

ALCOHOL AND TOBACCO
No interactions.

--   --

PREGNANCY
Discuss with your doctor.   Effect on pregnancy or fetus not established.

--   --

BREAST-FEEDING
Avoid drug or avoid nursing.   Drug passes in breast milk.

--   --

AGE FACTOR
1. Do not give to children.   1. Safety and effectiveness have not been estab-
                                                     lished for children under 12.

2. No problems have been seen in people over 60.

--   --

MISSED DOSE
May be taken up to two hours after scheduled time. If more than two hours have passed, wait until next dose, but do not double amount taken.

OVERDOSE
No overdose threat reported.

STOPPING DRUG
Must be taken for up to three weeks to determine efficacy. If drug works, discuss with your physician how long it should be used, at what frequencies, and how to discontinue drug once it is appropriate to do so.

OTHERS
Do not drive or operate machinery until you have determined how medication affects you.

Discuss with your doctor whether you should have periodic kidney function tests or other laboratory tests.

`drug or category:`

NIZATIDINE

`condition:`
ULCERS

warning

Tell your doctor if you have or have had:
- a previous allergic reaction to this medication
- allergic reactions to *Zantac, Tagamet,* or *Pepcid*
- liver or kidney disease

Tell your physician if you are taking aspirin in large quantities.

drugs

GENERIC	BRAND	RX
nizatidine	*Axid*	Yes

form/usage

CAPSULES: May be taken with milk.

Capsules may be opened.

when

For ulcer treatment, twice a day, 12 hours apart, or one dose before retiring. For prevention, once a day, before retiring.

side effects and adverse reactions

Rash, sore throat, irregular heartbeat, muscle pain, fever

Constipation or diarrhea, decline in libido, headache, hair loss, breast enlargement in men

what to do

Stop taking. Get in touch with doctor immediately.

Continue taking, but discuss with your doctor.

special precautions

DRUG INTERACTIONS
1. Antacids, metoclopramide

because

1. Decrease absorption of nizatidine.

DRUG INTERACTIONS
2. Alprazolam, anticoagulants, carbamazepine, chlordiazepoxide, diazepam, digitalis, flurazepam, glipizide, labetalol, methadone, metoprolol, metronidazole, morphine, phenytoin, procainamide, propafenone

3. Ketoconazole

4. Anticholinergics, encainide

2. Nizatidine increases their effect. May lead to toxicity in some cases.

3. Its effect is decreased.

4. Increases the effect of nizatidine.

DIET
Avoid foods high in protein.

Protein stimulates acid secretion.

ALCOHOL and TOBACCO
Avoid alcohol or use sparingly.

Avoid tobacco.

Alcohol stimulates acid production.

Nicotine interferes with drug.

PREGNANCY
Avoid drug, especially during first three months of pregnancy.

Nizatidine has caused severe birth defects in animal studies. No reported links between medication and human birth defects.

BREAST-FEEDING
Avoid drug or avoid nursing.

Medication passes into breast milk.

AGE FACTOR
1. Do not give to children under 12.

2. People over 60 and especially those who have difficulty chewing should use very carefully.

1. Safety and effectiveness have not been determined.

2. Drug can lead to aggregation of masses of undigested vegetables in stomach.

MISSED DOSE
Can be taken up to two hours after scheduled time; otherwise, wait until next scheduled dose, but do not double amount taken.

OVERDOSE
Get emergency medical help immediately in case of rapid heartbeat or breathing difficulties, or if person is delirious or confused.

(continued)

STOPPING DRUG

Do not stop taking even if you feel better until you have talked with your doctor.

Tell your physician immediately if ulcer symptoms return after you have stopped.

OTHERS

Patients on dialysis should take medication after treatment because dialysis can remove up to 14 percent of drug.

Do not drive or operate machinery until you have determined if drug makes you drowsy or affects reflexes in any way.

Periodic laboratory tests might be necessary to check kidney and liver function and blood counts.

RANITIDINE

condition:
ULCERS, EXCESSIVE ACID PRODUCTION

warning

May lead to confusion in elderly patients.
Tell your doctor if you have or have had:
- an allergic reaction to this drug, or to preservatives or dyes
- kidney or liver disease

Tell your doctor if you are taking an anticoagulant.

drugs

GENERIC	BRAND	RX
ranitidine	Zantac	Yes

form/usage

INJECTION, SYRUP, TABLETS: May be taken with milk.

Tablets may be crushed.

when

For active ulcer, take twice daily about 12 hours apart, preferably with or after meals (one dose after breakfast, one after dinner, for example).

As prevention, take one dose before going to bed.

side effects and adverse reactions

Diarrhea, rash, jaundice, confusion

Nausea, pain in stomach, constipation, dizziness

what to do

Stop taking. Get in touch with doctor immediately.

Continue taking, but discuss with your doctor.

(continued)

special precautions	because
DRUG INTERACTIONS	
1. Tamoxifen	**1.** Will lower tamoxifen's efficacy.
2. Antacids, ketoconazole	**2.** Will decrease absorption of ranitidine.
DIET	
No restrictions.	
ALCOHOL and TOBACCO	
Avoid alcohol or use very sparingly.	Drug can increase blood concentration of alcohol by one third.
Avoid tobacco.	Nicotine decreases effect of drug.
PREGNANCY	
Do not take if you are pregnant or are planning to conceive.	Impact on pregnancy or fetus has not been determined.
BREAST-FEEDING	
Avoid medication or avoid nursing.	Medication moves into breast milk. May affect baby.
AGE FACTOR	
1. Do not administer to children without physician's recommendation.	**1.** Effectiveness and safety in children has not been determined.
2. Adults over 60 should follow doctor's instructions carefully, especially if they have any problems chewing food well.	**2.** Drug may cause aggregation of undigested vegetables in stomach.
MISSED DOSE	
May be taken up to two hours after scheduled time. After two hours, wait until your next scheduled dose, but do not double amount taken.	
OVERDOSE	
Get emergency medical help immediately in case of coma or if patient has trouble breathing or has tremors.	

STOPPING DRUG

Should be taken for up to six weeks to determine efficacy. Do not discontinue without discussing with your doctor because you may need maintenance.

Advise your doctor immediately if you have a recurrence of ulcer symptoms after stopping.

OTHERS

May decrease sexual desire or cause impotence or enlarged breasts in males, though rarely.

Do not drive or operate machinery until you have determined if drug makes you dizzy.

Drug may affect metabolism of vitamin B_{12}. You may need periodic lab tests to determine if this is happening.

Lab tests to check liver function and blood count may also be required.

URSODIOL

condition:
GALLSTONES

warning

Tell your doctor if you have or have had:
- an allergic reaction to this medication or any medication containing bile acids
- biliary tract problems or pancreatitis

drugs

GENERIC	BRAND	RX
ursodiol (ursodeoxycholic acid)	*Actigall*	Yes

form/usage

TABLETS: May be taken with beverages or food to avoid stomach irritation.

Tablets may be crushed.

when

At meals.

side effects and adverse reactions

Diarrhea

what to do

Continue taking, but discuss with your doctor.

special precautions

DRUG INTERACTIONS
Aluminum-coated antacids, cholestyramine, clofibrate, colestipol, estrogens, progesterone

DIET
Doctor may put you on a weight-loss diet.

because

Decrease absorption or effect of ursodiol.

Weight and diet determine how fast drug can dissolve gallstones.

ALCOHOL and TOBACCO
No problems with alcohol expected except in patients with liver disease.

Avoid tobacco.

Tobacco may interfere with absorption of drug.

PREGNANCY
Discuss with your doctor.

Effect on pregnancy or fetus has not been established.

BREAST-FEEDING
Discuss with your doctor.

Not known if drug passes into breast milk.

AGE FACTOR
1. No specific information about effect on children, but drug probably works as it does in adults.

2. Not expected to cause adverse or side effects in older persons different from those in other adults.

MISSED DOSE
Take as soon as you remember. Otherwise, wait for next dose and **double amount taken**.

OVERDOSE
Get emergency medical help immediately if you have severe diarrhea.

STOPPING DRUG
Take full prescription even if it seems that you are feeling better.

OTHERS
You will need periodic laboratory tests to determine if drug is working and to make sure liver is not affected.

-32-

HORMONAL PREPARATIONS

Hormones are chemicals produced in the endocrine glands and tissues and secreted into the bloodstream to play a pivotal role in every bodily process. They control our sexual development, drive, and reproduction. They also control growth and the activities of all organs, including the brain. An intricate feedback system determines their levels in the bloodstream. Even a minute imbalance can cause grave problems, but most of the time, the endocrine system functions smoothly without any outside help. When it goes awry, however, doctors can turn to an array of natural and synthetic hormone products.

Estrogen and Progestin

Estrogen, the major female hormone, is the most widely prescribed hormone, used not only in oral contraceptives (see Chapter 26), but also to treat menopausal symptoms, to prevent or treat osteoporosis in older women, and to treat advanced prostate cancer in men. In recent years, an increasing number of doctors have started advocating long-term hormone replacement therapy for postmenopausal women, although this use remains somewhat controversial because it is still not

known whether estrogen in this setting increases the risk of breast cancer. Today's evidence, however, indicates that the benefits of hormone replacement—protection against osteoporosis, heart disease, and, perhaps, Alzheimer's disease—outweigh any cancer risk.

Estrogen is available as pills, injections, creams, and skin patches. *Ogen, Estrace, Estraderm, Estrogen, Premarin,* and others). In the early years of menopause, estrogen stops hot flashes, night sweats, vaginal dryness, and other symptoms. When given alone, estrogen causes a proliferation of endometrial tissue, which experts believe accounts for the increase in endometrial cancer among women taking estrogen alone. When progestin is added (as a separate prescription) it prompts a breakdown of the uterine lining, which is shed in bleeding similar to menstruation. This bleeding is lighter than that of ordinary menstruation, and after a few years of postmenopausal hormone therapy, it usually tapers off and stops. Even so, some women find the resumption of bleeding bothersome.

With or without progestin, postmenopausal hormone therapy can cause weight gain, breast tenderness, bloating, mood swings, and other relatively minor side effects.

In younger women, progestin (*Provera, Depo-*

Provera) may be prescribed to help regulate the menstrual cycle, or to treat endometriosis (in which the tissues that normally line the uterus grow outside it) or breast, kidney, or uterine cancer.

Progestin deficiency can cause fertility problems; in this setting, it is prescribed to promote implantation of the embryo in the uterine lining, and then to maintain the pregnancy.

Testosterone

Testosterone—the major male sex hormone—may be prescribed to initiate puberty in boys with delayed sexual development. It may also be prescribed for men who produce inadequate amounts of it. In unusual cases, it is given to women to treat some forms of breast cancer and severe cystic breast disease because it stops estrogen production, but its use is limited by its side effects—facial hair growth and other signs of masculinization—and the fact that there are safer alternative drugs to block estrogen production in women. Other anabolic steroids frequently are abused by athletes and others who use the hormones to build muscle tissue. This results in numerous serious side effects, including aggression, bone loss, heart disease, excessive fluid retention, liver cancer, and impaired fertility.

Some commonly prescribed forms are testosterone cypionate (*Depotest*), testosterone enanthate (*Testone* L.A.), and methyltestosterone (*Android, Metandren*).

Thyroid Hormones

The thyroid gland in the neck produces hormones that regulate body metabolism and numerous other functions. Too much thyroid hormone—hyperthyroidism, or Graves' disease—causes palpitations, weight loss, nervousness, weakness, fatigue, and intolerance to heat. An underactive thyroid, or hypothyroidism, is most serious in the newborn—unless detected and treated, it can lead to severe growth problems and a form of retardation called cretinism. Although thyroid hormones are sometimes misused for weight control and treatment of high cholesterol levels, they are indicated to treat various thyroid disorders—hypothyroidism; benign enlargement of the thyroid, or goiter; thyroid nodules; and cancer of the thyroid. In some cases of hyperthyroidism, the thyroid gland is destroyed by administering radioactive iodine or surgically removed, after which the patient must undergo lifelong thyroid hormone replacement.

Thyroid preparations, such as *Levothroid, Synthroid,* and others, are taken in tablet form or administered by injection. These are potent drugs that must be used as directed. They can cause serious problems when taken by people who do not need them. For example, they can aggravate existing cardiovascular problems, particularly in older people, and in excessive doses, they can bring on problems usually associated with an overactive thyroid.

Growth Hormones

Pituitary gland disorders and certain hereditary diseases can result in dwarfism, or failure to grow. In such cases, the use of growth hormones such as somatropin—which is produced in the pituitary gland—stimulates growth. Recent advances have made it possible to produce growth hormones using cloning techniques. As more of the hormone preparation is now available, there is growing concern that it will be misused; for example, given to children who are genetically programmed to be short, but are otherwise normal.

Long-term effects of using growth hormones for such purposes are unknown, but some studies suggest it may increase cancer risk by prompting uncontrolled growth of abnormal cells.

For information on corticosteroids and other adrenal hormones, see Chapters 16, 23, and 31.

drug or category:

ESTROGENS

condition:

MENOPAUSAL SYMPTOMS, ESTROGEN DEFICIENCIES, OSTEOPOROSIS, PROSTATE CANCER

warning

Do not use if you have had a previous allergic reaction to this compound in any form; if you have a history of blood clots, thrombophlebitis, cardiovascular disease, liver disease, or sickle-cell anemia; or if you are pregnant. Tell your doctor if you have or have had:

- breast cancer or cancer of the reproductive tract, or other diseases of the reproductive tract or breast
- asthma or high blood pressure
- gallbladder disease
- migraine headaches or epilepsy

drugs

GENERIC	BRAND	RX
estropipate	*Ogen*	Yes
estradiol	*Estrace, Estraderm*	
conjugated estrogens	*Premarin*, others	

form/usage

TABLETS, CAPSULES, VAGINAL CREAMS AND SUPPOSITORIES, INJECTION, SKIN PATCHES: Tablets may be crushed. Capsules may be opened. Either one can be taken with or without food.

Vaginal creams and skin patches should be used according to instructions on label.

when

At same time every day.

side effects and adverse reactions

Jaundice; calcium build up in blood; spasms; pain in stomach, side, or muscles; breast lumps; stomach cramps; rash

Depression; dizziness; migraine headaches; loss of appetite; gastrointestinal problems; swollen breasts, feet, or ankles

what to do

Stop taking. Get in touch with doctor immediately.

Continue taking, but discuss with your physician.

(continued)

special precautions	because
DRUG INTERACTIONS 1. Carbamazepine, phenobarbital, phenytoin, primidone, rifampin	1. Will decrease effect of estrogen.
2. Diabetes drugs	2. May cause wide fluctuations in blood sugar levels.
3. Tricyclic antidepressants	3. Adverse effects of antidepressants may be heightened and their effectiveness may be reduced.
4. Anticoagulants	4. Estrogen may hamper their effectiveness.
DIET No interaction, though it might be wise to restrict salt intake.	Salt may heighten tendency to retain fluids.
ALCOHOL AND TOBACCO No interaction with alcohol. Avoid smoking.	Smoking can increase risk of heart disease.
PREGNANCY Avoid drug.	Laboratory tests with animals as well as studies in humans show that estrogens can cause defects in the fetus and masculinization in the female fetus. Use of estrogen during pregnancy also puts a female child at greater risk for vaginal and cervical cancer.
BREAST-FEEDING Discuss with your doctor.	Estrogens migrate into breast milk in small amounts. May also suppress milk production.
AGE FACTOR 1. Not prescribed for children. 2. Should be given to women over 60 with caution and only if they run a high risk of developing bone loss.	2. Increased risk of blood problems, including thrombophlebitis as well as lung blood clots.

MISSED DOSE

You can take a missed dose up to 12 hours after the prescribed time. If longer than 12 hours, wait for next dose, but don't double the amount taken.

OVERDOSE

Get emergency medical help immediately in case of abnormal vaginal bleeding or if you have severe nausea or vomiting.

STOPPING DRUG

Drug should be stopped from time to time to determine if you still need it. However, it should be withdrawn slowly by reducing the dose gradually. Discuss with your physician.

OTHERS

Estrogens may cause milk production, breast tenderness and swelling, and an increase in vaginal secretions.

Tell physicians who order laboratory tests that you are taking estrogen. Hormone can affect results of several blood tests and liver function tests.

Estrogen in vaginal creams can be absorbed by the penis and lead to breast enlargement and tenderness in men.

May increase sensitivity to sun. If you go outdoors between 10 A.M. and 3 P.M., wear protective clothing and/or sunblock.

drug or category:

TESTOSTERONE

condition:
MALE HORMONE DEFICIENCY, BREAST PAIN IN WOMEN AFTER CHILDBIRTH,
APLASTIC ANEMIA; ALSO USED TO HELP IN GAINING WEIGHT

warning

Tell your doctor if you have had an allergic reaction to this medication, or to any preservatives or dyes.

drugs

GENERIC	BRAND	RX
testosterone cypionate	*Depotest*	Yes
testosterone enanthate	*Testone L.A.*	
methyltestosterone	*Android, Metandren,* others	

form/usage

TABLETS, CAPSULES, INJECTION: Take with food to avoid stomach upset.

when

Tablets and capsules should be taken at same time every day. Injection is administered once or twice a month, according to your physician's instructions.

side effects and adverse reactions

Sore throat, fever, jaundice, yellow eyes, vaginal bleeding, pain in scrotum, urination difficulties, gastrointestinal problems, severe mood changes

Heightened sexual desire, frequent erections, loss of appetite, bad breath, impotence, decrease in size of testicles, acne, enlarged clitoris, enlarged male breasts.

what to do

Stop taking. Get in touch with doctor immediately.

Continue taking, but discuss with your physician.

special precautions	**because**
DRUG INTERACTIONS	
1. Anticoagulants, oral antidiabetics, insulin	1. Testosterone increases their effect.
2. Chlorzoxazone, oxyphenbutazone, phenylbuta-zone, phenobarbital	2. Decrease impact of testosterone.
3. Any drug with capacity to induce liver damage	3. Testosterone will heighten damage.
DIET	
No restrictions, but tell your doctor or pharmacist if you are on a low-sugar or low-salt diet.	This drug may affect blood sugar levels and sodium levels. It could also increase water retention.
ALCOHOL AND TOBACCO	
No problems reported.	
PREGNANCY	
Avoid drug.	Causes fetal abnormalities.
BREAST-FEEDING	
Avoid drug or avoid nursing.	Drug passes into breast milk and may affect baby.
AGE FACTOR	
1. Not prescribed for children.	
2. People over 60 should use with caution.	2. In men testosterone increases the risk of prostate problems, including cancer. Drugs can increase cardiovascular problems.

MISSED DOSE

You can take a missed dose up to two hours after scheduled time. Otherwise, wait for next dose but do not double the amount taken.

OVERDOSE

Get in touch with a poison control center, emergency room, or doctor if you believe you have taken too much testosterone or have any of the following symptoms: severe headaches, changes in your vision, trouble talking, yellow eyes or skin, vomiting of blood, uncontrolled muscle spasms. No reports of acute overdosage have been reported.

(continued)

STOPPING DRUG
No problems reported discontinuing drug without finishing prescription or tapering off.

OTHERS
May increase sexual activity in males; increases risk of liver cancer; may cause excessive hair growth and voice changes in women.

PROGESTIN

IRREGULAR MENSTRUAL CYCLE; ENDOMETRIOSIS; BREAST, KIDNEY, AND UTERINE CANCER

warning

Tell your doctor if you have or have had:

- an allergic reaction to progestin medication, or to any preservatives or dyes
- kidney problems, asthma, or diabetes
- emotional problems, cardiovascular disease, or epilepsy

Do not take if you have or have had breast or reproductive tract cancer, circulatory problems, or abnormal vaginal bleeding, or if you are pregnant.

drugs

GENERIC	BRAND	RX
medroxyprogesterone	*Provera, Depo-Provera*, others	Yes

form/usage

TABLETS AND INJECTIONS: Take on an empty stomach. Can be taken with food.
Tablet may be crushed.

when

At same time every day.

side effects and adverse reactions

Pain in stomach or side, rash, vision problems, unusual vaginal bleeding, pain in lower part of legs

Swollen feet, fatigue, acne, enlarged clitoris, breast tenderness, sleeplessness, change in voice, change in menstrual cycle

what to do

Stop taking. Get in touch with doctor immediately.

Continue taking, but discuss with your physician.

special precautions

DRUG INTERACTIONS

1. Bromocriptine, oral antidiabetics, insulin

2. Phenobarbital, phenylbutazone

because

1. Progestin decreases their effect.

2. Lessen effectiveness of progestin.

(continued)

DRUG INTERACTIONS

3. Phenothiazine

3. Progestin increases its effect.

DIET

No restrictions, though it might be wise to restrict salt intake.

Salt may heighten tendency to retain fluids.

ALCOHOL and TOBACCO

No interactions with alcohol. Avoid tobacco.

Smoking, in combination with progestins, may cause blood clots.

PREGNANCY

Avoid medication. Do not become pregnant until at least three months after stopping drug.

May cause harm to fetus.

BREAST-FEEDING

Avoid drug or avoid nursing.

Drug passes into breast milk and may affect baby.

AGE FACTOR

1. Not prescribed for children.

2. Women over 60 may use—effects do not differ from those in younger women. However, watch for fluid retention.

MISSED DOSE

Take missed dose as soon as you remember it; however, if it is almost time for next dose, wait until then, but do not double amount taken.

OVERDOSE

Get emergency medical help immediately if you experience severe vomiting or nausea, painful or enlarged breasts, or vaginal bleeding.

STOPPING DRUG

Discuss with your doctor how you should stop taking drug.

OTHERS

Medication requires regular checkups so that dosage can be adjusted if necessary and side effects can be spotted.

Drug may have to be used for up to three months to determine efficacy in regulating menstrual cycle.

drug or category:

ANTIDIURETIC HORMONES

condition:
FLUID LOSS RELATED TO DIABETES, BED-WETTING

warning

Tell your doctor if you have or have had an allergic reaction to progestin medication or to any preservatives or dyes.

drugs

GENERIC	BRAND	RX
desmopressin	DDAVP, Stimate	Yes

form/usage

NASAL SPRAY, INJECTIONS: Use nasal spray pump or catheter according to directions with package.

when

At bedtime.

side effects and adverse reactions

Increased blood pressure, flushing

Headache, cramps

what to do

Stop taking. Get in touch with doctor immediately.

Continue taking, but discuss with your physician.

special precautions

DRUG INTERACTIONS
1. Carbamazepine, chlorpropamide, clofibrate
2. Demeclocycline, lithium, norepinephrine

DIET
No restrictions.

because

1. Will increase impact of desmopressin.
2. Will decrease effectiveness of desmopressin.

ALCOHOL AND TOBACCO
Avoid both.

May decrease effectiveness of drug.

PREGNANCY
Discuss with your doctor.

No reports of fetal damage in animal studies. Human studies have not been conducted.

BREAST-FEEDING
Discuss with your doctor.

Drug passes into breast milk. No reports of harm to baby.

AGE FACTOR
1. Administer to children only under close medical and adult supervision.

2. Adults over 60 years of age should use cautiously.

1. Children may react to medication more readily than adults.

2. Older patients are more likely to suffer side effects, including headaches and urinary and weight control problems.

MISSED DOSE
Depends on dosage frequency. Discuss with your doctor or pharmacist.

OVERDOSE
Get emergency medical help immediately in case of coma or if patient is confused or has seizures.

STOPPING DRUG
Discuss with your doctor.

OTHERS
All your doctors should know that you are taking this medication.

THYROID MEDICATIONS

condition:
THYROID HORMONE DEFICIENCIES, GOITER, THYROID CANCER

warning

Do not take if you have had a recent heart attack.
Drug may intensify angina.
Do not take to assist in weight control if your thyroid function is normal.
Tell your doctor if you have or have had:
• heart disease, high blood pressure, or adrenal gland problems
• an allergic reaction to progestin medication, or to any preservatives or dyes
Tell your doctor if you are taking asthma or anticoagulant medications.

drugs

GENERIC	BRAND	RX
liothyronine	*Cytomel,* others	Yes
liotrix	*Thyrolar*	

form/usage

INJECTIONS, TABLETS: Take on an empty stomach. Tablets may be crushed.

when

In the morning.

side effects and adverse reactions

Change in appetite, weight loss, nervousness, changes in menstrual cycle, leg cramps

what to do

Continue taking, but discuss with your physician.

special precautions

DRUG INTERACTIONS
1. Anticoagulants

because

1. May increase anticoagulant's effect.

DRUG INTERACTIONS

2. Digoxin

3. Cholestyramine

4. Oral antidiabetics and insulin

5. Tricyclic antidepressants

2. May decrease digoxin's effectiveness.

3. May decrease effectiveness of liothyronine.

4. May require adjustment of dosages.

5. Impact of antidepressants and liothyronine may be increased.

DIET

No restrictions.

ALCOHOL AND TOBACCO

No interactions reported.

PREGNANCY

No problems reported.

BREAST-FEEDING

Discuss with your doctor.

Drug appears in breast milk in minute amounts. No impact on baby if dose is carefully supervised.

AGE FACTOR

1. Avoid giving to children.

2. People over 60 should use cautiously.

1. Drug's impact on immature nervous system has not been fully explored.

2. Older people generally need much lower doses of thyroid hormone replacement than young adults. Overdosing problems may be severe.

MISSED DOSE

You can take missed dose up to 12 hours after scheduled time. Otherwise, wait for next dose, but do not double the amount taken.

OVERDOSE

Get in touch with poison control center, emergency room, or doctor if patient experiences palpitations, muscle cramps, shaking, nervousness, or irritability.

(continued)

STOPPING DRUG

Must be taken regularly and on schedule. Do not stop without discussing with your doctor.

OTHERS

Drug increases sensitivity to heat which may cause symptoms of overdose. Ask your doctor how you should take drug in summer.

May change menstrual pattern.

May be effective in treating sexual problems rooted in low thyroid function.

Periodic laboratory tests might be necessary to check thyroid and heart functions.

drug or category:

CALCITONIN

condition:

PAGET'S DISEASE, OSTEOPOROSIS IN POSTMENOPAUSAL WOMEN

warning

Tell your doctor if you have or have had:
- an allergic reaction to this medication, or to foreign proteins, or to any preservatives or foods
- a bone break that has not healed completely

drugs

GENERIC	BRAND	RX
calcitonin (human)	*Cibacalcin*	Yes
calcitonin (salmon)	*Calcimar*	

form/usage

INJECTION: Follow your doctor's instructions.

when

Follow your doctor's instructions.

side effects and adverse reactions

Flushed face; tingling in face, arms, or legs; dizziness; headache; breathing problems

Loss of appetite, other minor gastrointestinal problems, more frequent urination, stuffy nose

what to do

Stop taking. Get in touch with doctor immediately.

Continue taking, but discuss with your physician.

special precautions

DRUG INTERACTIONS
Calcium or vitamin preparations containing calcifediol or calcitriol

DIET
No interactions reported.

because

Interfere with calcitonin.

(continued)

ALCOHOL AND TOBACCO
No interactions reported.

PREGNANCY
Avoid drug or discuss with your doctor.

Drug has lead to decreased weight in newborn babies.

BREAST-FEEDING
Discuss with your doctor.

Drug may decrease milk production.

AGE FACTOR
1. Discuss with your doctor whether to give to children.

2. No special problems noted in adults over 60.

1. No studies done on safety or effectiveness.

MISSED DOSE
If you are on a twice-a-day schedule, you can take a missed dose up to two hours after scheduled time. Otherwise, wait for next dose but do not double the amount taken.

If you are taking the drug once a day and forget to take it, take missed dose when you remember it, then return to regular schedule. If you don't remember it until the following day, take only the dose scheduled for that day. Do not double the dose.

If you are taking the drug every other day, take missed dose when you remember it, then go back on schedule. If you do not remember it until the following day, take it then, wait a day, then return to your schedule. Do not double dose.

OVERDOSE
Get in touch with a poison control center, emergency room, or doctor if patient experiences severe gastrointestinal problems.

STOPPING DRUG
Discuss with your doctor.

OTHERS
Periodic laboratory tests might be necessary to check effect on levels of blood calcium and other minerals and of hydroxyproline in urine.

-33-

- - - - - - - - - - - - - - -

LAXATIVES

EACH YEAR, AMERICANS spend some $450 million on laxatives—products that experts contend are vastly overused. Contrary to popular belief, a daily bowel movement is not necessarily the norm; some perfectly healthy people may have two or three a day, while others who are equally healthy may have bowel movements only two or three times a week. So long as the stools pass easily and are reasonably regular, there is no problem.

The key to determining whether you are truly constipated is whether there is a change in bowel patterns. If you ordinarily have a bowel movement every day and suddenly find that you haven't had one for several days, perhaps you are constipated. Dry stool that is difficult to pass is also a sign of constipation.

Many factors can contribute to this condition—a change in diet, age, pregnancy, inactivity, the use of antacids and other drugs, hemorrhoids and other intestinal or rectal problems, and stress, among others. Most cases of constipation disappear on their own. However, if constipation, or any other unexplained change in bowel habits, persists for more than 10 to 14 days you should consult a doctor.

Before resorting to laxatives, try life-style changes to remedy the problem. For example, increase your intake of high-fiber foods—whole grain cereals and breads, fresh fruits, and raw or lightly processed vegetables are all good sources. Make sure you drink at least eight glasses of water or other nonalcoholic fluids a day. Include a long walk or some other physical activity in your daily regimen. Finally, don't put off going to the bathroom when you feel the urge to do so.

If you do take laxatives, make sure you follow the instructions carefully and don't overuse them, which can lead to a worsening of the condition. Overuse of laxatives can lead to dependency, in which your colon can no longer function normally. Some laxatives also irritate or damage the colon when overused; others can hinder absorption of medications and essential nutrients.

drug or category:

LAXATIVES

condition:
CONSTIPATION

warning

Do not take for more than one week.

Do not take if you have problems swallowing. If accidentally inhaled, some components of some laxatives could cause pneumonia.

Consult your doctor if you have any symptoms of appendicitis (severe pain in lower abdomen, nausea, constipation, fever), or if you have rectal bleeding.

Tell your doctor if you have or have had:

- an allergic reaction to laxatives, or to any preservatives or dyes
- a colostomy or any other surgery on your colon
- diabetes or heart or kidney disease
- high blood pressure or hemorrhoids

drugs

GENERIC	BRAND	RX
docusate	*Colace*	No (except for a few). Ask your doctor for advice.
lactulose	*Constilac, Portalac, others*	
psyllium hydrophilic mucilloid	*Metamucil, Reguloid, others*	
polycarbophil	*Fibercon*	
methylcellulose	*Citrucel, Cologel*	
phenolphthalein	*Ex-Lax, Espotabs, others*	
docusate and phenolphthalein	*Doxidan*	

form/usage

TABLETS, LIQUIDS, POWDERS, GRANULES, CHEWABLE WAFERS AND TABLETS: Follow directions of your doctor or the manufacturer.

All laxatives should be followed by ample supplies of water during the day.

when

Follow your doctor or the manufacturer's directions.

side effects and adverse reactions	**what to do**

Lactulose

1. Arrhythmias and muscle cramps

1. Stop taking. Get in touch with doctor immediately.

2. Confusion, fatigue, thirst, diarrhea

2. Continue taking, but discuss with your physician.

Psyllium, polycarbophil, methylcellulose, docusate

1. Asthma, skin problems

1. Stop taking. Get in touch with doctor immediately.

2. Swallowing problems

2. Continue taking, but discuss with your physician.

Phenolphthalein

1. Vomiting

1. Stop taking. Get in touch with doctor immediately.

2. Heart arrhythmias, confusion, cramps, painful urination, irritability

2. Stop taking. Get in touch with doctor immediately.

3. Anal itching, nausea, other mild stomach problems (such as belching, stomach cramps)

3. Continue taking, but discuss with your physician.

4. Change in urine color

4. Do nothing. This is a normal reaction.

special precautions	**because**

DRUG INTERACTIONS

1. Do not take any laxative within two hours of another medicine.

1. Laxatives may decrease or prevent absorption.

2. Neomycin

2. Effect of both drugs is increased.

3. Digitalis, aspirin drugs

3. Psyllium, polycarbophil, and methylcellulose reduce their effect.

Phenolphthalein and docusate may cause digitalis toxicity.

4. Tetracyclines

4. Polycarbophil reduces their effect.

5. Antacids

5. Antacids may cause phenolphthalein tablets to dissolve too quickly and irritate gastrointestinal tract.

(continued)

DRUG INTERACTIONS

6. Diuretics and high blood pressure medications

7. Mineral oil

8. Danthron

9. Do not combine laxatives.

---

6. Phenolphthalein in combination with these drugs may lead to dangerously low potassium levels.

7. Docusate increases absorption.

8. Could cause liver damage.

9. Could heighten laxative effect dangerously. Could cause poisoning.

DIET

1. Generally, avoid or use drug only if absolutely necessary if you are on a low-salt or low-sugar diet.

2. Avoid milk with phenolphthalein.

---

1. Some laxatives have large amounts of sodium or sugar and may aggravate high blood pressure (hypertension).

2. Milk may cause tablet to dissolve too quickly and irritate gastrointestinal tract.

ALCOHOL AND TOBACCO

No reports of adverse reactions.

PREGNANCY

Avoid drug or take under doctor's supervision.

Some laxatives are high in salt or sugar and could aggravate high blood pressure; others contain minerals that may cause difficulty if you have liver problems. Mineral oil will interfere with proper absorption of nutrients. Castor oil may cause contractions of uterus.

BREAST-FEEDING

Avoid drug or avoid nursing.

Components of laxatives pass into breast milk in tiny amounts and should not affect child; however, there have been reports of diarrhea in breast-fed infants.

AGE FACTOR

1. Do not give to children under six unless prescribed by a doctor.

2. People over 60 should avoid or take very cautiously.

1. Constipation may be caused by a problem the child is not explaining properly.

2. Some laxatives if taken too often will affect coordination or cause dizziness.

MISSED DOSE
Docusate, docusate and phenolphthalein psyllium, polycarbophyl, methylcellulose, and phenolphthalein:
Take when you remember, but do not take next dose for 12 hours. Then resume recommended schedule.

Lactulose
Can be taken up to eight hours before retiring; otherwise, wait till next dose, but do not double the amount taken. Do not make up for missed dosage before going to bed.

OVERDOSE
Get emergency medical help immediately if phenolphthalein causes vomiting. In case of overdose of other laxatives, **get in touch with a poison control center, emergency room, or doctor.**

STOPPING DRUG
Not necessary to finish bottle or pills if constipation ends.

OTHERS
Do not drive or operate machinery until you have determined how medication affects you.

-34-

EYE AND EAR MEDICATIONS

Glaucoma

Glaucoma is an insidious eye disorder that afflicts an estimated 5 to 10 million Americans, mostly over the age of 40. Glaucoma occurs when the aqueous humor, a fluid in the interior of the eye, builds up, putting pressure on the optic nerve. If untreated, this pressure can destroy the optic nerve and cause blindness. In fact, glaucoma is responsible for up to 15 percent of all cases of blindness in the United States.

In some instances of acute glaucoma, the person experiences sudden, severe eye pain, headache, and nausea. More often, however, the disease comes on silently, and there are no significant symptoms until the eye has suffered permanent damage; this condition is called open-angle glaucoma. Fortunately, glaucoma can be easily detected before it causes blindness by having periodic eye examinations that include tonometry, a relatively easy and painless test that measures internal eye pressures.

Once glaucoma is diagnosed, it usually can be controlled by the use of eye drops such as timolol maleate (*Timoptic*) and dipivefrin (*Propine*). Timolol—a beta-blocking drug—reduces the formation of the aqueous humor and also promotes flow of the liquid from the eye. Dipivefrin also promotes

the outflow of aqueous humor. Although these medications are generally safe, they can produce eye pain, mental confusion, stomach upset, and, in very rare cases, hallucinations. Timolol may also lower blood pressure and slow the heartbeat. Thus, it is important to see an ophthalmologist and primary care physician regularly to make sure that the drugs are working properly and not causing adverse effects on other organs.

Eye Infections

The eyes, especially the conjunctiva, the tissue forming a protective covering over the eyeball, are vulnerable to infection and inflammation. Conjunctivitis, or pink eye, may be caused by bacteria, viruses, or irritants. Other parts of the eye, such as the cornea, also may become infected. The use of contact lenses, especially the extended-wear type, may promote corneal infections and ulceration leading to vision loss. Some eye infections, such as ocular herpes, can damage sight.

Bacterial eye infections are treated with antibiotic eye ointments or drops such as gentamicin (*Garamycin*), tetracycline (*Achromycin*), and a combination of neomycin, polymixin B, and bacitracin (*Neosporin*). Some antibiotic eye preparations are combined with a steroid to counter eye inflammation. Ocular herpes is treated with vidarabine (*Vira-A*) eye ointment.

Hay Fever and Eye Irritations

Red, itchy, and teary eyes are a common manifestation of hay fever and other allergies. Compresses sometimes alleviate minor allergy symptoms, but in more severe cases, antihistamines such as naphazoline (*Naphcon-A*) and oxymetazoline (*Visine L.R.*), which reduce the inflammatory response by constricting the small blood vessels that serve the eyes, provide more lasting relief. Such medications can stop the itching and watering within two to ten minutes. On rare occasions, however, they may cause temporary vision problems, dizziness, and perhaps even some changes in heartbeat rhythm. Use them as directed, and avoid such medications if you have glaucoma, in which case they may cause blindness. If compresses and antihistamine drops are insufficient, corticosteroid (or adrenocorticoid) eye drops such as dexamethasone (*Decadron*) and prednisolone, (*Pred Forte*), may be considered. These medications, which are also used to treat other eye inflammations, are highly effective, but should not be used long-term because they increase the risk of glaucoma, cataracts, and bacterial infections.

Dry eyes, caused by either environmental factors or reduced tear production, are another source of eye irritation. Nonprescription products provide relief but also should be used judiciously because they contain preservatives that can cause eye damage if used excessively.

Ear Problems

Ear infections are among the most common childhood diseases, with the middle ear the most frequent target, resulting in otitis media. Contrary to popular belief, not all ear infections require antibiotic treatment. Studies show that children whose ear infections are treated with antibiotics fare no better than those given a placebo. Many pediatric experts argue that overly hasty antibiotic treatment for earaches actually increases the chances of recurrent infections because the bacteria in the ear canal can develop resistance to the drugs. Thus, if your child complains of an earache, wait a couple of days. If the earache persists for more than 48 hours, check with your pediatrician. If there is no fever or obvious sign of infection, many pediatricians adopt a wait-and-see approach.

Simple earaches often can be alleviated with a heating pad, acetaminophen for children, or a few drops of warm olive oil placed in the ear. If medication is needed, benzocaine or a combination of benzocaine and antipyrine may be tried, but check with your doctor first.

If pain persists and there are other indications for antibiotic therapy, a medication such as chloramphenicol (*Chloromycetin*) or a combination of neomycin, polymyxin B, and hydrocortisone (*Cortisporin, Pediotic*) may be prescribed.

Swimmer's ear, or outer ear infection, is another common problem, especially among people who spend a lot of time in the water. Excessive sweating and improper placement of a hearing aid can contribute to the problem. Both bacteria and fungi can cause these ear infections. *VōSol* drops (hydrocortisone and acetic acid) are sometimes prescribed for this condition.

Prevention is the best approach. Keeping the ear dry is critical. If water gets in your ear, tip your head to let it run out, and then dry the ear with a hairdryer set on low and held 10 to 12 inches from your ear. To keep water out of your ear, wear ear plugs when swimming or shampooing your hair.

drug or category:

ADRENOCORTICOIDS

condition:

EYE IRRITATION AND DISCOMFORT

warning

Tell your doctor if you have or have had:
• an allergic reaction to this medication, or to any preservatives or foods
cataracts or glaucoma, diabetes (patients with these illnesses are more likely to develop cataracts
with steroid use)
• herpes eye infections, eye tuberculosis, or any other eye infection

drugs

GENERIC	BRAND	RX
dexamethasone	*Decadron*	Yes
prednisolone	*Pred Forte*	

form/usage

when

OINTMENT, SOLUTION, SUSPENSION: For drops and solutions, ask your doctor to recommend proper procedure.

For ointment: Tilt head toward ceiling. Pull lower lid away from eye, creating a pocket. Squeeze a little bit of ointment into pocket. Close eye for a minute or two. Don't blink or squeeze. Do not touch tube tip with hands. Wipe clean with tissue.

As recommended by your doctor.

side effects and adverse reactions

what to do

Eye pain, enlarged pupils, vision problems

Stop taking. Get in touch with doctor immediately.

Burning or stinging, watery eyes

Continue taking, but discuss with your physician.

special precautions

DRUG INTERACTIONS
No interactions reported, but check with doctor if you are using any other eye preparations.

DIET
No interactions reported.

ALCOHOL and TOBACCO
No interactions reported.

PREGNANCY
Avoid drug.

BREAST-FEEDING
No interactions reported.

AGE FACTOR
1. Use cautiously in children and under medical supervision.

2. Drug is not expected to cause reactions in older people any different from those in young adults.

MISSED DOSE
Apply when you remember.

OVERDOSE
No overdose problems reported.

STOPPING DRUG
Discontinue when problem clears up.

because

Drug has caused fetal abnormalities in animal experiments.

1. Medication is more likely to cause side effects in children.

(continued)

OTHERS

Don't use without consulting doctor and making sure that your problem is not related to viral or bacterial infection. These illnesses do not respond to steroids.

If your condition does not clear up within three or four days, check with your doctor.

If medication is working, but you have been told to use it for several weeks, check with your doctor periodically.

drug or category:

TIMOLOL

condition:
GLAUCOMA

warning

Tell your doctor if you have or have had:
- an allergic reaction to this medication, or to demecarium, echothiophate, isoflurophate, or any preservatives or foods
- a respiratory illness, including asthma and emphysema (**There have been reports of deaths due to respiratory difficulties after timolol was used.**)
- diabetes (because medication may affect blood sugar levels)
- heart disease, myasthenia gravis, or thyroid disease

If you are going to have surgery (including extensive oral procedures), tell the doctor that you are taking these medications.

drugs

GENERIC	BRAND	RX
timolol maleate	*Timoptic*	Yes

form/usage

DROPS, OINTMENT: Recommended procedures may be awkward for you. Ask your doctor to go through process with you.

when

As suggested by your physician.

side effects and adverse effects

Vision changes, unexplained sweating, severe gastrointestinal problems, eye pain, eye twitching, headaches

Contraction of pupils

what to do

Stop taking. Get in touch with doctor immediately.

Do nothing. This is a normal reaction.

(continued)

special precautions	because
DRUG INTERACTIONS	
1. Cyclopentolate, physostigmine	1. Reduce effectiveness of timolol.
2. Pesticides containing organic phosphates	2. Timolol will increase their absorption into body.
3. Myasthenia gravis medications and topical anesthetics	3. May have toxic effects.
4. Atropine	4. May damage eyes. Discuss with your physician.
DIET No interactions reported.	
ALCOHOL AND TOBACCO No interactions reported.	
PREGNANCY Discuss with your doctor.	Drug increases risk of fetal death in animal experiments. No studies in humans.
BREAST-FEEDING Discuss with your doctor.	Medication will migrate into breast milk and could affect child.
AGE FACTOR	
1. Use cautiously in children.	1. Children are very sensitive to side effects of this drug.
2. People over 60 should use cautiously.	2. Adverse and side effects may be worse in older people.
MISSED DOSE Apply as soon as you remember.	
OVERDOSE No overdose problems reported.	

STOPPING DRUG

Do not stop taking even if you feel better until you have talked with your doctor. You may have to come off drug slowly.

OTHERS

Do not drive or operate machinery until you have determined how medication affects you.

drug or category:

DIPIVEFRIN

condition:
GLAUCOMA

warning

Tell your doctor if you have or have had:
- an allergic reaction to this medication, or to preservatives or food additives
- eye diseases other than glaucoma

If you are going to have surgery (including extensive oral procedures), tell the doctor that you are taking these medications.

drugs

GENERIC	BRAND	RX
dipivefrin	*Propine*	Yes

form/usage

DROPS: Recommended procedures may be awkward for you. Ask your doctor to go through process with you.

when

As suggested by your physician.

side effects and adverse reactions

Eye pain, vision problems, unexplained sweating, fainting, rapid heartbeat

Mild headaches, burning or itching sensation in eyes

what to do

Stop taking. Get in touch with doctor immediately.

Continue taking, but discuss with your physician.

special precautions

because

DRUG INTERACTIONS
No interactions reported with drugs taken by mouth, injection, or suppository. However, check with your doctor if you are taking other eye medications.

DIET

No interactions reported.

ALCOHOL AND TOBACCO

No interactions reported.

PREGNANCY

No negative interactions reported.

BREAST-FEEDING

No problems reported.

AGE FACTOR

1. Children are not reported to react differently to this medication than adults. However, it should be administered to them under strict medical supervision.

2. People over 60 should use cautiously.

2. Adverse and side effects may be worse in older people.

MISSED DOSE

Apply when you remember.

OVERDOSE

No overdose problems reported.

STOPPING DRUG

Do not stop taking even if you feel better until you have talked with your doctor. You may have to come off drug slowly.

OTHERS

Do not drive or operate machinery until you have determined how medication affects you.

EYE LUBRICANTS (ARTIFICIAL TEARS)

condition:

DRY EYES

warning

Tell your doctor if you have or have had an allergic reaction to this medication, or to preservatives or food additives.

drugs

GENERIC	BRAND	RX
hydroxypropyl methylcellulose	*Gonak, Just Tears*, others	Some

form/usage

DROPS: Recommended procedures may be awkward for you. Ask your doctor to go through process with you.

when

According to your doctor's instructions; usual schedule is three to four times a day.

side effects and adverse reactions

New eye irritation

what to do

Stop taking. Get in touch with doctor immediately.

special precautions

DRUG INTERACTIONS
No problems reported with any drug taken by mouth, injections, or suppository, but check with your doctor if you are using other eye medications.

DIET
No interactions reported.

ALCOHOL AND TOBACCO
No interactions reported.

because

PREGNANCY
No negative interactions reported.

--   --

BREAST-FEEDING
No problems reported.

--   --

AGE FACTOR

1. Do not use in children.   1. Safety and efficacy in children not established.

2. No problems reported in adults older than 60.

--   --

MISSED DOSE
Apply when you remember.

OVERDOSE
No overdose problems reported.

STOPPING DRUG
Discontinue when condition ends.

OTHERS
If condition persists or gets worse, check with your doctor.

ANTIBIOTICS

EYE INFECTIONS

warning

Tell your doctor if you have or have had an allergic reaction to this medication or any antibiotics, or to any preservatives or food additives.

drugs

GENERIC	BRAND	RX
gentamicin	*Garamycin*	Yes
tetracycline	*Achromycin*	
neomycin, polymyxin B, bacitracin	*Neosporin*	

form/usage

OINTMENT, CREAM, DROPS: For drops: Wash hands. Tilt head toward ceiling. Pull lower lid away from eye, creating a pocket. Drop medicine into pocket. Close eye for a minute or two. Don't blink or squeeze. If you miss, you can try again.

For ointment: Wash hands. Squeeze a little bit of medication into pocket between lower eyelid and eye.

Do not touch tip of eye dropper or applicator. Clean them with a tissue.

when

Discuss with your physician.

side effects and adverse reactions

Blurred vision for a minute or two after applying medicine

what to do

Continue taking, but discuss with your physician.

(continued)

special precautions

because

DRUG INTERACTIONS
No interactions reported.

DIET
No restrictions.

ALCOHOL AND TOBACCO
No interactions reported.

PREGNANCY
No negative interactions reported.

BREAST-FEEDING
No problems reported.

AGE FACTOR
No special age considerations.

MISSED DOSE
Use as soon as you remember.

OVERDOSE
No overdose problems reported.

STOPPING DRUG
Discontinue when infection has disappeared.

OTHERS
If your infection does not clear up in a month, discuss with your doctor.

drug or category:

NAPHAZOLINE

condition:

MINOR EYE IRRITATIONS

warning

Tell your doctor if you have or have had an allergic reaction to this medication, or to any preservatives or food additives.

drugs

GENERIC	BRAND	RX
naphazoline	*Naphcon-A*, others	Some
oxymetazoline	*Visine L.R.*, others	

form/usage

EYE DROPS: Recommended procedures may be awkward for you. Ask your doctor to go through process with you.

when

Discuss with your physician.

side effects and adverse reactions

Vision problems, dilation of pupils, lower body temperature, headache, gastrointestinal problems, reduced heartbeat, eye irritations

what to do

Stop taking. Get in touch with doctor immediately.

special precautions

because

DRUG INTERACTIONS
No interactions reported with drugs taken by mouth, injection, or suppository. Check with your doctor, however, if you are using other optical preparations.

DIET
No interactions reported.

ALCOHOL AND TOBACCO
No problems reported with alcohol or tobacco.

PREGNANCY
Studies relating to pregnancy have not been done.

BREAST-FEEDING
No problems reported.

AGE FACTOR
1. Not recommended for use in children.

2. No problems reported in adults over 60.

1. Use of drug may result in CNS depression leading to coma and marked hypothermia.

MISSED DOSE
Apply when you remember.

OVERDOSE
No overdose problems reported.

STOPPING DRUG
Discontinue when problem clears up.

OTHERS
Check with your doctor if condition persists or gets worse.

EAR MEDICATIONS

INFECTIONS

warning

Tell your doctor if you have or have had:
- an allergic reaction to this medication or other antibiotics, or to any preservatives or foods
- any other ear infection or problem, including herpes

Do not use with any other ear medications unless directed to do so by your doctor.

Do not use for more than ten days, unless directed to do so by your doctor.

drugs

GENERIC	BRAND	RX
neomycin, polymyxin B, hydro-cortisone	Cortisporin, Pediotic, others	Yes
colistin, neomycin, and hydrocor-tisone	Coly-Mycin S Otic	
chloramphenicol	Chloromycetin	

form/usage

SOLUTIONS, SUSPENSIONS: Lie down or sit so that the opening of the infected ear is up.

If giving to an adult, pull ear lobe up and back (toward opening); if giving to a child, pull ear lobe down and back.

Drop in medicine.

Hold position for five minutes.

Put cotton plug in ear (ask your doctor if you should put some medicine into cotton).

when

Follow your doctor's suggestion.

side effects and adverse reactions

Itching or burning in ear

what to do

Stop taking. Get in touch with doctor immediately.

special precautions	**because**
DRUG INTERACTIONS No interactions reported.	
DIET No interactions reported.	
ALCOHOL AND TOBACCO No interactions reported.	
PREGNANCY Avoid drug.	Adrenocorticoids have caused fetal abnormalities in animal experiments. There have been no studies in humans.
BREAST-FEEDING No problems reported.	
AGE FACTOR No problems related to age reported.	
MISSED DOSE Apply when you remember.	
OVERDOSE No overdose problems have been reported.	
STOPPING DRUG Do not stop taking even if you feel better until prescription is finished or you have talked with your doctor.	

drug or category:

ANTIPYRINE AND BENZOCAINE

condition:

EAR PAIN

warning

Use for pain only. Will not cure infection.
• Tell your doctor if you have or have had an allergic reaction to these medications or to any topical anesthetic.

drugs

GENERIC	BRAND	RX
antipyrine and benzocaine	*Auralgan*, others	Yes

form/usage

DROPS: Put bottle under warm running water to warm solution.

Lie down or sit so that the opening of the ear is up.

If giving to an adult, pull ear lobe up and back (toward opening); if giving to a child, pull ear lobe down and back.

Drop in medicine.

Hold position for five minutes.

Put cotton plug in ear (ask your doctor if you should put some medicine into cotton).

Do not touch drop dispenser. Wipe with clean tissue.

when

Follow your doctor's suggestion.

side effects and adverse reactions

Itching or burning

what to do

Stop taking. Get in touch with doctor immediately.

special precautions

because

DRUG INTERACTIONS
No interactions reported.

DIET
No interactions reported.

ALCOHOL and TOBACCO
No interactions reported.

PREGNANCY
No interactions reported.

BREAST-FEEDING
No interactions reported.

AGE FACTOR
No problems related to age reported.

MISSED DOSE
Apply when your remember.

OVERDOSE
No overdose problems reported.

STOPPING DRUG
You can stop using when pain ends.

HYDROCORTISONE AND ACETIC ACID

SWIMMER'S EAR

warning

Tell your doctor if you have or have had an allergic reaction to this or similar medications, or to any preservatives or food additives.

Don't use with other ear medications unless told to do so by your doctor.

drugs

GENERIC	BRAND	RX
hydrocortisone and acetic acid	VōSol	Yes

form/usage

DROPS: Warm drops by holding bottle under warm running water.

If giving to an adult, pull ear lobe up and back (toward opening); if giving to a child, pull ear lobe down and back.

Drop in medicine.

Hold position for five minutes.

Put cotton plug in ear (ask your doctor if you should put some medicine into cotton).

Do not touch drop dispenser. Wipe with clean tissue.

when

Follow your doctor's recommendations.

side effects and adverse reactions

Itching or burning in ear

what to do

Stop taking. Get in touch with your doctor immediately.

special precautions	because
DRUG INTERACTIONS No interactions reported.	
DIET No interactions reported.	
ALCOHOL AND TOBACCO No interactions reported.	
PREGNANCY No negative interactions reported.	
BREAST-FEEDING No problems reported.	
AGE FACTOR No problems related to age reported.	
MISSED DOSE Apply when you remember.	
OVERDOSE No overdose problems reported.	
STOPPING DRUG Stop using when problem clears up.	

-35-

SKIN, MOUTH, AND HAIR PREPARATIONS

Problems affecting the skin, mouth, and hair may seem trivial compared to severe diseases, but they can make life miserable and, in some instances, even pose a threat to health or point to a serious underlying disease.

Acne

Acne—our most common skin problem—typically starts in adolescence and can persist well into adulthood. The more virulent forms can be disfiguring, but even milder outbreaks can cause embarrassment and emotional problems for a teenager. Hormones play a key role in the development of acne; in women especially, any hormonal change—menstruation, pregnancy, the use of oral contraceptives, and menopause—can provoke a flare-up of acne. Hormones step up the production of sebum, a fatty substance produced in the skin's sebaceous glands. Sebum lubricates the skin and also carries dead skin cells to the surface. Too much sebum, however, clogs the skin pores, setting the stage for an overgrowth of the bacteria that normally reside in the hair follicles; this results in black heads, white heads, and cystic pimples.

Most acne can be controlled with nonprescription medications, which may take the form of cleansing soaps, creams, gels, lotions, facial masks, and solutions. These include:

- **Benzoyl peroxide.** This is the key ingredient for some of the most popular acne medications (*Benoxyl, benzac, Clearasil,* and others). It works by loosening dead skin cells, thereby unclogging the blocked pores. It also has a mild antibiotic effect. Because benzoyl peroxide may cause skin irritation, dermatologists recommend starting with the lowest concentration—2.5 or 5 percent—and going on to greater strengths if needed. Don't overuse this medication, because skin irritation itself can worsen acne.

- **Salicylic acid, triclosan, alcohol, and sulfur.** These ingredients, found in products such as *Clearasil, Fostex, Oxy,* and others, are also mild peeling agents that loosen dead cells and help unclog pores.

- **Topical antibiotics,** Lotions, gels, and other topical preparations containing clindamycin (*Cleocin T*), erythromycin (*Erycette, EryDerm, Erygel*), and tetracycline (*Topicycline*) are prescribed for acne that is not controlled by benzoyl peroxide and other nonprescription products. They kill bacteria on the skin and also fight inflammation. Tretinoin (*Retin-A*), a topical drug derived from vitamin A, promotes peeling of dead skin cells, thereby unblocking clogged pores. It may cause some irritation and an initial flare-up of acne; otherwise it is a safe drug. However, it should not be used with benzoyl peroxide products because the combination can cause excessive peeling and irritation.

- **Isotretinoin** (*Accutane*). This drug is also derived from vitamin A. It is an oral drug and one of the most effective antiacne medications. But it is recommended only for severe cystic acne because of its risk of side effects such as depression, gastrointestinal reactions, and headaches. More seriously, it can cause severe birth defects. The drug should never be taken if there is any possibility of pregnancy, and it should be stopped at least three months before attempting to conceive.

Dermatitis and Eczema

These itchy conditions are often triggered by contact with an allergen or irritant. Household cleaners, cosmetics, jewelry, various chemicals, certain fibers, and stress are among the many things that can trigger dermatitis. Topical adrenocorticoids such as hydrocortisone acetate (*Cortaid* and others) usually bring prompt relief. If not, oral steroids may be considered. (See chapters 16, 23, and 31.)

Psoriasis

This skin disease is characterized by a rapid turnover of skin cells, resulting in inflamed patches of thick, scaly lesions. In some cases, psoriasis is

accompanied by arthritis. There is no cure for psoriasis, but the condition can usually be controlled by a combination of treatments, including judicious exposure to the sun. Drugs used to treat psoriasis include:

- **Topical adrenocorticoids** (*Cortaid, Medrol,* others), which counteract inflammation
- **Coal tar products** (*Tegrin, Denorex,* others), which help remove the layers of scaly, thickened skin
- **Salicylic acid** (*Clearasil, Noxzema,* others), which also promotes peeling
- **Psoralens**, such as methoxsalen (*Oxsoralen Lotion*), which is used in conjunction with light treatments
- **Etretinate** (*Tegison*), an oral derivative of vitamin A, which promotes peeling
- **Methotrexate** (*Rheumatrex*), an anticancer drug that slows down the turnover of skin cells

All of these drugs have potentially serious side effects and should be used only under a doctor's careful supervision.

Hair Problems

BALDNESS

In 1988, an antihypertensive drug called minoxidil (*Loniten*) was introduced to treat high blood pressure associated with organ damage. Before long, one of its side effects—unwanted hair growth—became apparent. Minoxidil never gained wide use as an antihypertensive agent, but its manufacturer decided to capitalize on the hair growth side effect. Minoxidil was reformulated into a topical medication and reintroduced as *Rogaine*, a prescription drug to treat baldness.

Rogaine is not exactly the answer to baldness; about 50 to 60 percent of men using it achieve moderate to good regrowth. Recent studies show that the best results are achieved by men who start using it during early hair loss to prevent further balding. The drug is also being promoted for women with thinning hair. A major drawback is that the drug must be used continuously; once it is stopped, you will probably shed the new hair within a few months. Its cost—about $50 a month—is another drawback. Because some of the drug is absorbed through the scalp, it may lower blood pressure, a factor that must be taken into consideration if you are taking other antihypertensive drugs.

Mouth Problems

Various mouth sores and fever blisters can be disconcertingly painful. The cause of canker sores is unknown—stress, food allergies or sensitivities, hormonal changes, and injuries (such as biting the inside of one's mouth) seem to trigger attacks. Most clear up in a few days—in the meantime, a benzocaine anesthetic preparation (*Orabase-B*) lessens the pain.

Cold sores are caused by the herpes simplex virus. The blisters usually disappear within 7 to 14 days, but commonly recur. If you are continuously bothered by cold sores, you may want to discuss an antiviral preparation like acyclovir (*Zovirax*) with your doctor. This drug reduces recurrences and also shortens the course of flare-ups (see Chapter 19).

Lice and Scabies

Humans are hosts to any number of parasites, including various mites, lice, and other insects. Scabies, caused by the itch mite *Sarcoptes scabiei* var. *hominis*, produces an intensely itchy rash wherever the female mite invades the skin to lay her eggs—usually in the folds of skin on the trunk.

Lice infestations are also common, especially outbreaks of head lice among schoolchildren. These outbreaks have nothing to do with cleanliness; instead, they are spread when people share combs, hairbrushes, hats, even headphones. They also can be picked up from upholstered seats in movie theaters, trains, and other public places.

Pubic lice, or crabs, are somewhat larger than head lice, and are most often spread by sexual contact or sharing towels and other personal items. To get rid of these parasites, you not only have to get rid of those on the body, you also must eliminate them from your carpets, rugs, upholstered furniture, mattresses, clothing, bedding, and other items that may harbor the insects or their eggs. This can be done by vacuuming; laundering with hot, soapy water; dry-cleaning; or moving out for several weeks to remove the insects' source of food—human blood.

As for getting rid of lice on your person, this is best done by using an antilice shampoo. In the past, lindane products such as *Kwell* were the drug of choice, but newer pyrethrin products are now preferred. Pyrethrins are natural substances obtained from chrysanthemums that are safe for humans but lethal to lice and many other pests. They have fewer side effects than lindane, which can cause dizziness, intestinal disturbances, and sometimes seizures. Over-the-counter products containing pyrethrins include *Rid* and *R&C Shampoo*.

TRETINOIN

ACNE

warning

Tell your doctor if you have or have had an allergic reaction to this medication, or to preservatives or food additives.

Do not use harsh soaps, preparations that contain alcohol, or acne preparations that have benzoyl peroxide, resorcinol, salicylic acid, or sulfur on area where you use tretinoin.

drugs

GENERIC	BRAND	RX
tretinoin	*Retin-A*	Yes

form/usage

CREAM, GEL, TOPICAL SOLUTION: wash and dry affected areas; then wait half an hour.

Gel or cream: Rub in enough to cover affected area.

Solution: Put medication on gauze pad or cotton, but don't soak. Rub over affected areas.

when

Same time every day.

side effects and adverse reactions

Severe reactions on skin, including blistering, crusting, swelling, burning

Feeling of warmth on skin, change in color of skin, peeling

what to do

Stop using. Get in touch with doctor immediately.

Continue using, but discuss with your physician.

(continued)

special precautions	**because**
DRUG INTERACTIONS	
1. Other antiacne topical medications, harsh soaps or cleaners, medicated makeup	1. Skin irritation may result.
2. Etretinate	2. Possible toxicity.
DIET	
No interactions reported.	
ALCOHOL AND TOBACCO	
No interactions reported.	
PREGNANCY	
Avoid drug.	Minor skull formation effects reported in animals. No adequate studies have been done in humans.
BREAST-FEEDING	
No problems reported.	
AGE FACTOR	
Not recommended for infants, children, or adults over 60.	Safety and efficacy have not been established in children or older adults.
MISSED DOSE	
Apply when you remember.	
OVERDOSE	
No overdose problems reported.	
STOPPING DRUG	
Do not stop taking even if your skin is better until you have talked with your doctor.	
OTHERS	
Don't stay in sun or under sunlamp too long. Your skin may be more prone to sunburn when using tretinoin.	

ISOTRETINOIN

condition:
CYSTIC ACNE

---

warning

Drug is considered highly toxic and should not be used unless other medications have been tried unsuccessfully, and then only if acne is severe.

Tell your doctor if you have or have had:

- an allergic reaction to this medication, or to any preservatives or foods
- a history of alcohol or drug abuse
- a family history of high triglyceride levels
- diabetes

Do not take vitamin A or any vitamin combinations that contain vitamin A while you are taking this medication.

Do not donate blood until 30 days have passed since your last dose.

---

drugs

GENERIC	BRAND	RX
isotretinoin	Accutane	Yes

---

form/usage

CAPSULES: May be taken with food or beverage.

Capsules may be opened.

when

Twice a day.

---

side effects and adverse reactions

Abdominal or eye pain, vision problems, severe gastrointestinal problems, bleeding from rectum, jaundice, skin reactions, burning eyes, nosebleeds

Muscle, bone, and joint pain; hair loss; fatigue; itchiness

Dry mouth

what to do

Stop taking. Get in touch with doctor immediately.

Continue taking, but discuss with your physician.

Try sugarless candy or gum. If condition persists, discuss with your doctor or dentist.

(continued)

special precautions	because
DRUG INTERACTIONS	
1. Etretinate, high doses of vitamin A	1. Toxicity.
2. Tetracyclines	2. May raise pressure in brain and cause symptoms resembling brain tumor.
DIET	
No interactions reported.	
ALCOHOL AND TOBACCO	
Avoid both.	Alcohol could cause increase in blood triglycerides. Tobacco may interfere with absorption of medication.
PREGNANCY	
Avoid drug.	Drug is considered highly dangerous to fetus. Do not use while pregnant. Do not use if you are likely to become pregnant within one month. It is recommended that women have pregnancy test two weeks before starting drug and that medication not be started unless a highly effective contraceptive has been used for at least one month beforehand.
BREAST-FEEDING	
Avoid drug or avoid nursing.	Medication will migrate into breast milk and could affect child. Discuss with your doctor. If you do take isotretinoin, keep a close eye on baby for any possible side effects.
AGE FACTOR	
1. Not recommended for children.	1. Side effects likely to be stronger in children.
2. People over 60 should use cautiously.	2. Adverse and side effects may be worse in older people.
MISSED DOSE	
You can take a missed dose up to two hours after scheduled time. Otherwise, wait for next dose. **Double the amount taken.**	

OVERDOSE
No overdose problems reported.

STOPPING DRUG
Medication often works after one treatment. If a second one is recommended, wait eight weeks before resuming.

OTHERS
You should have periodic checkups to assess blood counts, and blood cholesterol and triglyceride levels. Eye exams and liver and kidney function tests may also be a good idea.

May increase sensitivity to sun. If you go outdoors between 10 A.M. and 3 P.M., wear protective clothing and/or sunblock.

drug or category:

MUPIROCIN

condition:
INFECTIONS OF THE SKIN

warning

Tell your doctor if you have or have had an allergic reaction to this medication, or to preservatives or food additives.

drugs

GENERIC	BRAND	RX
mupirocin	*Bactroban*	Yes

form/usage

OINTMENT: Wash infected area thoroughly and dry completely.
Rub in a small amount of ointment.
Affected area may be covered.

when

Usually three to four times a day.

side and adverse effects

Overly dry, itchy, and swollen skin

what to do

Stop taking. Get in touch with doctor immediately.

special precautions

DRUG INTERACTIONS
Any other topical drug

DIET
No restrictions.

ALCOHOL AND TOBACCO
No restrictions.

because

May increase sensitivity to both mupirocin and the other medication.

PREGNANCY
No negative interactions reported.

BREAST-FEEDING
No problems reported.

AGE FACTOR
No restrictions.

MISSED DOSE
Apply when you remember.

OVERDOSE
No overdose problems likely.

STOPPING DRUG
Stop when infection clears up; however, discuss with your doctor.

OTHERS
Do not store where there is heat or humidity.

BENZOYL PEROXIDE

condition:

ACNE

warning

Tell your doctor if you have or have had an allergic reaction to this medication, or to preservatives or food additives.

drugs

GENERIC	BRAND	RX
benzoyl peroxide	*Benoxyl, benzac, Clearasil, Desquam-X*, others	Some

form/usage

when

CLEANSING SOAP, CREAMS, GELS, LOTIONS, FACIAL MASKS, STICK: Wash affected area according to instructions on package.

Rub in creams, gels, and lotions gently.

After applying mask, leave in place for 15 to 25 minutes, then wash off with warm water and dry.

Discuss with doctor.

side effects and adverse reactions

what to do

Rash, peeling, very dry skin

Mild but painful skin irritation

Stop taking. Get in touch with doctor immediately.

Continue taking, but discuss with your physician.

special precautions

because

DRUG INTERACTIONS
Other acne preparations or medications to peel skin

Will irritate skin.

DIET

Avoid foods with cinnamon if taking *Desquam-X*.

Could cause skin rash.

ALCOHOL AND TOBACCO

No interactions reported.

PREGNANCY

Discuss with your doctor.

No human or animal tests done. Medication, however, is absorbed into body.

BREAST-FEEDING

Discuss with you doctor.

Not known if drug migrates into breast milk.

AGE FACTOR

1. Do not use in infants or children.

1. No information on the drug's safety in children is available.

2. No problems reported when used by adults over 60 years of age.

MISSED DOSE

Apply when you remember.

OVERDOSE

No overdose problems reported.

STOPPING DRUG

Discontinue when acne clears up. If acne persists for more than two to four weeks, consult your doctor.

OTHERS

May bleach hair and clothing.

Avoid getting into eyes, nose, mouth, or on back of neck.

drug or category:

CLINDAMYCIN

condition:
ACNE

warning

Tell your doctor if you have or have had an allergic reaction to this medication, or to preservatives or food additives.

Drug may be absorbed into body, even though it is applied on skin. **May cause severe gastrointestinal problems, fever, loss of weight.**

drugs

GENERIC	BRAND	RX
clindamycin	*Cleocin T*	Yes

form/usage

GEL, SOLUTION, SUSPENSION: Wash affected area thoroughly and dry. However, do not wash area too often during the day. Discuss with your dermatologist.

Half an hour after washing, apply medication according to instructions in package.

when

As directed by your dermatologist.

side effects and adverse reactions

Gastrointestinal problems, fever, loss of weight

Peeling, itching, redness, stinging, or burning

what to do

Stop taking. Get in touch with doctor immediately.

Continue taking, but discuss with your physician.

special precautions

DRUG INTERACTIONS
Antidiarrhea medications.

because

Some diminish effectiveness of clindamycin, others worsen the diarrhea caused by the drug.

DIET
No interactions reported.

ALCOHOL AND TOBACCO
No interactions.

PREGNANCY
Use with caution or avoid.

No evidence of problems in animal experiments, but there are no adequate studies with humans.

BREAST-FEEDING
Discuss with doctor.

Not known if drug migrates to milk.

AGE FACTOR
Do not give to children.

Safety in children under 12 not established.

MISSED DOSE
Take up to two hours after scheduled dose, otherwise wait until next dose. Do not double dosage.

OVERDOSE
Get emergency help or contact poison control center if user has severe diarrhea, vomiting, or nausea.

STOPPING DRUG
Discuss with your doctor, even if your problems seem to have cleared up.

OTHERS
Be sure to keep medication out of mouth, nose, or eyes because it can cause painful burning. If medication does enter these areas, wash out with cool water.

drug or category:

BENZOCAINE

condition:

MOUTH AND DENTAL PAIN

warning

Tell your doctor if you have or have had:

- an allergic reaction to this medication or to any preservatives or food additives
- any mouth infections or disorders

Tell your doctor if you are taking:

- medications for myasthenia gravis or glaucoma
- any sulfa medications

drugs

GENERIC	BRAND	RX
benzocaine	*Orabase-B*	Some

form/usage

AEROSOL, JELLIES: As directed by your doctor or dentist, or the package.

Use cotton-tipped applicator or spray on affected places.

Avoid swallowing. Don't chew gum or eat or drink for up to one hour after applying.

when

As directed by package. Do not use more often than prescribed.

side effects and adverse reactions

Swelling in mouth, on skin, or in throat; vision problems; unexplained sweating; ringing in ears; changes in heartbeat; nervousness or restlessness

Stinging or tenderness in mouth, skin reactions

what to do

Stop taking. Get in touch with doctor immediately.

Continue taking, but discuss with your physician.

special precautions	because
DRUG INTERACTIONS No interactions reported.	
DIET No interactions reported.	
ALCOHOL AND TOBACCO Avoid both.	Alcohol increases risk of side effects. Tobacco irritates mouth tissues.
PREGNANCY No negative interactions reported.	
BREAST-FEEDING No problems reported.	
AGE FACTOR 1. Children should use lower-strength over-the-counter products only. 2. People over 60 should use prescription-strength formulations cautiously.	1. Prescription-strength benzocaine could cause some side effects. 2. Adverse and side effects may be worse in older people, who may react more strongly to local anesthetics.
MISSED DOSE Apply when you remember. Do not double dose.	
OVERDOSE **Get emergency medical help immediately** if patient has seizures or vision problems, is dizzy, or can't be kept awake.	
STOPPING DRUG Medication may be discontinued when problem clears up.	
OTHERS Do not drive or operate machinery until you have determined how medication affects you.	

drug or category:

ADRENOCORTICOIDS—LOW POTENCY

condition:

SKIN IRRITATIONS

warning

Tell your doctor if you have or have had:

- an allergic reaction to this medication, or to any preservatives or foods
- diabetes, a skin infection, ulcers, or tuberculosis

Do not use for acne.

drugs

GENERIC	BRAND	RX
hydrocortisone acetate	*Cortaid*, others	Yes
methylprednisolone	*Medrol*	

form/usage

OINTMENT, CREAM, LOTION, SOLUTIONS (SPRAY AND AERO-SOL), SUSPENSION: Do not bandage unless your doctor has recommended you do so. If you use a plastic wrapping, do not do so for more than two weeks.

Wash hands after using medication.

when

As recommended by your doctor.

side effects and adverse reactions

Unusual skin problems, including burning, blisters, itching, and pain

what to do

Continue taking, but discuss with your physician.

special precautions

DRUG INTERACTIONS
Antibiotics, antifungals

because

Medication will decrease their effectiveness.

DIET
No interactions reported.

ALCOHOL AND TOBACCO
No interactions reported.

PREGNANCY
Avoid drug.

Drug has caused fetal abnormalities in animal experiments.

BREAST-FEEDING
No interactions reported.
Do not apply to breasts.

AGE FACTOR
1. Children and teenagers who use this medication over long periods of time should do so under medical supervision.

2. Drug has not been reported to cause unusual problems in adults over 60.

1. Medication is absorbed through the skin and can affect development.

MISSED DOSE
Apply when you remember.

OVERDOSE
No overdose problems reported.

STOPPING DRUG
Discontinue when problem clears up, but discuss with your doctor.

OTHERS
Do not use topical steroids for long periods. They may affect the thickness of the outer layers of the skin. Discuss with your doctor or pharmacist if you are likely to use this drug for more than two weeks.

ADRENOCORTICOIDS— MEDIUM/HIGH POTENCY

condition:
SKIN IRRITATIONS, PSORIASIS

warning

Tell your doctor if you have or have had an allergic reaction to this medication, or to any preservatives or foods.

drugs

GENERIC	BRAND	RX
betamethasone	*Diprosone, Valisone*	Yes
fluocinolone	*Synalar*, others	
fluocinonide	*Lidex, Fluocin*	

form/usage

CREAMS, OINTMENTS, SOLUTION, GELS, TOPICAL AEROSOL:
Read instructions that come with medication.

Do not place bandages over treated site unless directed to do so by your doctor.

when

According to your doctor's or the package instructions.

side effects and adverse reactions

Skin reactions, including pain, redness, blistering, peeling, acne

what to do

Continue taking, but discuss with your physician.

special precautions

DRUG INTERACTIONS
Antibiotics and antifungal medications

DIET
No restrictions.

because

Effectiveness of antibiotics and antifungals will be decreased.

ALCOHOL AND TOBACCO
No restrictions.

PREGNANCY
Discuss with your doctor.

No studies in humans. In animal tests medications applied in high doses have caused fetal abnormalities.

BREAST-FEEDING
Do not apply to breasts before nursing.

It is not known whether topical use of adrenocorticoids results in sufficient absorption to yield detectable quantities in breast milk.

AGE FACTOR
1. Infants: Do not use with plastic pants or diapers.

2. All children: Use medication only under medical supervision.

3. People older than 60 should use cautiously.

1. Could cause an increase in the amount absorbed into body.

2. Prolonged use can cause growth problems.

3. Greater likelihood of side and adverse effects.

MISSED DOSE
Apply when you remember, unless it is nearly time for next dose. In that case, just apply the scheduled dose, but do not double the amount put on.

OVERDOSE
No overdose problems expected.

STOPPING DRUG
Stop when your skin is better. No need to finish prescription.

OTHERS
Do not use topical steroids for long periods. They may affect the thickness of the outer layer of the skin. Discuss with your doctor or pharmacist if you are likely to use drug for more than two weeks.

ADRENOCORTICOIDS—TOPICAL

RECTAL IRRITATIONS

warning

Tell your doctor if you have or have had an allergic reaction to this medication, or to any preservatives or foods. Do not use if your hemorrhoids are bleeding or if you have an infection around rectum.

drugs

GENERIC	BRAND	RX
hydrocortisone	*Anusol HC, Corticaine,* others	Some

form/usage

CREAM, OINTMENT, SUPPOSITORIES: Follow directions on package.

when

As directed on package or by your doctor.

side effects and adverse reactions

Bloody urine, reduced heartbeat, new irritations to rectal area and other skin symptoms around anus, nervous feelings

Painful urination, vision problems, swelling of feet

what to do

Stop taking. Get in touch with doctor immediately.

Continue taking, but discuss with your physician.

special precautions

DRUG INTERACTIONS
Sulfa medications

DIET
No restrictions.

ALCOHOL AND TOBACCO
No restrictions.

because

Effectiveness of sulfa medications will be decreased.

PREGNANCY
Avoid drug.

Drug has caused fetal abnormalities in animal experiments when used in high doses because it is absorbed through the skin. No human studies have been performed.

BREAST-FEEDING
No problems reported.

AGE FACTOR
1. Use cautiously in children.

1. Prolonged use could interfere with growth because drug is absorbed into body.

2. People over 60 should use cautiously.

2. Adverse and side effects may be worse in older people.

MISSED DOSE
Apply when you remember.

OVERDOSE
No overdose problems expected.

STOPPING DRUG
Stop when itching abates.

drug or category:

SELENIUM SULFIDE

condition:
DANDRUFF

warning

Tell your doctor if you have or have had:
- an allergic reaction to this medication, or to preservatives or food additives
- any serious scalp problems in addition to dandruff, including blisters or open sores

drugs

GENERIC	BRAND	RX
selenium sulfide	*Selsun Blue, Head & Shoulders Intensive Treatment Lotion* and *Intensive Treatment Lotion* 2-in-1, others	Some

form/usage

LOTION: As directed on package.

when

As directed on package. Do not use more often.

side effects and adverse reactions

Irritation or other scalp problems that were not present before medication was applied

Dry or itchy scalp

what to do

Stop using. Get in touch with doctor immediately.

Continue using, but discuss with your physician.

special precautions

DRUG INTERACTIONS
Do not use with other medicated shampoos unless directed by doctor.

because

Could cause severe scalp irritation.

DIET

No interactions reported.

ALCOHOL AND TOBACCO

No interactions reported.

PREGNANCY

No negative interactions reported.

BREAST-FEEDING

No problems reported.

AGE FACTOR

No problems related to age reported.

MISSED DOSE

Apply when you remember.

OVERDOSE

No overdose problems reported.

STOPPING DRUG

Stop using when dandruff abates. You may want to discuss with your doctor, however, if you have a persistent problem.

drug or category:

ALLANTOIN, PADIMATE O

condition:

HERPES INFECTIONS IN MOUTH; ALSO HELPS PREVENT COLD SORES,
SUN AND FEVER BLISTERS

warning

Tell your doctor if you have or have had an allergic reaction to this medication, or to preservatives or food additives.

drugs

GENERIC	BRAND	RX
allantoin, padimate O	*Herpecin-L, Herpecin-C*	For *Herpecin-L*

form/usage

LIP BALM STICK: Apply as directed.

when

For herpes, once an hour. Apply liberally.

If using for protection against sun, apply before and after exposure, after swimming, and before going to bed.

For chapped lips, use as needed.

side effects and adverse reactions

Irritation of mouth tissues

what to do

Continue taking, but discuss with your physician.

special precautions

DRUG INTERACTIONS
No interactions reported.

because

DIET
No restrictions.

ALCOHOL AND TOBACCO
No interactions reported.

PREGNANCY
No restrictions

BREAST-FEEDING
No problems reported.

AGE FACTOR
1. Should not be given to children under the age of two.

2. No problems reported with older adults.

1. Drugs containing sunscreens are not recommended for children under two.

MISSED DOSE
Apply when you remember.

OVERDOSE
No overdose problems reported.

STOPPING DRUG
Stop when your symptoms abate. Discuss with your doctor if you have a persistent problem.

OTHERS
If you are sensitive to any of the drug's ingredients, such as petroleum and titanium dioxide, discontinue use.

drug or category:

LINDANE

condition:

SCABIES, LICE INFESTATIONS

warning

Tell your doctor if you have or have had:
- an allergic reaction to this medication, or to any preservatives or foods
- a seizure disorder

Medication is poisonous. Avoid spilling or using near mouth. Avoiding using in areas where there is a rash, sores, or broken skin. If you are applying this medication to another person, use rubber or disposable gloves.

drugs

GENERIC	BRAND	RX
lindane	*Kwell*, others	Yes

form/usage

SHAMPOO, LOTION, CREAM: Follow your doctor's instructions.

Be sure to remove all creams, ointments, etc., from skin before using lindane.

If you wash prior to using, make sure you are completely dry.

If you are using **for scabies**, be sure entire body (including soles of feet) is covered.

Take shower or bath eight hours later to remove completely.
If you are using **for head lice,** do not use in a bath; keep on your head only and avoid having shampoo run down your body.

Be sure to keep shampoo in hair for at least four minutes. Run a fine-tooth comb through hair several times after washing to remove remaining lice eggs or lice egg shells.

when

Follow your doctor's instructions.

side effects and adverse reactions

Skin reactions

what to do

Stop using. Get in touch with doctor immediately.

special precautions	because
DRUG INTERACTIONS Myasthenia drugs, cholinesterase inhibitors	May cause increased toxicity.
DIET No interactions reported.	
ALCOHOL AND TOBACCO No interactions reported.	
PREGNANCY Avoid drug or discuss with your doctor.	Drug could cause fetal abnormalities in humans.
BREAST-FEEDING Avoid drug or avoid nursing for at least two days after you have used medication.	Medication will migrate into breast milk and could affect child. Discuss with your doctor.
AGE FACTOR Children and adults over 60 should use with caution.	Increased sensitivity to medication, which is absorbed into body.
MISSED DOSE Apply as soon as you remember.	

OVERDOSE
Get emergency medical help immediately if person has seizures or changes in heart rate, vomits, has cramps, or suffers dizziness.

STOPPING DRUG
Discontinue when lice or scabies disappear.

OTHERS
Clean thoroughly or discard clothing worn by the affected person since lice eggs in garments may reinfect the wearer.

drug or category:

PYRITHIONE ZINC

condition:

DANDRUFF, SEBORRHEIC DERMATITIS

warning

Tell your doctor if you have or have had:

- an allergic reaction to this medication, or to preservatives or food additives
- sores, blisters, or open lesions on scalp

drugs

GENERIC	BRAND	RX
pyrithione zinc	*Head & Shoulders Dry Scalp Lotion* and *Dry Scalp Lotion 2-in-1, Sebex,* others	No

form/usage

BAR, CREAM, AND LOTION SHAMPOOS: Follow instructions on package.

when

Follow instructions on package.

side effects and adverse reactions

Irritation of scalp or skin on face

what to do

Stop using and get in touch with your doctor.

special precautions

DRUG INTERACTIONS

Other antidandruff or antiseborrhea shampoos

because

May increase scalp and skin irritation. Discuss with your doctor.

DIET

No restrictions.

ALCOHOL AND TOBACCO

No restrictions.

PREGNANCY

No negative interactions reported.

BREAST-FEEDING

No problems reported.

AGE FACTOR

No restrictions.

MISSED DOSE

Use when you remember.

OVERDOSE

No overdose problems expected.

STOPPING DRUG

Stop when dandruff or seborrhea disappear.

drug or category:

MINOXIDIL

condition:

MALE BALDNESS AND FEMALE PATTERN HAIR LOSS

warning

Tell your doctor if you have or have had:
- an allergic reaction to this medication, or to preservatives or food additives
- any scalp diseases
- cardiovascular disease or hypertension

drugs

GENERIC	BRAND	RX
minoxidil	*Rogaine*	Yes

form/usage

SOLUTION: Shampoo hair and dry completely; do not use hair dryer. Then apply according to physician's instruction.

when

Follow your doctor's recommendation. If you use at night, put on at least half an hour before going to bed.

side effects and adverse reactions

Heartbeat irregularities

Burning scalp, headache, dizziness, fainting, tingling or numbness in extremities, weight gain

what to do

Get emergency medical help immediately.

Stop taking. Get in touch with doctor immediately.

special precautions

DRUG INTERACTIONS
Topical steroids, petrolatum, or retinoids

because

May interfere with proper absorption of medication.

DIET
No interactions reported.

ALCOHOL AND TOBACCO
No interactions reported.

PREGNANCY
Avoid drug.

While drug has not caused fetal defects in animal experiments, it has caused pregnancy difficulties.

BREAST-FEEDING
Avoid drug or avoid nursing.

It is unknown whether topical Minoxidil passes into breast milk.

AGE FACTOR
1. Not prescribed for children.

2. No special problems reported in adults older than 60.

MISSED DOSE
Apply when you remember. Do not double dose.

OVERDOSE
No overdose problems reported.

STOPPING DRUG
Discontinue at will; however, within a few months you will lose whatever hair has grown back.

OTHERS
Periodic exams to check on water retention and heart function may be advisable.

-36-

DIETARY SUPPLEMENTS

Who should take nutrition supplements and in what dosages remains a topic of considerable debate and conflicting opinion. Nutrition experts agree that a varied and balanced diet based on the new Food Pyramid and five basic food groups—starches, fruits, vegetables, meats, and dairy products—will fulfill the Recommended Dietary Allowances (RDAs) listed below. They also agree that a multiple vitamin and mineral pill that supplies 100 percent of the RDA, while not necessary, will not do any harm. Disagreement arises, however, over whether certain nutrients should be taken in higher doses. For example, a number of recent studies show that high doses of vitamin E may protect against heart disease and colon cancer. Similar claims (with less supporting evidence) are being made for vitamins C and beta carotene, a precursor of vitamin A.

Vitamins A, E, and C, as well as the mineral zinc, are all antioxidants—substances that protect against free radicals, the detrimental by-products of oxygen metabolism. Researchers theorize that antioxidants can retard aging and prevent disease by blocking free radical molecules. Before rushing out to stock up on high-dose antioxidants, however, pause to consider that when taken in pharmaco-logical amounts, these vitamins take on the properties and risk of side effects of drugs. For example, it is well known that excessive intake of vitamin A causes birth defects, liver damage, and other problems, including death. Vitamin C in large amounts causes kidney and bladder problems. Vitamin D is also toxic in sustained high doses. Beta carotene appears to be safe, because the excess is excreted from the body. Researchers here and abroad are working to document what, if any, benefits can be derived from high-dose supplements. In the meantime, let common sense be your guide.

If you do take high-dose antioxidant vitamins, do not exceed 200 to 400 international units (IU) of vitamin E, 25,000 IU of beta carotene, and 1 gram of vitamin C a day. Even those amounts may be too high, especially if you have a medical problem that can be worsened by these drugs. For example, vitamin E has an antiplatelet effect, and may worsen a bleeding problem. Vitamin C can exacerbate kidney stones and produce diarrhea in AIDS patients. High-dose niacin (vitamin B_3), sometimes prescribed to lower cholesterol levels (see Chapter 24) can cause liver damage and should be avoided by people with liver disease.

If you are taking a high-dose vitamin or mineral

supplement under your doctor's supervision for a medical problem, periodically check with your physician for tests to make sure the compounds are not causing serious damage.

The following tables, from the Food and Nutrition Board of the National Academy of Sciences—National Research Council, give the Recommended Dietary Allowances for some key vitamins and minerals.

VITAMINS A, D, AND E

DIETARY SUPPLEMENTS

warning

These vitamins should be taken only by people whose diets are seriously lacking in them or by those in whom illness prevents proper absorption of them.

The ability of these vitamins in high doses to slow down aging or to cure or prevent ailments like cancer, heart disease, arthritis, or impotence, has not been proven by rigorous scientific experimentation in humans. Vitamins A, D, and E are fat-soluble vitamins, which means that they are stored in the body in tissues containing fat. Thus, in high concentrations these vitamins could prove toxic and could cause death.

Tell your doctor if you have or have had:

- an allergic reaction to these vitamins
- cystic fibrosis, cardiovascular disease, or diabetes
- diarrhea or other intestinal problems
- liver, kidney, pancreas, or thyroid disease

form/usage

CAPSULES, SOLUTIONS, TABLETS (REGULAR OR CHEWABLE) INJECTIONS: As supplements only if your diet does not contain sufficient amounts because of dietary restrictions or if you have been fed intravenously for long periods of time.

Should be taken under a doctor's supervision.

when

As directed by your doctor, then at the same time every day.

side effects and adverse reactions

Vitamin A: Bulge in baby's soft spot; vision problems; frequent urination; stomach, joint or bone pain

Vitamin D: Psychotic reactions, severe stomach pains, fever, pink eye

Vitamin E: Blurred vision, diarrhea

what to do

Stop using. Get in touch with doctor immediately.

side effects and adverse reactions	what to do
Vitamin A: Minor gastrointestinal problems, mild headache, skin reactions, loss of hair	Continue taking, but discuss with your physician.
Vitamin D: Pain in muscles or bone, mild gastrointestinal problems, cloudy urine, increased sensitivity to light	
Vitamin E: Minor gastrointestinal problems, fatigue, lower leg discomfort, breast enlargement, dizziness, headaches	

special precautions	because
DRUG INTERACTIONS	
Vitamin A	
1. Anticoagulants	1. Increases effect of anticoagulants.
2. Calcium supplements, cholestyramine, colestipol, mineral oil, neomycin, vitamin E	2. Decrease vitamin A absorption or effectiveness.
3. Oral contraceptives	3. Increase vitamin A absorption.
Vitamin D	
1. Anticonvulsants, cholestyramine, colestipol, cortisone, mineral oil, neomycin, phenobarbital, rifampin	1. Decrease absorption or effect of vitamin D.
2. Antacids with magnesium	2. Excessive intake of magnesium.
3. Calcium channel blockers	3. Decreases their effectiveness.
4. Digitalis	4. May cause heart rhythm disturbances.
5. Phosphorus preparations	5. May cause buildup of phosphorus.
6. Calcium supplements	6. Excessive buildup of calcium.
Vitamin E	
1. Anticoagulants	1. May increase anticoagulant effect.
2. Cholestyramine, colestipol, mineral oil, neomycin	2. Decrease effect or absorption of vitamin E.
3. Iron supplements	3. Possible decreased effect of iron supplements or vitamin E.

(continued)

DIET
No interactions reported.

--   --

ALCOHOL and TOBACCO
No interactions reported.

--   --

PREGNANCY
Avoid amounts exceeding recommended daily allowance.

Can cause fetal defects.

BREAST-FEEDING
Avoid amounts exceeding recommended daily allowance.

Some forms of vitamin preparations can pass into breast milk and prove toxic to baby.

--   --

AGE FACTOR
1. Avoid giving to children in doses higher than recommended allowance.

2. Older people should use cautiously.

1. Children may react more adversely to high doses of these vitamins.

2. Older people are more likely to have side effects, particularly when taking vitamin D.

--   --

MISSED DOSE
Take when you remember.

OVERDOSE
Get in touch with a poison control center, emergency room, or doctor if patient experiences vision problems, jaundice, severe gastrointestinal problems, seizures, heart rhythm changes, extreme mood changes, skin reactions, or an increased need to urinate.

STOPPING DRUG
If you are taking any of these vitamins under a doctor's orders, do not stop taking until you have talked with your doctor.

OTHERS
If you are taking vitamin D in high doses, you should have periodic liver and kidney function tests and tests for blood levels of calcium and phosphate.

drug or category:

VITAMINS B$_2$ (RIBOFLAVIN), B$_9$ (FOLIC ACID), AND B$_{12}$ (CYANOCOBALAMIN)

condition or use:
DIETARY SUPPLEMENTS

warning

These vitamins should be taken only by people whose diets are seriously lacking them, by those in whom illness prevents proper absorption of them from food, and by people with high cholesterol levels.

The ability of these B vitamins in high doses to cure allergies, anemia, migraine headaches, mental illness, skin afflictions, sterility, and other illness has not been proven in rigorous scientific experiments.

Tell your doctor if you have or have had:

- an allergic reaction to these vitamins, or to any preservatives or foods
- liver disease, pernicious anemia, or kidney failure

form/usage

TABLETS, INJECTIONS: According to your doctor's instructions.

when

According to your doctor's instructions.

side effects and adverse reactions

what to do

Vitamin B$_{12}$

Severe allergic reaction (anaphylactic shock)

Get emergency medical help immediately.

Vitamins B$_9$ and B$_{12}$

Skin reactions, irritation of bronchial tubes

Stop taking. Get in touch with doctor immediately.

Vitamin B$_{12}$

Diarrhea

Continue taking, but discuss with your physician.

Vitamins B$_2$ and B$_9$

Intensely yellow urine

No action necessary.

(continued)

special precautions	because

DRUG INTERACTIONS
Vitamin B$_2$

1. Anticholinergics

2. Tricyclic antidepressants, phenothiazines, probenecid

Vitamin B$_9$

1. Anticonvulsants

2. Pain relievers, chloramphenicol, oral contraceptives, steroids, methotrexate, para-aminosalicylic acid, pyrimethamine, sulfasalazine, triamterene, trimethoprim

Vitamin B$_{12}$

1. Anticonvulsants, chloramphenicol, cholestyramine, cimetidine, colchicine, famotidine, histamine antagonists, neomycin, extended-release potassium supplements, ranitidine

2. Para-aminosalicylic acid

3. Vitamin C

DIET
No interactions reported.

ALCOHOL and TOBACCO
Vitamin B$_2$

Avoid both.

Vitamin B$_{12}$

Avoid alcohol.

---

because column:

1. May increase absorption of vitamin.

2. May decrease vitamin's absorption

1. Vitamin may result in increased seizures.

2. Will diminish vitamin's effectiveness.

1. Will decrease absorption of B$_{12}$.

2. Vitamin will decrease its effect.

3. Vitamin C will destroy B$_{12}$. Take the vitamins at least two hours apart.

Both interfere with vitamin's absorption.

Alcohol may decrease absorption of vitamin.

PREGNANCY
Vitamins B$_2$ and B$_9$

Avoid high doses.

Have caused fetal abnormalities in animal experiments. There have been reports of increased risk of fetal deformations in humans.

Vitamins B$_{12}$

No interactions reported.

BREAST-FEEDING
Vitamins B$_2$ and B$_9$

Avoid drug or avoid nursing.

Vitamins will migrate into breast milk and could affect child. Discuss with your doctor.

Vitamins B$_{12}$

No interactions reported.

AGE FACTOR
No special problems in children or adults over 60.

MISSED DOSE
Take when you remember. Take next dose as scheduled, but don't double amount taken.

OVERDOSE
Vitamin B$_2$
Get in touch with a poison control center, emergency room, or doctor if urine is very dark in color or if patient experiences gastrointestinal problems.

Vitamin B$_9$ or B$_{12}$
Not likely to cause any overdose problems. If any listed side effects or adverse reactions seem particularly severe, call doctor or get in touch with poison control center or emergency room.

STOPPING DRUG
Vitamin B$_2$
May be discontinued any time.

Vitamin B$_9$ or B$_{12}$
If doctor has prescribed, do not stop taking until you have talked with him or her.

drug or category:

VITAMIN B$_3$ (NIACIN, NICOTINIC ACID)—FOR NIACIN AS AN ANTICHOLESTEROL DRUG, SEE CHAPTER 24.

condition or use:
DIETARY SUPPLEMENT

warning

This vitamin should be taken only by people whose diets are seriously lacking it, by those in whom illness prevents proper absorption of it from food, and by people with high cholesterol levels.

The ability of this vitamin in high doses to prevent or cure drug abuse, cardiovascular disease, and other problems has not been proven by rigorous scientific experimentation in humans.

High doses of these vitamins should be taken under medical supervision only.

Drug can cause fainting or lightheadedness if you rise from a chair or bed too quickly.

Tell your doctor if you have or have had:

• an allergic reaction to this medication, or to preservatives or food additives
• bleeding problems, diabetes, glaucoma, gout, liver disease, ulcers, or low blood pressure

form/usage

TABLETS (INCLUDING EXTENDED-RELEASE), INJECTIONS, SOLUTIONS, EXTENDED-RELEASE CAPSULES: As recommended by your doctor.

Extended-release capsules and tablets should be taken whole. Extended-release tablets, however, can be cut in half if they are scored (marked by a line down the middle).

when

As recommended by your doctor.

side effects and adverse reactions

Severe gastrointestinal problems, skin reactions, vision problems, dizziness when getting up from sitting or lying position

Flushing of face, dry skin

what to do

Stop taking. Get in touch with doctor immediately.

Continue taking, but discuss with your physician.

special precautions	because
DRUG INTERACTIONS	
1. Antidiabetic drugs, probenecid, sulfinpyrazone	1. High-dose niacin reduces effectiveness of these drugs.
2. Beta-blockers, mecamylamine, methyldopa, pargyline	2. Will result in excessive lowering of blood pressure
DIET	
No interactions reported.	
ALCOHOL and TOBACCO	
Avoid both.	Alcohol could lower blood pressure to dangerous levels.
	Tobacco diminishes effect of niacin.
PREGNANCY	
Avoid high doses.	Could cause fetal damage.
BREAST-FEEDING	
Avoid high doses.	Could pass into breast milk and be harmful to baby.

MISSED DOSE

Take when you remember. Wait four hours till next dose. Return to prescribed schedule. Do not double dose.

OVERDOSE

Get in touch with a poison control center, emergency room, or doctor if patient experiences severe gastrointestinal problems, fainting, or unexplained sweating.

STOPPING DRUG

May be discontinued at any time.

OTHERS

Periodic laboratory tests might be necessary to check effect on some body functions, including sugar levels.

drug or category:

VITAMIN C

condition or use:
DIETARY SUPPLEMENT

warning

This vitamin should be taken only by people whose diets are seriously lacking it or by those in whom illness prevents proper absorption of it from food.

The ability of this vitamin in high doses to slow down aging and cure or prevent ailments like cancer, heart disease, arthritis, or impotence has not been proven by rigorous scientific experimentation in humans.

High doses of this vitamin should be taken under medical supervision only.

Tell your doctor if you have or have had an allergic reaction to vitamin C or to preservatives or food additives.

High doses of vitamin C can aggravate sickle-cell anemia and cause anemia in people with glucose-6-phosphate dehydrogenase deficiency.

Consistent use of high doses has been associated with formation of kidney stones.

form/usage

TABLETS (INCLUDING CHEWABLE, EFFERVESCENT, AND EXTENDED-RELEASE), INJECTIONS, SYRUPS, EXTENDED-RELEASE CAPSULES:

As recommended by your doctor.

when

As recommended by your doctor.

side effects and adverse reactions

Mild gastrointestinal problems, kidney stones

Headaches, flushing in face

what to do

Stop taking. Get in touch with doctor immediately.

Continue taking, but discuss with your physician.

special precautions

DRUG INTERACTIONS
1. Amphetamines, anticholinergics, oral anticoagulants, tricyclic antidepressants, mexiletine, quinidine, phenothiazines

because

1. The effectiveness of these drugs may be reduced.

DRUG INTERACTIONS

2. Aspirin and aspirin-related drugs, barbiturates, cellulose sodium phosphate, oral contraceptives

2. Drugs will decrease vitamin C's effectiveness.

3. Estrogens

3. Increased estrogen side or adverse effects if vitamin C is taken in doses over 1 gram.

4. Iron supplements

4. Vitamin C may increase their absorption.

DIET
No interactions reported.

ALCOHOL and TOBACCO
No negative interactions reported.

PREGNANCY
No negative interactions reported, but discuss with your doctor.

Taking high doses of vitamin C may result in birth of vitamin-dependent baby.

BREAST-FEEDING
No problems reported, but discuss with your doctor.

It is unknown whether vitamin C passes into breast milk.

AGE FACTOR
Children and adults over 60 should avoid taking large doses.

Can cause kidney and bladder problems; increases iron absorption, which can result in liver and heart damage.

MISSED DOSE
Take when you remember.

OVERDOSE
Get in touch with a poison control center, emergency room, or doctor in case of severe gastrointestinal problems of dizziness.

STOPPING DRUG
May be discontinued at any time.

(continued)

OTHERS
High concentrations of vitamin C in body may interfere with results of tests for blood in stool or for sugar in urine.

VITAMIN D ANALOGS

condition:
CALCIUM DEFICIENCIES RESULTING FROM ILLNESS, INCLUDING KIDNEY DISEASE

warning

Vitamin supplements should be taken only by people whose diets are seriously lacking these vitamins or by those in whom illness prevents proper absorption of them from food.

The ability of vitamin D analogs to treat illnesses like arthritis, vision deficiencies, and nervous problems has not been proven by rigorous scientific experimentation in humans.

Tell your doctor if you have or have had:
- an allergic reaction to vitamin D or to any preservatives or foods
- diarrhea or other intestinal problems
- liver, pancreas, cardiovascular, or kidney disease
- sarcoidosis

drugs

GENERIC	BRAND	RX
calcifediol	*Calderol*	Some
calcitriol	*Rocaltrol*	

form/usage

CAPSULES: May be taken with liquids.

when

Follow your doctor's instructions.

side effects and adverse reactions

Psychotic reactions, severe stomach pains, fever, pink eye

Pain in muscles or bone, mild gastrointestinal problems, cloudy urine, increased sensitivity to light

what to do

Stop taking. Get in touch with doctor immediately.

Continue taking, but discuss with your physician.

special precautions

DRUG INTERACTIONS
1. Antacids with magnesium

because

1. Could increase level of magnesium to dangerous level.

(continued)

DRUG INTERACTIONS

2. Other vitamin D products

2. Could raise vitamin D to excessive levels.

3. Anticonvulsants, cholestyramine, colestipol, cortisone, mineral oil, neomycin, phenobarbital, rifampin

3. Decrease absorption or effect of vitamin D.

4. Calcium channel blockers

4. Decreases effectiveness of blockers.

5. Digitalis

5. May cause heart rhythm disturbances.

6. Phosphorus preparations

6. Buildup of phosphorus.

DIET
No interactions reported.

ALCOHOL and TOBACCO
No interactions reported.

PREGNANCY
Avoid drug.

Drug can increase risk of fetal deformations in humans.

BREAST-FEEDING
Discuss with your doctor.

Small amounts of vitamin D pass into breast milk; however, no problems have been reported in nursing babies.

AGE FACTOR
1. Give cautiously to children. Do not give them high doses.

1. Children are especially sensitive to vitamin D analogs. In high doses these compounds could interfere with proper growth.

2. People over 60 should use cautiously.

2. Adverse and side effects may be worse in older people.

MISSED DOSE
You can take a missed dose up to 12 hours after scheduled time. Otherwise, wait for next dose but do not double the amount taken.

OVERDOSE

Get in touch with a poison control center, emergency room, or doctor if patient experiences severe gastrointestinal problems, pain in muscles and bones, increase in urination and clouding of urine, severe mental disturbances, increase in blood pressure, or skin reactions.

STOPPING DRUG

Do not stop taking even if you feel better until you have talked with your doctor. You may have to come off drug slowly.

drug or category:

VITAMIN K

condition:

GENERALLY GIVEN TO BABIES TO PREVENT BLEEDING PROBLEMS AND TO SOME PEOPLE
WHO HAVE BLEEDING PROBLEMS BECAUSE THEY TAKE ANTICOAGULANTS

warning

Vitamin K supplements should be taken only by people whose diets are seriously lacking this vitamin or by those in whom illness prevents proper absorption of it from food.

The ability of vitamin K in high doses to cure certain illnesses has not been proven in rigorous scientific experiments.

Tell your doctor if you have or have had:

• an allergic reaction to vitamin K, or to preservatives or food additives
• G6PD deficiency, liver problems, cystic fibrosis, diarrhea, or other intestinal illnesses

Tell any doctors and dentists you consult that you are taking this drug.

drugs

GENERIC	BRAND	RX
menadiol	*Synkayvite*	Yes
phytonadione	*AquaMEPHYTON, Konakion, Mephyton*	

form/usage

TABLETS, INJECTIONS: May be taken with food or liquid. Tablets may be crumbled.

when

According to your doctor's instructions.

side effects and adverse reactions

Skin reactions

Flushing of face, funny taste in mouth

what to do

Stop taking. Get in touch with doctor immediately.

Continue taking, but discuss with your physician.

special precautions	because
DRUG INTERACTIONS	
1. Anticoagulants	1. Vitamin decreases their effectiveness.
2. Cholestyramine, colestipol, neomycin	2. Decreases vitamin K's absorption or effect.
3. Dapsone	3. May increase risk of adverse blood reaction.

DIET
No interactions reported.

ALCOHOL and TOBACCO
No interactions reported.

PREGNANCY
No negative interactions reported.

BREAST-FEEDING
No problems reported.

AGE FACTOR
No problems reported in adults over 60 or in children.

MISSED DOSE
You can take a missed dose up to 12 hours after scheduled time. Otherwise, wait for next dose but do not double the amount taken.

OVERDOSE
Get in touch with a poison control center, emergency room, or doctor if patient experiences serious gastrointestinal problems.

STOPPING DRUG
Discuss with your doctor.

OTHERS
Periodic laboratory tests might be necessary to check how vitamin is affecting your blood's clotting time.

RECOMMENDED DIETARY ALLOWANCES (REVISED 1989)

FOOD AND NUTRITION BOARD,
NATIONAL ACADEMY OF SCIENCES—NATIONAL RESEARCH COUNCIL

The allowances, expressed as average daily intakes over time, are intended to provide for individual variations among most normal persons as they live in the United States under usual environmental stresses. Diets should be based on a variety of common foods in order to provide other nutrients for which human requirements have been less well defined.

FAT-SOLUBLE VITAMINS

vitamin A

WHO	AGE (YEARS)	HOW MUCH (µG RE)*
Infants	0.0–0.5	375
	0.5–1.0	375
Children	1–3	400
	4–6	500
	7–10	700
Males	11–14	1,000
	15–18	1,000
	19–24	1,000
	25–50	1,000
	51+	1,000
Females	11–14	800
	15–18	800
	19–24	800
	25–50	800
	51+	800
Pregnant		800
Nursing	1st 6 months	1,300
	2nd 6 months	1,200

vitamin D

WHO	AGE (YEARS)	HOW MUCH (µG)**
Infants	0.0–0.5	7.5
	0.5–1.0	10
Children	1–3	10
	4–6	10
	7–10	10
Males	11–14	10
	15–18	10
	19–24	10
	25–50	5
	51+	5
Females	11–14	10
	15–18	10
	19–24	10
	25–50	5
	51+	5
Pregnant		10
Nursing	1st 6 months	10
	2nd 6 months	10

*RE = retinol equivalents; 1 RE = 1 µg retinol or 6 µg beta carotene.
**As cholecalciferol; 10 µg cholecalciferol = 400 IU vitamin D.

vitamin E

WHO	AGE (YEARS)	HOW MUCH (mg αTE)*
Infants	0.0–0.5	5
	0.5–1.0	4
Children	1–3	6
	4–6	7
	7–10	7
Males	11–14	10
	15–18	10
	19–24	10
	25–50	10
	51+	10
Females	11–14	8
	15–18	8
	19–24	8
	25–50	8
	51+	8
Pregnant		10
Nursing	1st 6 months	12
	2nd 6 months	11

vitamin K

WHO	AGE (YEARS)	HOW MUCH (μg)
Infants	0.0–0.5	5
	0.5–1.0	10
Children	1–3	15
	4–6	20
	7–10	30
Males	11–14	45
	15–18	65
	19–24	70
	25–50	80
	51+	80
Females	11–14	45
	15–18	55
	19–24	60
	25–50	65
	51+	65
Pregnant		65
Nursing	1st 6 months	65
	2nd 6 months	65

*αTE = alpha-tocopherol equivalents; 1 α-TE = 1 mg d-alpha-tocopherol.

WATER-SOLUBLE VITAMINS

vitamin C

WHO	AGE (YEARS)	HOW MUCH (mg)
Infants	0.0–0.5	30
	0.5–1.0	35
Children	1–3	40
	4–6	45
	7–10	45
Males	11–14	50
	15–18	60
	19–24	60
	25–50	60
	51+	60
Females	11–14	50
	15–18	60
	19–24	60
	25–50	60
	51+	60
Pregnant		70
Nursing	1st 6 months	95
	2nd 6 months	90

thiamin (vitamin B_1)

WHO	AGE (YEARS)	HOW MUCH (mg)
Infants	0.0–0.5	0.3
	0.5–1.0	0.4
Children	1–3	0.7
	4–6	0.9
	7–10	1.0
Males	11–14	1.3
	15–18	1.5
	19–24	1.5
	25–50	1.5
	51+	1.2
Females	11–14	1.1
	15–18	1.1
	19–24	1.1
	25–50	1.1
	51+	1.0
Pregnant		1.5
Nursing	1st 6 months	1.6
	2nd 6 months	1.6

riboflavin (vitamin B₂)

WHO	AGE (YEARS)	HOW MUCH (µg)
Infants	0.0–0.5	0.4
	0.5–1.0	0.5
Children	1–3	0.8
	4–6	1.1
	7–10	1.2
Males	11–14	1.5
	15–18	1.8
	19–24	1.7
	25–50	1.7
	51+	1.4
Females	11–14	1.3
	15–18	1.3
	19–24	1.3
	25–50	1.3
	51+	1.2
Pregnant		1.6
Nursing	1st 6 months	1.8
	2nd 6 months	1.7

niacin (vitamin B₃)

WHO	AGE (YEARS)	HOW MUCH (mg NE)*
Infants	0.0–0.5	5
	0.5–1.0	6
Children	1–3	9
	4–6	12
	7–10	13
Males	11–14	17
	15–18	20
	19–24	19
	25–50	19
	51+	15
Females	11–14	15
	15–18	15
	19–24	15
	25–50	15
	51+	13
Pregnant		17
Nursing	1st 6 months	20
	2nd 6 months	20

*NE = niacin equivalent. 1 NE = 1 mg of niacin or 60 mg of dietary tryptophan.

vitamin B₆

WHO	AGE (YEARS)	HOW MUCH (MG)
Infants	0.0–0.5	0.3
	0.5–1.0	0.6
Children	1–3	1.0
	4–6	1.1
	7–10	1.4
Males	11–14	1.7
	15–18	2.0
	19–24	2.0
	25–50	2.0
	51+	2.0
Females	11–14	1.4
	15–18	1.5
	19–24	1.6
	25–50	1.6
	51+	1.6
Pregnant		2.2
Nursing	1st 6 months	2.1
	2nd 6 months	2.1

Folate

WHO	AGE (YEARS)	HOW MUCH (μG)
Infants	0.0–0.5	25
	0.5–1.0	35
Children	1–3	50
	4–6	75
	7–10	100
Males	11–14	150
	15–18	200
	19–24	200
	25–50	200
	51+	200
Females	11–14	150
	15–18	180
	19–24	180
	25–50	180
	51+	180
Pregnant		400
Nursing	1st 6 months	280
	2nd 6 months	260

vitamin B$_{12}$

WHO	AGE (YEARS)	HOW MUCH μg)
Infants	0.0–0.5	0.3
	0.5–1.0	0.5
Children	1–3	0.7
	4–6	1.0
	7–10	1.4
Males	11–14	2.0
	15–18	2.0
	19–24	2.0
	25–50	2.0
	51+	2.0
Females	11–14	2.0
	15–18	2.0
	19–24	2.0
	25–50	2.0
	51+	2.0
Pregnant		2.2
Nursing	1st 6 months	2.6
	2nd 6 months	2.6

MINERALS

Calcium

WHO	AGE (YEARS)	HOW MUCH (mg)
Infants	0.0–0.5	400
	0.5–1.0	600
Children	1–3	800
	4–6	800
	7–10	800
Males	11–14	1,200
	15–18	1,200
	19–24	1,200
	25–50	800
	51+	800
Females	11–14	1,200
	15–18	1,200
	19–24	1,200
	25–50	800
	51+	800
Pregnant		1,200
Nursing	1st 6 months	1,200
	2nd 6 months	1,200

Phosphorus

WHO	AGE (YEARS)	HOW MUCH (mg)
Infants	0.0–0.5	300
	0.5–1.0	500
Children	1–3	800
	4–6	800
	7–10	800
Males	11–14	1,200
	15–18	1,200
	19–24	1,200
	25–50	800
	51+	800
Females	11–14	1,200
	15–18	1,200
	19–24	1,200
	25–50	800
	51+	800
Pregnant		1,200
Nursing	1st 6 months	1,200
	2nd 6 months	1,200

Magnesium

WHO	AGE (YEARS)	HOW MUCH (mg)
Infants	0.0–0.5	40
	0.5–1.0	60
Children	1–3	80
	4–6	120
	7–10	170
Males	11–14	270
	15–18	400
	19–24	350
	25–50	350
	51+	350
Females	11–14	280
	15–18	300
	19–24	280
	25–50	280
	51+	280
Pregnant		320
Nursing	1st 6 months	355
	2nd 6 months	340

Iron

WHO	AGE (YEARS)	HOW MUCH (mg)
Infants	0.0–0.5	6
	0.5–1.0	10
Children	1–3	10
	4–6	10
	7–10	10
Males	11–14	12
	15–18	12
	19–24	10
	25–50	10
	51+	10
Females	11–14	15
	15–18	15
	19–24	15
	25–50	15
	51+	10
Pregnant		30
Nursing	1st 6 months	15
	2nd 6 months	15

Zinc

WHO	AGE (YEARS)	HOW MUCH (mg)
Infants	0.0–0.5	5
	0.5–1.0	5
Children	1–3	10
	4–6	10
	7–10	10
Males	11–14	15
	15–18	15
	19–24	15
	25–50	15
	51+	15
Females	11–14	12
	15–18	12
	19–24	12
	25–50	12
	51+	12
Pregnant		15
Nursing	1st 6 months	19
	2nd 6 months	16

Iodine

WHO	AGE (YEARS)	HOW MUCH (µg)
Infants	0.0–0.5	40
	0.5–1.0	50
Children	1–3	70
	4–6	90
	7–10	120
Males	11–14	150
	15–18	150
	19–24	150
	25–50	150
	51+	150
Females	11–14	150
	15–18	150
	19–24	150
	25–50	150
	51+	150
Pregnant		175
Nursing	1st 6 months	200
	2nd 6 months	200

Selenium

WHO	AGE (YEARS)	HOW MUCH (μg)
Infants	0.0–0.5	10
	0.5–1.0	15
Children	1–3	20
	4–6	20
	7–10	30
Males	11–14	40
	15–18	50
	19–24	70
	25–50	70
	51+	70
Females	11–14	45
	15–18	50
	19–24	55
	25–50	55
	51+	55
Pregnant		65
Nursing	1st 6 months	75
	2nd 6 months	75

OTHER VITAMINS AND MINERALS (TRACE ELEMENTS)

The following figures are provided in the form of ranges of recommended intakes because there is less information on which to base allowances.

The toxic levels for many trace elements may be only several times usual intakes. Therefore, the upper levels given in the table below should not be exceeded.

biotin (vitamin)

WHO	AGE (YEARS)	HOW MUCH (µg)
Infants	0.0–0.5	10
	0.5–1.0	15
Children	1–3	20
	4–6	25
	7–10	30
	11+	30–100
Adults		30–100

pantothenic acid (vitamin)

WHO	AGE (YEARS)	HOW MUCH (mg)
Infants	0.0–0.5	2
	0.5–1.0	3
Children	1–3	3
	4–6	3–4
	7–10	4–5
	11+	4–7
Adults		4–7

Copper (Trace Element)

WHO	AGE (YEARS)	HOW MUCH (mg)
Infants	0.0–0.5	0.4–0.6
	0.5–1.0	0.6–0.7
Children	1–3	0.7–1.0
	4–6	1.0–1.5
	7–10	1.0–2.0
	11+	1.5–2.5
Adults		1.5–3.0

Manganese (Trace Element)

WHO	AGE (YEARS)	HOW MUCH (mg)
Infants	0.0–0.5	0.3–0.6
	0.5–1.0	0.6–1.0
Children	1–3	1.0–1.5
	4–6	1.5–2.0
	7–10	2.0–3.0
	11+	2.0–5.0
Adults		2.0–5.0

Fluoride (Trace Element)

WHO	AGE (YEARS)	HOW MUCH (mg)
Infants	0.0–0.5	0.1–0.5
	0.5–1.0	0.2–1.0
Children	1–3	0.5–1.5
	4–6	1.0–2.5
	7–10	1.5–2.5
	11+	1.5–2.5
Adults		1.5–4.0

Chromium (Trace Element)

WHO	AGE (YEARS)	HOW MUCH (µg)
Infants	0.0–0.5	10–20
	0.5–1.0	20–60
Children	1–3	20–80
	4–6	30–120
	7–10	50–200
	11+	50–200
Adults		50–200

Molybdenum (Trace Element)

WHO	AGE (YEARS)	HOW MUCH (µg)
Infants	0.0–0.5	15–30
	0.5–1.0	20–40
Children	1–3	25–50
	4–6	30–75
	7–10	50–150
	11+	75–250
Adults		75–250

Index